T0344662

Tissue and Cell
Clinical Use

Tissue and Cell Clinical Use

AN ESSENTIAL GUIDE

EDITED BY

Ruth M. Warwick, MB, ChB, FRCP, FRCPath
Honorary Research Fellow
University of Bristol
Bristol, UK

Scott A. Brubaker, CTBS
Chief Policy Officer
American Association of Tissue Banks
McLean, VA, USA

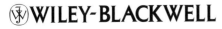
A John Wiley & Sons, Ltd., Publication

This edition first published 2012 © 2012 by Blackwell Publishing Ltd

Blackwell Publishing was acquired by John Wiley & Sons in February 2007. Blackwell's publishing program has been merged with Wiley's global Scientific, Technical and Medical business to form Wiley-Blackwell.

Registered office: John Wiley & Sons, Ltd, The Atrium, Southern Gate, Chichester, West Sussex, PO19 8SQ, UK

Editorial offices: 9600 Garsington Road, Oxford, OX4 2DQ, UK
   The Atrium, Southern Gate, Chichester, West Sussex, PO19 8SQ, UK
   111 River Street, Hoboken, NJ 07030-5774, USA

For details of our global editorial offices, for customer services and for information about how to apply for permission to reuse the copyright material in this book please see our website at www.wiley.com/wiley-blackwell

The right of the author to be identified as the author of this work has been asserted in accordance with the UK Copyright, Designs and Patents Act 1988.

All rights reserved. No part of this publication may be reproduced, stored in a retrieval system, or transmitted, in any form or by any means, electronic, mechanical, photocopying, recording or otherwise, except as permitted by the UK Copyright, Designs and Patents Act 1988, without the prior permission of the publisher.

Designations used by companies to distinguish their products are often claimed as trademarks. All brand names and product names used in this book are trade names, service marks, trademarks or registered trademarks of their respective owners. The publisher is not associated with any product or vendor mentioned in this book. This publication is designed to provide accurate and authoritative information in regard to the subject matter covered. It is sold on the understanding that the publisher is not engaged in rendering professional services. If professional advice or other expert assistance is required, the services of a competent professional should be sought.

The contents of this work are intended to further general scientific research, understanding, and discussion only and are not intended and should not be relied upon as recommending or promoting a specific method, diagnosis, or treatment by physicians for any particular patient. The publisher and the author make no representations or warranties with respect to the accuracy or completeness of the contents of this work and specifically disclaim all warranties, including without limitation any implied warranties of fitness for a particular purpose. In view of ongoing research, equipment modifications, changes in governmental regulations, and the constant flow of information relating to the use of medicines, equipment, and devices, the reader is urged to review and evaluate the information provided in the package insert or instructions for each medicine, equipment, or device for, among other things, any changes in the instructions or indication of usage and for added warnings and precautions. Readers should consult with a specialist where appropriate. The fact that an organization or Website is referred to in this work as a citation and/or a potential source of further information does not mean that the author or the publisher endorses the information the organization or Website may provide or recommendations it may make. Further, readers should be aware that Internet Websites listed in this work may have changed or disappeared between when this work was written and when it is read. No warranty may be created or extended by any promotional statements for this work. Neither the publisher nor the author shall be liable for any damages arising herefrom.

Library of Congress Cataloging-in-Publication Data

Tissue and cell clinical use : an essential guide / edited by Ruth M. Warwick, Scott A. Brubaker.
   p. ; cm.
   Includes bibliographical references and index.
   ISBN 978-1-4051-9825-7 (hardcover : alk. paper)
   I. Warwick, Ruth M. II. Brubaker, Scott A.
   [DNLM: 1. Tissue Transplantation.   2. Cell Transplantation.   3. Transplantation–standards.
4. Transplantation, Homologous.   WO 660]

   617.9'54–dc23

                           2012009761

A catalogue record for this book is available from the British Library.

Wiley also publishes its books in a variety of electronic formats. Some content that appears in print may not be available in electronic books.

Cover images: Left hand image courtesy of editors, remainder © Getty Images.
Cover design by Sarah Dickinson.

Set in 9.25/12 pt Meridien by Toppan Best-set Premedia Limited
Printed and bound in Singapore by Markono Print Media Pte Ltd

1 2011

Contents

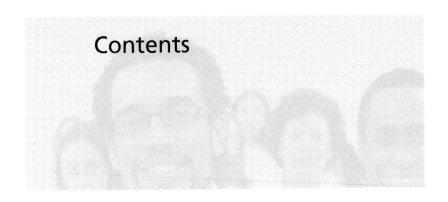

Contributor List

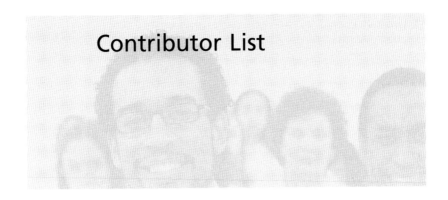

Joseph M. Biber, MD
Fellow, Cornea Service
Cincinnati Eye Institute
Cincinnati, OH, USA

Nikola Biller-Andorno, MD, PhD
Professor of Biomedical Ethics
Institute of Biomedical Ethics
University of Zurich
Zurich, Switzerland

Cesar V. Borlongan, PhD
Professor and Vice-Chairman for Research
Center of Excellence for Aging and Brain Repair
Department of Neurosurgery
University of South Florida College of Medicine
Tampa, FL, USA

Scott A. Brubaker, CTBS
Chief Policy Officer
American Association of Tissue Banks
McLean, VA, USA

Linda C. Cendales, MD
Assistant Professor of Surgery
Division of Plastic Surgery and the Emory Transplant Center
Emory University
Atlanta, GA, USA

Jeremy R. Chapman, OAM, MD, FRACP, FRCP
Director of Renal Medicine
Centre for Transplant and Renal Research
Westmead Millienium Institute
University of Sydney
Westmead Hospital
Sydney, NSW, Australa

Christopher R. Chapple, BSc, MD, FRCS (Urol), FEBU
Consultant Urological Surgeon
Royal Hallamshire Hospital;
Honorary Senior Lecturer of Urology
University of Sheffield;
Visiting Professor of Urology
Sheffield Hallam University
Sheffield, UK

Gabriel L. Converse, PhD
Director of Bioengineering
Cardiac Regenerative Surgery Research Laboratories
The Ward Family Center for Congenital Heart Disease and the
Department of Cardiac Surgery
Children's Mercy Hospital and Clinics
Kansas City, MO, USA

Mauro Costa, MD
Clinical Director
Preconceptional and Prenatal Medicine Unit
Galliera Hospital
Genoa, Italy

Jeffery Dattilo, MD
Associate Professor of Surgery and
Program Director for Vascular Surgery Fellowship
Vanderbilt University Medical Center;
Chief, Vascular Surgery
Veterans Affairs Hospital
Nashville, TN, USA

Francesco Dazzi, MD, PhD
Professor of Stem Cell Biology
Haematology Centre
Department of Medicine
Imperial College
London, UK

P. Dominic F. Dodd, MD, FRCSEd
Consultant Vascular Surgeon
Sheffield Vascular Institute
Sheffield, UK

Stephen B. Dunnett, DSc, PhD, MA, BA(Hons), BSc(Hons), FMedSci, FLSW
Full Professor
The Brain Repair Group, School of Biosciences
Cardiff University
Cardiff, UK

Peter Dziewulski, FRCS(Plast)
Consultant Plastic and Reconstructive Surgeon
Clinical Director, Burn Service
St Andrews Centre for Plastic Surgery and Burns
Chelmsford, UK

Ted Eastlund, MD
Division of Transfusion Medicine and Department of Pathology
University of New Mexico
Albuquerque, NM, USA

Tarek El-Toukhy, MBBCh, MSc, MD, MRCOG
Consultant in Reproductive Medicine and PGD
Guy's and St. Thomas' Hospital NHS Foundation Trust;
Honorary Senior Lecturer
King's College London
London, UK;
Associate Professor of Obstetrics and Gynaecology
Cairo University
Cairo, Egypt

Deirdre Fehily, PhD
Inspector and Technical Advisor, Tissues and Cells
National Transplant Centre
Rome, Italy

Stefano Ferrari, PhD
Head of R&D
The Veneto Eye Bank Foundation
Venice, Italy

Glenn Greenleaf, BA
LifeCell Corp.
Branchburg, NJ, USA

Eva-Lisa Heinrichs, MD, PhD
Chief Medical Officer
Orteq Ltd
London, UK

Edward J. Holland, MD
Professor of Ophthalmology
University of Cincinnati;
Cornea Service
Cincinnati Eye Institute
Cincinnati, OH, USA

Danny Holtzclaw, DDS, MS
Diplomate, American Board of Periodontology;
Diplomate, International Congress of Oral Implantologists;
Private Practice, Periodontics
Austin, TX, USA

Richard A. Hopkins, MD
Professor of Surgery
University of Missouri-Kansas City School of Medicine;
Director, Cardiac Regenerative Surgery Research Laboratories
Section of Cardiovascular Surgery
Children's Mercy Hospitals and Clinics
Kansas City, MO, USA

Nicole J. Horwood, PhD
University Research Lecturer
Kennedy Institute of Rheumatology
University of Oxford
London, UK

Rachael Hough, BmedSci, BMBS, MD, FRCP, Frcpath
Consultant Haematologist and Clinical Lead of the Children and
Young People's Cancer Service
University College Hospital
London, UK

Moustapha Kassem, MD
Professor, Consultant
Endocrinology and Metabolism
University Hospital of Odense
Odense, Denmark

Ian Kerridge, BA, BMed(Hons), MPhil(Cantab), FRACP, FRCPA
Director and Associate Professor of Bioethics
Centre for Values, Ethics and the Law in Medicine
Sydney Medical School
University of Sydney;
Haematologist and BMT Physician
Haematology Department
Royal North Shore Hospital
Sydney, NSW, Australia

Katie Kinzer, AB
Research Specialist
Division of Transplantation
Department of Surgery
University of Illinois at Chicago
Chicago, IL, USA

Joan C. Monllau, MD, PhD
Knee Unit
IMAS – Hospitals del Mar and Esperança
Universitat Autònoma de Barcelona
Barcelona, Spain

Praveen V. Mummaneni, MD
Associate Professor and Vice-Chairman
Department of Neurosurgery
University of California
San Francisco, CA, USA

Jose Oberholzer, MD
Chief, Division of Transplantation
C. & B. Frese and G. Moss Professor of Transplant Surgery, Bioengineering and
Endocrinology
University of Illinois at Chicago
Chicago, IL, USA

Eduardo J. Ortiz-Cruz, MD
Department of Orthopaedic Surgery
Chief of Bone and Soft Tissue Tumour Unit
Hospital Universitario La Paz;
MD Anderson Cancer Center
Madrid, Spain

David Otterburn, MD
Assistant Professor of Surgery
Division of Plastic Surgery
Emory University
Atlanta, GA, USA

John R. Pepper, MD
Professor and Consultant Cardiac Surgeon
Royal Brompton Hospital and Harefield NHS Trust;
National Heart and Lung Institute
Imperial College London
London, UK

Diego Ponzin, MD
Director
The Veneto Eye Bank Foundation
Venice, Italy

Amish N. Raval, MD
Assistant Professor of Medicine
Division of Cardiovascular Medicine
Director of Clinical Cardiovascular Regenerative Medicine
University of Wisconsin School of Medicine and Public Health
Madison, WI, USA

Hans-Oliver Rennekampff, MD
Professor of Plastic Surgery
Associate Director Burn Center
Department of Plastic, Hand and Reconstructive Surgery
Medical School Hannover
Hannover, Germany

Scott A. Rodeo, MD
Co-Chief, Sports Medicine and Shoulder Service;
Professor, Orthopaedic Surgery
Weill Medical College of Cornell University;
Attending Orthopaedic Surgeon
The Hospital for Special Surgery
New York, NY, USA

Patrick Salmon, PharmD, PhD
Scientist-Lecturer
Department of Neurosciences
Faculty of Medicine
Centre Médical Universitaire
Geneva, Switzerland

Paul R. Sanberg, PhD, DSc
Executive Director
Center of Excellence for Aging and Brain Repair
Department of Neurosurgery
University of South Florida College of Medicine
Tampa, FL, USA

Ranil de Silva, PhD, MRCP
Senior Lecturer in Clinical Cardiology
National Heart and Lung Institute
Imperial College London
Royal Brompton and Harefield NHS Foundation Trust
London, UK

Ulrich Stock, MD
Professor and Deputy Chief of Cardiothoracic Surgery
University Hospital Frankfurt
Frankfurt, Germany

William W. Tomford, MD
Professor of Orthopedic Surgery
Harvard Medical School;
Director, MGH Bone Bank;
Attending Surgeon
Department of Orthopaedic Surgery
Massachusetts General Hospital
Boston, MA, USA

Tolga Fikret Tözüm, DDS, PhD
Associate Professor
Department of Periodontology
Faculty of Dentistry
Hacettepe University
Ankara, Turkey

René Verdonk, MD, PhD
Head, Department of Orthopaedic Surgery and Traumatology
Ghent University Hospital
Ghent, Belgium

John E. Wagner, MD
Professor and Director
Blood and Marrow Transplant Program
Department of Pediatrics
University of Minnesota
Minneapolis, MN, USA

Ruth M. Warwick, MB, ChB, FRCP, FRCPath
Honorary Research Fellow
University of Bristol
Bristol, UK

Alexander E. Weber, MD
Orthopaedic Surgery Resident
Department of Orthopaedic Surgery
University of Michigan
Ann Arbor, MI, USA

Diane Wilson, BSN, MSN/MHA
Chief Operating Officer
Community Tissue Services
Dayton, OH, USA

Steven E. Wolf, MD
Betty and Bob Kelso Distinguished Chair in Burns and Trauma
Professor and Vice Chairman for Research
Department of Surgery
University of Texas Health Science Center at San Antonio;
Chief, Clinical Research
United States Army Institute of Surgical Research
San Antonio, TX, USA

Jau-Ching Wu, MD
Attending Surgeon
Department of Neurosurgery, Neurological Institute
Taipei Veterans General Hospital;
School of Medicine, National Yang-Ming University
Taiwan

Walid Zaher, MD, MSc, MHPE
Lecturer, Specialist
Department of Anatomy and Stem Cell Unit
College of Medicine
King Saud University
Riyadh, Kingdom of Saudi Arabia;
Regenerative Medicine Fellow
Institute of Clinical Research (KMEB)
University Hospital of Odense
Odense, Denmark

Foreword

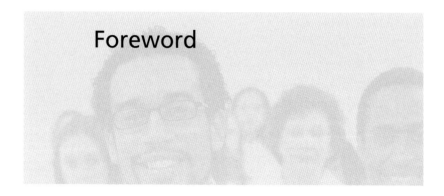

Clinical allograft transplantation of various body parts has a long and some-times disturbing history. Many authors have commented on the old histori-cal events surrounding Saints Cosmas and Damian, who were from the Turkish region and practiced medicine. It was said that they were beheaded by the Emperor Diocletian in the third century AD because they were Catho-lics. However, they returned in the fifth century to perform the "Miracle of Black Leg" as a remarkable treatment for the soon-to-become Roman Emperor, Justinian, for a cancer of his extremity. The origin of the black limb that they transplanted was from a Moor who had died that morning, and the transplant was performed after amputation of Justinian's limb. The success of the procedure was certainly questionable but several events occurred as a result. First, almost every artist of the Renaissance became intrigued by the procedure, which resulted in hundreds of remarkable artworks displaying it. Secondly Cosmas and Damian were canonized in 570 and became saints. Finally, the alleged site of the operative procedure was in a church in the Roman Forum, which is now titled the Basilica Cosma e Damiano. Thus, the concept of transplantation from one individual to another has caught the imagination of generations during the past 14 centuries. Slowly, evidence has accrued about its benefits but, along with much success, we are now venturing into gathering information to manage and prevent adverse outcomes. Understanding biology continues to evolve.

The first clinical bone allograft transplantation was in 1881, when William MacEwen used the technique to treat a 3-year-old child with osteomyelitis of the humerus. Eric Lexer in 1908 reported four such procedures about the knee and in 1925 described a reasonable success rate with 34 joints. Since then numerous programs have reported many allograft transplants, includ-ing those of Volkov in Russia, Frank Parrish in Houston, Texas, Carlos

Ottolenghi in Buenos Aires, Istituto Rizzoli in Bologna, the Mayo Clinic and Bill Tomford, Henry Mankin, and Francis Hornicek at the Massachusetts General Hospital. Development of the National Naval Tissue Bank in 1991 by George Hyatt and Kenneth Sell was of considerable value, and its remarkable capacity to train numerous individuals led to the development of tissue banks in a variety of centers. It was Curtiss and his group who demonstrated that freezing the tissue improved outcome, and Friedlaender and Strong showed that patients with MHC class II antigens did better than those with class I or those with mismatch. There were additional benefits to improved survival of the cartilage of joint allografts from the use of glycerol and dimethylsulfoxide. Careful clinical follow-up with outcome reporting and collation provide evidence for advancement in this important, developing field. My personal interest has been in orthopedics but it is clearly only one of a variety of disciplines that have benefited from allograft use. This volume seeks to describe the clinical use of many different cell and tissue allografts to address multiple conditions.

It should be apparent to the readers of this volume that the difficulties associated with variation in cellular elements, tissue structure, bacterial contamination, and very slow regeneration result in complications and in some cases, significant system failures. It is not just the bone and other tissue allografts that have the remote but discrete possibility of developing this array of problems: all forms of allograft transplantation, including organ transplantation and haemopoietic stem cell transplants, can develop serious complications and result not only in failure of the system but potentially threaten the life of the graft recipient. Other recipients, who might receive an allograft from the same donor or the same batch of materials, can also be at risk. It is noteworthy that this book contains descriptions of recent advances in vigilance and surveillance of substances of human origin and I commend this.

The information provided by the authors in this volume clearly defines the clinical advantages and the potential and real problems associated with allograft transplant of all sorts, including those in new and developing fields such as complex tissue grafts of the hand and face as well as in my own area of large bone segments. The chapters offer the readers a major opportunity to review the advantages and as well as problems that have resulted. Ultimately, it is the balance between the advantages and the disadvantages that lead to patient benefit in the long term. This will improve the success of allografting, whether it is a stem cell or large allograft.

As a performer and caring physician for many patients with allograft bone transplants and as a teacher, it is my privilege and my honor to have the opportunity to introduce the subject with this foreword. I am hopeful that some of this discussion will increase the depth of understanding of the excellent presentations by the multiple outstanding authors of the chapters, and that this important didactic book, with its case studies and learning points in each chapter, will continue the critically important task of teaching and educating professionals working in, and regulating, diverse fields associated with tissue and cell allografting.

Henry J. Mankin MD
Senior Research Consultant, Orthopaedic Oncology Service
Massachusetts General Hospital;
Edith M. Ashley Professor Emeritus of Orthopaedics
Harvard Medical School
Boston, MA, USA

Preface

This book on the use of donated tissues and cells is the third in a series of three. The first was published in 2009. Its 13 chapters focused on the human dimensions of donation, addressing the topic from the history of the discipline, through donor recruitment and consent, medical and behavioral history taking, to the role of donor testing and the management of test results. Case studies demonstrated the diversity of the field in different cultural and economic realities, and issues relating to the care of the professionals who undertake rewarding but sometimes arduous, emotional duties were discussed. The first book also covered aspects relating to the donation of hemopoietic stem cells, the reproductive context, and the role of clinical governance in tissue and stem cell banks.

The second book is published in parallel with this third book and covers all aspects of recovery and processing of tissues and cells, including collection of reproductive donations and hemopoietic stem cells, and the training of staff in these disciplines. The foreword to the first book was written by Professor Rafael Matesanz from the Spanish National Transplant Organisation in Madrid. Dr Matesanz describes two things that should always be strictly linked to assure a solid foundation for a transplant system to offer the best opportunities and results for patients: technical quality standards and ethics. This is true for the donation aspects and for the use of donated tissues and cells. We invited international experts to collaborate with us in developing this book so that our readers would have access to a broad reference from the expert surgeons and physicians using tissues and cells, with evidence from the literature on the clinical benefits of these invaluable donations.

This volume is designed in a similar format to its sister books. It has 20 chapters and includes cases and learning points. We cover the same fields as the first two books and deal with the application of tissues and cells by those working in the clinical field. Similarly, this volume has a cross-continental editorship and chapters co-authored by experts in their field with representation from all over the world in an attempt to provide a global perspective. We are especially honored that Dr Henry Mankin has written the foreword to this third book. He has commented on the long history of the use of allografts and the advances that have made their use an essential part of the armamentarium of doctors in many specialties. This is an important point from him because he has been recognized as an innovator and expert clinician in the use of allografts in orthopedics, in which he has been working for over 50 years. He started orthopedic residency at the Hospital for Joint Diseases in New York City and later became orthopedist-in-chief at Massachusetts General Hospital and a professor at Harvard. He has several specialty interests including in Gaucher's disease and in the use of major bone allografts. He has developed a computerized system for following the 18 000 tumor cases that he and his unit have treated over many years. The more than 600 papers published by his team is an extraordinary literature on the evidence of benefit from the use of donated bone. He has recognized in his foreword that although allografts carry many advantages, there are also risks associated with their use. We have structured this book in a way that allows clinicians to weigh up these two opposing aspects of allografts and to make informed choices on when to use them. Information is provided on how to recognize adverse reactions and to collaborate with the clinical allograft network to promote maximum safety.

The book starts with a chapter on the ethics of the use of allografts, a subject fundamental to the continuing support of the donating public. We follow with chapters on clinical governance in hospitals, dental surgeries, and other establishments that use allografts. In Chapter 3 existing vigilance and surveillance schemes for tissues and cells from around the world are described. Vigilance activity is generally so recent in this field that most of the references that have been provided are web based. This reflects an important new development in the field that will undoubtedly increase safety of allografts, which is especially important in the context of global distribution. Chapter 4 reviews transmission of disease by organs, tissues, and cells. This is followed in Chapters 5–20 with specific descriptions of the use of allografts in surgical specialties such as vascular, cardiac, and orthopedic surgery, as well as neurosurgery, sports medicine, dentistry, burns, and the use of skin substitutes for a variety of other applications. There is a chapter on ophthalmic use of tissues and cells, and in the innovative areas of complex composite vascular tissue grafting such as hand and face transplantation, which has received huge lay press interest. A specific chapter describes the rapidly evolving work in the use of hemopoietic stem cells and mesenchymal stem cells. Our authors also relate areas of recent developments in the use of stem cells, with a chapter covering embryonic or neural stem cells and the central nervous system with a particular focus on Parkinson's disease, multiple sclerosis, spinal cord damage, and stroke. To round out this exciting innovative approach to therapy, there is a chapter on pancreatic islet cells and another on cardiac stem cells. We are most grateful to Dr Stephen Minger for reviewing the stem cell chapters. We finish with a chapter on the use of donated gametes in the assisted reproduction sector.

We hope that this set of three sister books provides a comprehensive overview from experts in their fields, of all the multidisciplinary aspects of donation, recovery, and use of donated materials of human origin. Our aim is that they will help inform both professionals and regulators on recent developments in this diverse and unique field of medicine. Ultimately these books are about the generosity of donors, the skills of the professionals, and communities of individuals working together for the benefit of patients around the globe.

Ruth M. Warwick
Scott A. Brubaker

1 Ethical Issues Regarding the Use of Human Tissues and Cells

Nikola Biller-Andorno[1], Diane Wilson[2], Ian Kerridge[3], and Jeremy R. Chapman[3]
[1]University of Zurich, Zurich, Switzerland
[2]Community Tissue Services, Dayton, OH, USA
[3]University of Sydney, Sydney, NSW, Australia

Introduction

Over the past two decades the use of human tissues and cells for transplantation has steadily increased. In the United States (USA), for example, 2,141,960 tissue grafts were distributed by American Association of Tissue Banks (AATB)-accredited tissue banks in 2007 (2007 AATB Annual Survey Results, Tissue Banks in the United States, May 2010). The AATB reported that tissue donor recoveries in the USA have continued to rise with every survey [1] (Figure 1.1).[1] Other countries, such as Spain and Slovakia, have also witnessed a rapid increase in donation of tissues. It is not clear, however, if this increase is in every case a response to need, a consequence of required death referral[2] or of other process improvements, or if tissue referral, procurement, and processing are growing as business opportunities.

The field of hematopoietic stem cell (HSC) transplantation has witnessed remarkable development from a highly experimental and risky procedure in the 1970s to a continuing complex procedure with inherent risks but is now a widely applied therapy for a variety of lethal conditions of the bone marrow [2].

---

[1]Contributing to this was the establishment of first person consent registries in many states, and most important was a change in federal law that required all deaths or imminent deaths to be referred to the local organ procurement organization or a tissue bank. These organizations approach families for consent or authorization using specially trained personnel and they provide call centers that handle all referrals.
[2]In the USA per Centers for Medicare & Medicaid Services (CMS) Final Rule – the Conditions of Participation.

Tissue and Cell Clinical Use: An Essential Guide, First Edition. Edited by Ruth M. Warwick and Scott A. Brubaker.
© 2012 Blackwell Publishing Ltd. Published 2012 by Blackwell Publishing Ltd.

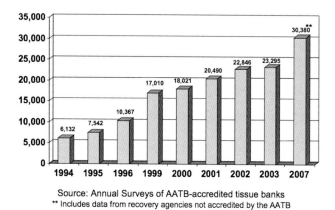

Tissue Donors Recovered

Source: Annual Surveys of AATB-accredited tissue banks
** Includes data from recovery agencies not accredited by the AATB

Figure 1.1 Increasing number of tissue donors in the USA [1]. (Reproduced by permission of American Association of Tissue Banks, 2007 AATB Annual Survey Results, Tissue Banks in the United States, May 2010.)

This dynamic development is in part due to scientific advances, such as in histocompatibility matching, immunosuppression, and prophylactic treatment of infections. Another reason for the rapidly expanding activities in human cells and tissues for transplantation (HCTT) is the increasing international exchange of these human donations. Collaborative efforts from more than 60 registries of unrelated volunteer bone marrow and other types of HSC donor have expanded the pool of potential donors for these patients from their immediate and extended family through to close to 14 million people globally. The success of some tissue banking systems has led to excess supply and allowed export of certain tissues to countries in need. The export of corneas retrieved in the USA, for instance, has grown from 7% (of the total number of corneas available for transplantation) in 1990 to 29% in 2000 [3]. Anecdotal reports state that 10–15% of the tissue distributed by USA tissue banks (excluding eye banks) is sent outside of the USA. The Canadian Council for Donation and Transplantation report in their surveys that more than 80% of the tissue used in Canada is imported from the USA.[3]

However, data on global use and exchange of tissues are patchy with poor levels of traceability. On the other hand, the unrelated HSC programs are quite tightly controlled by the bone marrow donor registries and cord blood banks, and both activity levels and adverse events data are reported annually

---

[3]Supply of Human Allograft Tissue in Canada. April 2003, CCDT. http://www.organsandtissues.ca/s/wp-content/uploads/2011/11/Supply-Allograft.pdf. Accessed April 2012.

by the World Marrow Donor Association (WMDA) (http://www.worldmarrow. org). The World Health Organization (WHO) has also accumulated data on various organ and tissue transplantation rates derived from government sources in its Global Knowledge of Transplantation (http://www.who.int/ transplantation/knowledgebase/en).

The idea of transplanting tissues has a longstanding history. A frequent reference is to the legend of Saints Cosmas and Damian, who attempted to transplant a limb from a deceased moor to a white nobleman in the 3rd century AD. Van Meekeren, a Dutch surgeon, reported in 1668 the first successful bone transplant performed on a Russian soldier where a piece of canine skull was used to fill the defect in an injured soldier's skull. When this transplant was discovered he was excommunicated because the treatment was seen as un-Christian. To return to the good graces of the Church, the soldier asked for the bone to be removed but the graft had already incorporated and healed [4]. Centuries later the surgeon Alexis Carrel expressed his view of the need for organ and tissue transplantation when he stated, "if it were possible immediately after death . . . to transplant the tissues and organs . . . no elemental death would occur, and all the . . . parts of the body would continue to live. A supply of tissues . . . would be constantly ready for use . . . and could be sent to surgeons who need them" [5].

From these early times, tissue banking organizations have now grown to many hundreds of establishments providing millions of tissue grafts for transplantation annually, often with excellent success. The early Bone Marrow Registries have grown to more than 70 organizations, and perhaps 200 cord blood banks exist globally. But even if medical advances have allowed cell and tissue transplantations to become standard procedures that are readily accepted by many patients across nations, cultures, and religions, new scientific and ethical challenges have emerged.

One of these challenges is the development of a solid evidence base for clinical and policy decisions regarding HCTT. What is the need and demand for each tissue in each country every year? Can communities be self-sufficient from the tissue donations from their own population? When are cell or tissue transplants the best treatment option, and when is a product being used just as a convenient solution? For example, when is a human heart valve better or worse than a mechanical or a porcine valve? How can governments ensure that precious and rare tissues and cells be optimally used? These issues gain particular importance once donated substances of human origin are highly processed and start to be considered as tradable goods like any other.

The challenge of maintaining both confidentiality and transparency is a responsibility that exists through every step in donation, banking, allocation, and transplantation of human cells and tissues. There has been a longstanding effort in organ transplantation to establish and promote transparency about the availability and allocation of human organs. In tissue transplantation, some health authorities are uncertain of the number of tissue establishments operating in their country, let alone the number of donated, transplanted, exported or imported tissue [6]. Transparency, however, is a key requirement for public trust. This trust is regularly challenged, for example, when bodies or component tissues are reported by the media to have been sold by Funeral Home Directors or when a young patient dies after a dubious experimental stem cell treatment. A clear and well-implemented framework of ethical principles may help avoid such scandals. Detailing how respect for autonomy, stewardship, and fair access to treatment by these special donations is going to be achieved and maintained, together with applying appropriate quality and safety standards, is an important basis for the future development of HCTT.

This chapter outlines major ethical principles and issues of HCTT. It does not enter into issues arising from tissue or cell donation as these have been treated extensively elsewhere [7]. Cell and tissue transplantation are considered separately, as they are in fact two rather distinct fields, while the use of germ line tissues and cells are covered in Chapter 20. The complexity of issues that will need consideration if and when the decision is made to use human embryonic stem cells and induced pluripotent stem cells (IPS) cells has yet to be defined as the science turns slowly from fiction to fact.

A normative framework for HCTT

There are several general ethical rules and principles that cut across the various fields of cell and tissue transplantation and, indeed, organ transplantation. The principle of respect for autonomy requires that any donation be based on informed, voluntary consent. In the case of a deceased donor who in life has not opted out from donation, this may suffice as authorization, but even in presumed consent systems the donor's family is usually asked for approval, acknowledging the psychological implications a donation may have for them. Also their cooperation is desired for providing a medical and behavioral history.

The concept of stewardship is also inspired by respect for autonomy of the donor: it wishes to honor the intention of the donor – to help another suffering person with his or her gift, a part of one's own body. Charging unjustifiable fees for processing the cells or tissues or otherwise turning the gift into a commodity just like any other would be incompatible with the idea of serving as the steward of a human tissue or cell gift that one was entrusted with.

Stewardship also requires making optimal use of the donated material. Using the donation in the most efficacious way can also be argued for within the principle of beneficence. Quality and safety requirements, on the other hand, follow from the ethical principle of non-maleficence: risks to the (live) donor, the recipient and third parties are to be minimized. The principle of

---

Box 1.1 Elements of a normative framework for HCTT

An international consensus has emerged on the following ethically relevant rules and concepts
Transparency (while protecting privacy of donor and recipient)
Evidence-based standards for procurement, processing and clinical use
Quality, safety, and efficacy
Informed and voluntary consent for donation as well as for receiving a
  transplant
Stewardship and non-commercialization
Equitable access and fair allocation

Underlying general ethical principles
Respect for autonomy – beneficence – non-maleficence – justice

---

non-maleficence could also be used to argue against paying donors or their families, as this may encourage dishonesty about the medical history, with the consequence of possible harm to the donor during the donation and to the recipient from an unsuitable product.

Paying for donation could also be considered as being in conflict with the principle of justice. More donors or families with low socio-economic status would respond to financial incentives for donation, whereas high prices for the respective cell and tissue products would favor transplantation of affluent individuals and patients from high resource countries. If human cells and tissue are to be considered not as a commodity but as a community resource their distribution becomes a justice concern, requiring criteria and processes for defining equitable access and fair allocation.

International guidance documents – such as the World Medical Association Statement on Human Organ Donation and Transplantation [8], the Council of Europe's Additional Protocol to the Convention on Human Rights and Biomedicine [9], the European Directive 2004/23/EC [10] and the WHO Guiding Principles on Human Cell, Tissue and Organ Transplantation (2010) [11] – concur on these fundamental principles and rules (Box 1.1).

Ethical issues of HCTT

Once a normative framework of HCTT has been defined, the practical challenge lies in specifying the meaning of these overarching principles and rules in the light of ethical issues that arise in the different stages of donation and transplantation activities – from procurement to processing, testing, storage, allocation and distribution.

Table 1.1 Central ethical issues in the regulation of human cell (HC) and human tissue (HT) transplantation. (Reproduced with permission from Schulz-Baldes A, Biller-Andorno N, Capron AM (2007) International perspectives on the ethics and regulation of human cell and tissue transplantation. Bulletin of the World Health Organization 85, 941–948.)

Issue	Agreement	Disagreement
Consent for HC/HT removal	• No HC/HT removal without consent • Informed consent for donation from living donors • Disclosure of possible limitations to withdrawing consent	• Informed versus presumed consent in deceased donation? • Role of the next of kin ("family veto") in deceased donation? ○ Obligation to inform about possible profit-making, international circulation or cosmetic applications?
Confidentiality of donor data	• Confidentiality of donor data (with exceptions)	
Unpaid HC/HT donation	• Unpaid donation • Removal of financial disincentives for donation ○ Only not-for-profit institutions in donation discussions and the promotion of donation	
Fair HC/HT procurement	• Fair criteria for donor identification and selection	○ Binding priority of organ over HC/HT recovery?
Stewardship for donated HC/HT	• Obligation to honour and realize donor intent • Option to veto HC/HT use for research or education • No discriminatory restrictions of HC/HT use ○ Stewardship, effectiveness, accountability, fair pricing, responsiveness to local and/or national needs and fair allocation are more important than institutional for-profit/not-for-profit structure	○ Option to veto HC/HT use abroad or for cosmetic applications?
Quality and safety management	• Necessity of quality and safety management • Long-term follow-up of donors and recipients	• Balance between quality, safety and HC/HT availability in resource-poor settings?

Table 1.1 (*Continued*)

Issue	Agreement	Disagreement
Fair distribution of processed HC/HT	• Need for allocation criteria and prioritization rules despite limited scarcity ○ General priority of HC/HT use for life-saving over life-enhancing and cosmetic purposes ○ General priority of local and/or national self-sufficiency	○ Scope of allocation criteria and prioritization rules: institutional, national, subregional? ○ Institutional reciprocity as an allocation criterion? ○ For-profit organizations in HC/HT distribution? ○ General priority of subregional self-sufficiency? ○ International HC/HT circulation to subsidize public health care?
Consent for HC/HT transplantation	• No HC/HT transplantation without voluntary and informed consent	○ Obligation to inform recipients about profit-making and international circulation? ○ Limits of consent for medically contested uses?

• normative agreement or disagreement was analogous to that for organ transplantation;
○ normative agreement or disagreement was specific for HC/HT transplantation.

Whereas some ethical issues are highly specific to a certain kind of intervention or graft, there are also several cross-cutting themes. Table 1.1 shows issues that emerged at the 2006 International Symposium on Ethical and Policy Issues of Human Cell and Tissue Transplantation that was organized by the University of Zurich in collaboration with WHO, outlining areas of agreement and disagreement among meeting participants.

The question of financial incentives, although related to the donation, will be considered, as it relates to the larger context of commercialization of cell and tissue transplantation. The focus, however, will be on selected issues regarding processing, access and allocation and recipient consent in HCTT, respectively.

Ethical issues: tissue transplantation

Tissue transplantation comprises a heterogeneous group of grafts and procedures, including the transplantation of vessels, heart valves, bone allografts, tendons, skin, corneas, and complex tissues, such as hands and face. These grafts are used in a variety of disciplines, for example: orthopedics and sports medicine, neurosurgery, ophthalmology, craniofacial, urology, cardiothoracic, vascular, dentistry, and plastic surgery.

From an ethical point of view, there are several possible ways to categorize different allografts (Box 1.2). One relates to the degree of processing applied to the donation. There seem to be morally relevant differences between

---

Box 1.2 Ethically relevant criteria for distinguishing tissue transplants

Tissue transplants may be distinguished according to the following ethically relevant criteria
Degree of processing
Link to individual donor as source of transplant
Temporary versus permanent transplants
Medical purpose (life saving versus enhancing)
Therapeutic alternatives
Established versus experimental therapy
Preservation methods and storage conditions
Need for immunosuppression (hand and face transplantation)
Availability of the type of tissue and size matching criteria
Living donor versus deceased donor

---

allografts such as an entire bone versus a screw that contains a small amount of bone powder: whereas we would think of the bone segment primarily as a part of an individual donor's body we might be more inclined to consider the screw as a commercial, although somewhat special, product.

Another psychologically relevant distinction relates to how obviously the donor is the source of the graft. This particular issue is relevant in composite grafts; receiving a recognizable hand or face may trigger more far-reaching questions about the relationship between body and identity. Similarly, the questions of permanence of the graft, whether it is transient or permanent will affect the degree to which the recipient will need to confront the task of integrating the graft into his or her own body and sense of self.

Some transplanted tissues have an important impact on quality of life or even survival (such as skin allografts for burn victims), whereas others may achieve only moderate improvements or aim at enhancing an already fair quality of life (such as a knee replacement for arthritis). Some tissue transplantations, such as autologous bone, are the clear gold standard for a certain indication, whereas in other cases comparable or even superior therapeutic alternatives may exist. Some transplants (for example, human embryonic stem cells) remain highly experimental, whereas others, such as cryopreserved heart valves, have been used successfully for decades.

Tissue grafts differ in the way they are preserved and the subsequent environmental storage conditions which they need. This can affect concepts for allocation as these will need to be quite different if a tissue can only be stored short-term vis-à-vis a graft that can be stored for a long period. For instance, tissues with a short preservation time need to be used quickly and cannot be transported over long distances. Another important factor affecting access to therapy using transplantation relates to the need for costly immunosuppression, which is required for some vascularized complex tissues such as hand and face transplantation. There may be limited availability of some graft types, especially where size matching (e.g., pediatric allograft heart valves) is required and this needs to be taken into account in determining rules for allocation.

Finally, whereas most tissues are donated by deceased donors, some may be retrieved from living donors. These include a femoral head, which can be donated when hip replacement surgery is undertaken. In such cases, the procedure resulting in the donation is to the benefit of the donor/patient and therefore poses no intrinsic risk from the donation.

Retrieval and processing

The amount of tissues retrieved differs considerably among populations. Some countries such as Sri Lanka and the USA have corneas donated in excess of domestic demand, whereas other countries import corneas to meet a considerable part of their need. What countries should aim for in regard to donation and/or self-sufficiency is a controversial ethical question. Should they strive for self-sufficiency, i.e., to procuring enough tissues to cover the needs of their own population or should they aim for the maximum number of donations to facilitate export of surplus tissues for other needy populations? And if they export what should the rules be: export to those populations with the greatest need, as a humanitarian action, or to those who have the ability to reimburse processing fees? Can a commercial company export donations to another jurisdiction when the needs of the donating population have not been met? What if no transplant program for the respective material exists in the country where the donations are made that would serve the donating population? Or, conversely, do countries carry a responsibility for their donation rates, given that they could simply import tissues if that country was not self-sufficient?

Such queries raise, of course, the underlying question of whether tissue grafts or products are commercial items, commodities that can be traded according to the rules of the market, or if they retain something of their special nature as a gift. Given the business potential of the tissue market the economic implications of this question are considerable. The monetary value of the human body after donation varies between different tissue banks. It has been reported that the value can exceed (USAD) US$220,000, but more commonly quoted figures are between US$30,000 and US$50,000, with an average of 50–60 grafts made available for distribution per donor [13]. The variability is usually a result of different processing methods and the types of tissue produced. Medical devices, demineralized bone matrices, or dermal implants can yield higher reimbursement to processing facilities than do traditional grafts such as femoral heads and cancellous bone. This provides an incentive for driving donations to financially more attractive products, such as acellular dermis for wound healing or reconstructive surgery uses (abdominal wall, bladder sling, dura replacement, etc.) rather than skin used for burns therapy.

If the concept of tissue establishments acting as stewards of a generous donation they were entrusted with is to be taken seriously, it seems problematic to simply consider human tissues as marketable products, just like equipment or furniture. As exchanges with donor family organizations have revealed, some relatives have been offended by the commercialization of the precious gift donated to tissue banks. Families may be asked to make the decision to donate at a time in their lives when they have just lost a loved one. The process of giving the "final gift" from their relative requires a lot of thought and is emotionally demanding. Families have been upset and distraught upon the discovery that tissue establishments to which they entrusted a family member's donation may have profited from their gift. The use of terms like "products" and "sales", in relation to tissue allografts, can be offensive.

The challenge is to find an appropriate way to appreciate the gift and to act in accordance with the concept of stewardship. This should be accomplished without hampering the development of a dynamic, innovative field as well as the efficient, state-of-the-art recovery, processing, storage and distribution of tissues for the benefit of patients who are potential tissue or cell recipients. Beyond the moral dimension there is also a pragmatic reason for honoring donations: if tissue banking is perceived by the population as reckless profiteering and exploiting peoples' altruism and goodwill this can be expected to have a negative impact on a population's willingness to donate.

How can the delicate balance between legitimate professionalism and unwanted commercialization be achieved? One precondition is certainly transparent pricing, so that fees can be examined and justified. The WHO Guiding Principles [11] have offered a clear criterion: whereas covering verifiable costs and expenses does not fall under the prohibition on sale or purchase, charging excess fees (independently from the market situation) should not be allowed (Box 1.3). To implement this requirement the operational schemes of both for profit and not-for-profit organizations would need to be discussed in detail. This is likely to lead to questions such as the following. What maximum level of remuneration would be appropriate for an employee in a not-for-profit organization? Are shareholder models compatible with the principle of non-commercialization?

Ethical issues about procurement of human tissue do not only relate to commercialization. Another question is the prioritization of body parts to be recovered. Usually, vascularized organs would come first, as the donor pool is more limited. However, relevant criteria include the clinical need of the recipient and the possibility of death without the graft, rather than the nature of the body part. There have been some concerns, however, that the recovery of certain grafts may put a high psychological demand on donors

> **Box 1.3 WHO Guiding Principles on human cell, tissue, and organ transplantation, endorsed by the 63rd World Health Assembly (2010) [11]**
>
> **Guiding Principles on non-commercialization**
> **WHO Guiding Principle 5**
>   Cells, tissues, and organs should only be donated freely, without any monetary payment or other reward of monetary value. Purchasing, or offering to purchase, cells, tissues, or organs for transplantation or their sale by living persons, or by the next of kin in the case of deceased persons, should be banned.
>   The prohibition on sale or purchase of cells, tissues and organs does not preclude reimbursing reasonable and verifiable expenses incurred by the donor, including loss of income, or paying the costs of recovering, processing, preserving and supplying human cells, tissues or organs for transplantation.
> **WHO Guiding Principle 8**
>   All health care facilities and professionals involved in cell, tissue, or organ procurement and transplantation procedures should be prohibited from receiving any payment that exceeds the justifiable fee for the services rendered.

or their families. Such grafts include uterus, face, limb, or hand donation. If the public feels repelled by these types of donations and transplants, the psychological demands may result in a negative impact on overall donation rates.

One way to overcome such qualms might be by providing financial incentives for donation. Implementing such policy would, however, exploit the difficult economic situation of some families who would be more vulnerable to responding to such a reward.

Another topic that has frequently been discussed is the use of donated tissues for cosmetic/reconstructive purposes. Whereas it is clear that the different uses of tissues should be disclosed to donor families when consent for donation is requested, it needs to be appreciated that the term "cosmetic use" is a broad and somewhat vague term and can be misleading. Is the use of cartilage to repair a congenital defect of a child's ear considered to be a reconstructive or cosmetic procedure? The repair of facial scars from a traumatic accident might be seen as cosmetic use by some, but for the individual patient this type of procedure could be a major life enhancement, which could help restore their self-image. Involving the donor or donor family perspectives in the discussion regarding what constitutes appropriate use of donated body materials might be the appropriate way forward.

CASE STUDY 1.1

Directed use of tissue

Mr and Mrs Z were recently informed of the death of their only child KT. She was 17 years old and had just received her driver's license. KT lost control of her car on a slippery, icy road. Her parents are obviously distraught. Her mother had not wanted her driving to school this morning because of the hazardous roads but had agreed after a long argument. Their daughter was a beautiful, thoughtful young lady. KT was on the girls' track and field team and was planning on attending college with hopes of studying to be a doctor. She always wanted to help others. KT volunteered at the local children's hospital and assisted in the burn unit.

When she recently received her drivers' license she signed up to be an organ and tissue donor. Her parents were unaware of her wishes. There were no restrictions identified on her first person consent document. After discussing the donation process with the donation specialist, the parents decided to honor her daughter's wishes and allow organ and tissue donation. Her mother had read about some skin grafts being used for "profiting" and for "cosmetic" uses. The family insisted that her skin donation be used for children who were patients on burn units only.

Questions

1. Should the processing agency provide specific criteria to educate "consenting" specialists about all possible uses of donated tissue?

2. How can the tissue-processing establishment abide by the wishes of the family regarding these specific limitations for use?

3. How can it be expected that tissue distribution intermediaries and the hospital abide by the wishes of the family regarding these specific limitations for use? What if a surgeon uses the skin graft, which is made available in the hospital's inventory, for a breast reconstruction or repair of a facial deformity?

4. How can tissue establishment personnel know exactly what the family means by "cosmetic use," use for the treatment of "burns," or what they consider "profiting" to be? A less important issue may be what they believe the age of a "child" to be, but is that also a consideration to be addressed? Is there a limit to what wishes should be respected and which should not?

5. Because the tissue facility has the name and telephone number of the family do they have the right to call the family and explain more details and ask for permission for additional use?

6. How does "altruistic donation" relate to use of the gift (by whom and what for)?

7. What is "reasonable" regarding all of the above?

Access and allocation

Equitable access to tissue and cell transplants stands firm as an ethical principle. Its precise meaning and its practical implications are, however, far less clear. On a global scale, what does the different availability of certain tissues, which may be in part due to a differential willingness to donate, mean in terms of international solidarity? Should we think of human tissues as a global resource to be distributed according to need? That would mean, for instance, that skin could not be transformed into highly processed/higher cost products as long as there were burn victims worldwide needing cryopreserved allograft skin. Or are tissues transformed along the way into commodities that can legitimately be distributed according to a profit-maximizing strategy? So far, it is unclear at what level specific criteria for fair allocation should be defined, and what role for-profit tissue or cell establishments should have in the distribution of substances of human origin.

If the population of a certain country, which is underserved in terms of health care because of racial discrimination or economic difficulties, were hesitant to agree to postmortem donation, could they expect solidarity from other countries that did not have a similar viewpoint or situation? Alternatively should that country just be referred back to the principle of self-sufficiency or to the possibility of importing donated human substances even if the country might not have the resources to pay for them? Or what about a low-resource country that did not have significant transplantation activities for their populace but was exporting tissues with significant monetary gain? Would this be acceptable if the proceeds were invested into that country's health care system but unacceptable if the proceeds went to a private company that made considerable profit? There is an urgent need for further clarification of these types of ethical rules for cross-border circulation of human tissues.

Another issue is the trade-off between access and safety. When the supply is limited an argument might be made for lowering standards to have a larger pool of grafts available. The challenge on a policy level is to work against a downward spiral in terms of safety standards, but to uphold minimum and best practice standards and to decide on exceptions on a case-by-case basis. This should only be applicable when no other therapy or product exists and a patient will be harmed if the non-conforming allograft is not used.

Consent to receive

Recipient consent needs to follow standard rules for informed consent. Individuals need to be informed about the fact that they are receiving a human allograft, about the risks and benefits of the treatment, and about therapeutic alternatives. Instances of disease transmission would need to be reported, potentially infringing on the confidentiality of the intervention. The use of non-optimal grafts would also need to be explained when applicable, and the appropriate consent obtained. The same principle applies to the use of novel therapies.

CASE STUDY 1.2

Amputation of transplanted hand

A 48-year-old man had lost his right hand many years ago in an accident. When he received a transplanted hand and forearm from an anonymous donor, the victim of a motorcycle accident, doctors were surprised how quickly he regained function. As this was the first transplant of its kind, the case was followed closely by the press.

Two months after the transplant there were no signs of rejection, and the patient was not bothered by any adverse effects from the potent immunosuppressive drugs he needed. Psychologically, he was described as being "on top of the world." The patient had prepared for the operation with an intensive exercise program that made sure his muscles of his handless right arm were strong enough to carry out movements with his new hand. After the operation he was in fact able to bend each finger about 25 degrees and then straighten it and to move his whole wrist around in a circle. Later, the patient was able to write with a pen and hold a glass of water. The patient was reported as stating that the hand seemed like his own, not like somebody else's. He had made the promise to himself that when he had his new hand, it would not just be for him, "but for everyone."

Two years later, however, the patient asked for the hand to be taken off. He admitted to not having taken his medication regularly, leading to a rejection reaction. Doctors discovered that he had been convicted of fraud and served a prison term. "This guy is a very good con man," one of the doctors commented. The psychological testing that the patient had undergone before the transplant had concluded that he could be expected to be a cooperative patient. In the end the hand was removed in a 90-minute operation by one of the surgeons who had helped to attach it.

Questions
1. How can donor selection be improved to prevent such cases?
2. How can donor compliance be maximized?
3. Did the fact that hand transplants receive a lot of public interest and media attention have any impact on this case?
4. Is there a competitive drive between professionals in transplantation surgery (in particular with a view to "first ever" transplants), and if so, what is its potential impact on donor selection?
5. If the tissue had not been dependent on continued immunosuppression for its maintenance, should the wish of the patient have been respected?

Ethical issues: cell transplantation

Human cell transplantation covers a diverse field. It includes bone marrow, peripheral blood stem cells (PBSC), umbilical cord blood, HSCs (autologous, related, and unrelated), mesenchymal stem cells, pancreatic islet cells, embryonic stem cells, induced pluripotent stem cells, and gametes. The common characteristic of all of these is that live human cells with uniform features are being provided to replace lost function in the recipient.

Ethically relevant distinctions can be made regarding the kind of cell (somatic versus germ line cell), the source (adults/children, embryos, deceased bodies, umbilical cord), the invasiveness of the collection process and associated risks (bone marrow aspiration and general anesthesia, peripheral blood drawing, apheresis procedures) and the clinical application.

Retrieval and processing

The retrieval of bone marrow or peripheral blood HSCs are well-established procedures, involving several stages of informed consent: for joining a donor registry, for further medical screening and testing if selected, and finally, to proceed with the donation. Still, being an HSC donor does come with certain risks, in particular the use of mobilization medicines required for PBSC donation, which need to be carefully monitored and weighed against the benefits of the procedure.

Another set of ethical issues arises when the donor decides to withdraw their offer, particular when this occurs at a moment when the recipient's own bone marrow has already been destroyed in preparation of the transplant.

CASE STUDY 1.3

Brotherly love

Mrs X was diagnosed with leukemia after a nose bleed that would not stop. A few weeks later she was ready for a bone marrow transplant. She was fortunate that she had a brother who despite living in another country was tested quickly and turned out to be a perfect tissue-type match. A medical work up in his own country revealed that he was a suitable donor and he flew to the city where his sister lived. The transplant was confirmed and the patient underwent preconditioning to destroy her bone marrow before the transplant. The day planned for the donation arrived and her brother did not arrive for admission. He was found to be at the airport on his way home. Mrs X's physician hurried to speak to him and explain that his sister would now die within a week because of the preconditioning therapy. He was aware of this and departed on the plane to his own country. His sister admitted that he had demanded more money than she and her husband could afford. They did not believe that he would carry out his threat to leave if the money was not deposited in his account before the donation. But he did.

Questions
1. How can this situation be avoided?
2. Is there anything that the transplant program can do to manage this risk to their patient?
3. What would you say to the prospective "donor" to convince them to proceed to the donation?
4. Could withdrawal from donation after preconditioning be made against the law/ethical standards?
5. What alternative options are available to the patient after preconditioning?
6. Is there a role for autologous bone marrow storage preconditioning?
7. Is there a role for unrelated HSC transplantation?

Recently, another issue has been amply discussed in the context of blood and organ donation. This is the payment of unrelated bone marrow donors to increase the number of willing individuals. This idea stems from the relatively poor availability of some individuals when they are selected for an actual donation even though they had registered to donate. It has been suggested that payment at this point might encourage both recruitment to the registries and to make the actual donation when the potential donor is called upon.

Relevant professional societies in the field, among them the National Marrow Donor Program and the WMDA, do not agree with the principle of payment for donation, for several reasons:

- The proposal is based upon the fallacy that nonavailability can be resolved by payment. In fact, payment would risk demolishing the structure of global altruistic HSC donation, possibly spreading to other fields of transplantation and leading in fact to reduced access to grafts.
- A vendor has motivation to disguise information that might jeopardize the sale of their cells. This would endanger the vendor if the hidden medical issue were of relevance to safety of cell collection and the recipient if the issue was related to risk of a transmissible disease.
- If payment was to be covered by the recipient this would make the feasibility of transplantation subject to the individual recipient's capacity to pay, even if health insurance coverage was available.
- During the phase of preconditioning before HSC transplant the patient passes the point of no return and becomes entirely dependent on receiving the transplantation. The patient thus immediately becomes increasingly vulnerable to a fiscally driven vendor's demands to increase the price.

Pricing is in itself a contentious issue. What is an appropriate price for a unit of PBSC? Such questions raise deeper philosophical and legal issues of ownership of the human body. Do I own my bone marrow and can I freely dispose of it through sale? These issues have been debated ever since John Moore famously claimed a share of the profits derived from patents on a cell line that was generated from his spleen tissue [14].

Whereas pricing is a hypothetical issue while the context remains donation, it becomes very real when it comes to processing and value adding to donated tissues and cells. A transparent justification of costs that is amenable to oversight would be highly desirable. Another issue for regulatory oversight is the control of quality, safety, and efficacy, with the aim of stopping unfounded and bogus therapeutic claims and dubious, experimental treatments. An open question that would need to be reviewed in each case, is a possible difference in risk management – an individual suffering from a certain condition may be more willing to take considerable risks for the slight chance of a cure and may differ in their judgment from the position held by the responsible regulatory authority.

Access and allocation

Although there is widespread consensus on the desirability of equitable access to HSC transplantation, it is quite clear this goal has not yet been achieved. Differential access to transplants results from two different but related issues. Some ethnic groups have very similar tissue types (human leukocyte antigen, HLA) and have relatively homogeneous genetics, thus they need to have fewer individuals on the registries to have a good chance of finding a donor match. The Japanese and Korean populations are examples of this phenomenon. Indian and North American Black populations have the opposite situation, with diverse, heterogeneous tissue types leading to low chances of finding a matched donor among the same number of potential volunteers. The second problem is actually recruiting broadly representative ethnic groups to the registries in sufficient numbers to provide for patients with each particular ethnic background.

Another concern is limited access of patients without sufficient resources or appropriate health insurance coverage. In resource-poor countries, access to "gold standard" treatment will be substantially limited. The cost of creating global registries of potential HSC donors has been large with tissue typing and infrastructure costs for the unrelated registry reaching perhaps US$300 for each of the currently 14 million registrants; adding up to a US$4.2 billion capital investment. These costs are being borne by multiple payers: individuals providing for their own costs of typing, charitable organizations, governments, etc. HSC transplants themselves are additionally very expensive procedures with hospital costs of approximately US$250,000 for each patient. The high expenses for an individual treatment tie into the more general debate on allocating scarce health care resources, raising the question of how much money a society is prepared to spend per quality adjusted life year (QALY). One advantage that HSC transplants have is the generally long-term survival once the initial high-risk period of the first year has passed. Once cured of the disease for which transplantation was performed, patients may expect a fairly normal lifespan. Thus the life years per patient procedure is higher than in many economic models of other health care interventions.

Private cord blood banking is another topical issue that has enjoyed some media and commercial popularity over recent years. Parents or grandparents are offered a "life insurance" to their offspring in the form of stored cord blood, without any proof of its clinical utility and for a considerable fee. Professional societies and several physicians have voiced their concern about this practice [15], requiring, at a minimum, full disclosure of the lack of proven benefit to potential users and the problems associated with adherence to usual volume, quality and safety standards. Some alternative models that are currently under discussion suggest public-private hybrids, allowing samples stored for autologous purposes to be used for allogeneic transplantation if needed and vice versa. Regulation may well assist in clarifying what claims may be made in this area.

Regulation, on the other hand, may also threaten to cause problems. Given the dependency on suitable HLA matches, international exchanges are frequently a necessity in unrelated bone marrow transplantation. But if donor centers around the world have to fulfill different national licensing requirements, then the cost and regulatory incompatibilities are highly likely to hinder access unless effective measures are put in place to avoid this. An international harmonization of requirements will be needed [16] to avoid a situation in which measures intended to improve safety actually imperil access.

Consent to receive

Consent to receive is very complex in HSC transplantation. Whereas it shares many features with consent to any other high risk procedure it still is an ethical challenge given the high mortality and morbidity, the need for third party consent for children, the absence of other choices in certain clinical diagnoses, the complexity of the information required to fully understand the intervention, and the question as to what one is actually consenting to (Box 1.4).

HSC transplantation is not simply a single event and is more akin to being cast over a waterfall with no choice as to the subsequent turn of events. The hematologist's task is to reduce the complexity in a way that is appropriate for the individual patient so that they can make a reasonably informed decision. What options are available will also depend on a country's health care resources. In rich countries, the range of options is enhanced by the possibility of using very expensive medication (such as imatinib mesylate, Gleevec®) that may reduce the need for HSC transplantation. This difference needs to be taken into account when discussing equitable access on a global scale.

Box 1.4 Making meaning of mortality statistics: deciding about HSC transplantation for refractory acute myeloid leukemia

Clinical options in refractory acute myeloid leukemia (i.e., all treatment fails to achieve remission)

Option 1. No transplant

Immediate mortality risk:	Very high (90% within 3 months)
Medium-term mortality risk:	100%
Long-term survival chances:	Nil

Option 2. Transplant

Immediate mortality risk:	High (20–40% mortality within 3 months)
Medium-term mortality risk:	Very high (75–85% 2-year mortality)
Long-term survival chances:	20%

For all these reasons, consent for receiving a transplant is a delicate procedure that requires a considerable level of professional expertise. On the one hand, there is certainly no point in confusing patients with details they cannot fully appreciate or in informing them about options that may not be within reach for them. On the other hand, not informing about possible implications may lead to difficult situations, not only with a view to the recipient but, in fact, also to the donor.

CASE STUDY 1.4

Inconvenient results

RM was 12 when diagnosed with leukemia. He weighed only 27 kg and despite having no siblings there was optimism that an unrelated donor would be found quickly. There were no obvious matches on the preliminary search but two cord blood units showed up on the search of the Bone Marrow Donors Worldwide database. One of the cord units was a good match and was transplanted a few weeks later. The delay in engraftment was a tense period for his parents but it all worked out well. A few months of anxiety and medications were followed by a progressive relaxation of restrictions and return to school. At one year after the transplant he had a check bone marrow biopsy to test for relapse. The good news for residual disease was that there was no evidence of relapse of his disease. The inconvenient result was that the bone marrow had been populated by the donor cord blood and those cells were abnormal. The cytogenetic diagnosis was Klinefelter's syndrome.

Questions

1. What should you tell the recipient? (There are no medical consequences of this diagnosis for the recipient.)
2. Should the possibility of such a transmission occurring have been raised during the recipient consent process?
3. Should the possibility of such an incidental diagnosis occurring have been raised as part of the consent for donation, including a discussion of feeding back such a finding?
4. What should you tell the mother of the donor of the cord blood? (There are consequences of the diagnosis for the child who has the genetic disorder. Although the diagnosis will in the end be made in the recipient, early diagnosis may help both timely medical therapy and adjustment.)
5. Should cord blood banks undertake cytogenetic testing of all cord blood units at storage, with the implication that all donors will be tested as a consequence of volunteering the donation?

Yet consent is not a sufficient requirement for transplantation. Patients may be desperate and willing to undergo or even demand exceedingly risky or unsuitable therapies. Medical indications and suitable oversight mechanisms are needed as an additional safeguard.

Conclusions and outlook

Whereas some ethical issues are specific to certain interventions, others cut across the field of HCTT, such as identifying and eliminating quackery, provision of fair, transparent pricing, and equitable access. To tackle these challenges, more data are needed on activities, on establishments, and on the effect of policies, e.g., access. Registries such as the European Registry for Organs, Cells and Tissues (EUROCET) begin to allow for an overview of what is happening in the field. Such data, as well as the development of common nomenclature, can facilitate the preparation of harmonized standards, which are essential in view of the importance of international exchange. In focusing on appropriate policy for cell and tissue transplantation, possible therapeutic alternatives should not be overlooked and preventive strategies should be strengthened, where possible.

There has been major progress over the past few years in spelling out some of the fundamental ethical principles governing the field of HCTT. Yet there is a striking gap between the level of principles and their implementation. A concrete challenge to be taken up as soon as possible consists of the need to integrate ethically relevant aspects into regulatory oversight. This is similar to what is happening in the area of clinical research, where "ethics audits," as a follow-up to the review committee's recommendations, are being increasingly discussed and realized [17].[4] Issues to be resolved in reporting or in inspections should go beyond a simple check on the consent form; they should include procedural and content aspects of consent: How were donors or their families approached? What information did they receive? Other issues that could be considered for good inspection practice might include transparency and appropriateness of pricing, or a justification of why a certain product was given priority over other options or why products were exported rather than used for the donating population. A formal system of reporting instances of "tissue trafficking" would be a useful step in implementing globally recognized ethical principles.

Yet another challenge ahead is the realization of access to evidence-based, cost-effective HCTT in low-resource countries. At the same time, patients in these countries may be particularly vulnerable to dubious treatments that are highly experimental or are offered mainly for the sake of profit. Fostering access to HCTT while taking account of public health priorities of each respective country and putting in place effective safeguards against abuses of this promising and dynamic field is an important task. It will require a joint effort from professional societies, health authorities, patient representatives, ethicists and international organizations such as the WHO.

KEY LEARNING POINTS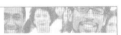

- Application of HCTT has expanded considerably over the past few years; cross-border circulation and global activities have intensified.

- Transparency, evidence-based standards, and an ethical framework are needed to allow for appropriate regulation and to maintain the public's trust.

- In tissue transplantation, major ethical challenges relate to stewardship of a gift rather than commercialization and commodification driven by desire to profit.

- Ethical issues surrounding cell transplantation include access to very costly treatments, and global harmonization of regulatory standards to enable international matching of HSCs, while countering activities that are of no proven benefit.

- Future challenges consist of building a solid database for policy decisions, closing the gap between ethical principles and their implementation, and working towards equitable access to well-proven, cost-efficient treatments, including for patients from low-resource countries.

---

[4]The International Ethical Guidelines for Biomedical Research Involving Human Subjects (CIOMS, 2002), for instance, state that Ethical Review Committees "should be required to monitor the implementation of an approved protocol and its progression, and to report to institutional or governmental authorities any serious or continuing non-compliance with ethical standards as they are reflected in protocols that they have approved or in the conduct of the studies." www.cioms.ch/publications/layout_guide2002.pdf, p. 29, accessed October 2011.

References

1. American Association of Tissue Banks 2007 Annual Survey of Accredited Tissue Banks in the United States, McLean, VA, American Association of Tissue Banks, 2010.
2. Apperley J, Carreras E, Gluckman E, Gratwohl A, Masszi T (eds). Hematopoietic Stem Cell Transplantation, European School of Hematology, Paris, 2008.
3. Aiken-O'Neill P, Mannis MJ. Summary of corneal transplant activity: Eye Bank Association of America. Cornea 2002;21:1–3.
4. De Boer H. The history of bone grafts. Clin Orthop Relat Res 1988;226:292–298.
5. Carrel A. Landmark article Nov 11, 1911: rejuvenation of cultures of tissues. J Am Med Assoc 1983;250:1085.
6. Office of the Inspector General (2001) Oversight of Tissue Banking, http://oig.hhs.gov/oei/reports/oei-01-00-00441.pdf (accessed February 16, 2010).
7. Rid A, Dinhofer L in Tissue and Cell Donation: An Essential Guide (eds Warwick RM, Fehily D, Brubaker SA, Eastlund T), Blackwell Publishing, Oxford, 2009, 67–97.
8. World Medical Association. Statement on Human Organ Donation and Transplantation, 2007.
9. Council of Europe. Additional Protocol to the Convention on Human Rights and Biomedicine concerning Transplantation of Organs and Tissues of Human Origin, ETS No. 186, 2002.
10. DIRECTIVE 2004/23/EC OF THE EUROPEAN PARLIAMENT and OF THE COUNCIL of 31 March 2004 on setting standards for quality and safety in the donation, procurement, processing, preservation, storage and distribution of human tissues and cells. Official Journal of the European Union L 102/48 07/04/2004.
11. World Health Organization. WHO Guiding Principles on Human Cell, Tissue and Organ Transplantation, WHA63/22, Annex 8, 2010.
12. Schulz-Baldes A, Biller-Andorno N. Capron AM. International perspectives on the ethics and regulation of human cell and tissue transplantation. Bull Wld Hlth Org 2007;85:941–8.
13. Youngner SJ, Anderson MW, Schapiro R. (eds) Transplanting Human Tissue: Ethics, Policy, and Practice, Oxford University Press, Oxford, 2004.
14. Supreme Court of California. Moore v. Regents of the University of California. 51 C3d 120, 1990.
15. Fox NS, Chervenak FA, McCullough LB Ethical considerations in umbilical cord blood banking. Obstet Gynec 2008;11:178–82.
16. Hug K. Banks, repositories and registries of stem cell lines in Europe: regulatory and ethical aspects. Stem Cell Rev 2009;5:18–35.
17. Council of International Organizations of Medical Sciences. International Ethical Guidelines for Biomedical Research Involving Human Subjects, Geneva, Council of International Organizations of Medical Sciences, 2002.

2 Clinical Governance by Physicians: Maintaining the Safety and Effectiveness of Cell and Tissue Transplantation

Ted Eastlund[1] and Ruth M. Warwick[2]
[1]University of New Mexico, Albuquerque, NM, USA
[2]University of Bristol, Bristol, UK

Introduction

The growing application of human tissue, cell, and organ transplantation has created unique roles and responsibilities for physicians. These donated substances of human origin include blood components, organs, tissues, and cells such as those used in hemopoietic transplantation and in assisted reproduction. They are donated altruistically, are sometimes in short supply, and can carry the risk of transmitting disease from donor to recipient. Their clinical use creates expectations and obligations that are more comprehensive than those associated with the use of implantable nonbiologic, sterilized medical devices (Table 2.1).

The clinician and the recipient have the expectation that the allograft will be available when needed and will be safe and effective. The expectation of donors and donor families is that their privacy and autonomy will be maintained and respected, and that their donation will be used wisely and provided fairly for the benefit of patients. Use for research or for education should not occur without their permission and many might expect their donation will not be used for commercial gain.

Clinicians have an important leadership role in meeting these expectations and obligations through participation in an oversight system of processes called good clinical governance.

Tissue and Cell Clinical Use: An Essential Guide, First Edition. Edited by Ruth M. Warwick and Scott A. Brubaker.
© 2012 Blackwell Publishing Ltd. Published 2012 by Blackwell Publishing Ltd.

Table 2.1 Cell and tissue allografts as human-derived materials

Altruistically donated for public use, requiring fair access by patients in need.

Potentially in short supply requiring judicious use based on evidence-based medicine.

Perishable, requiring proper storage and inventory management to avoid wastage.

Potentially dangerous with risk of transmitting disease, requiring informed recipient consent and a post-transplant surveillance and biovigilance system.

This chapter focuses on the essential roles of clinicians in clinical governance to improve quality of care in tissue and cell transplantation, which includes the oversight and handling of tissue allografts within health care facilities. The models and clinical governance issues described here for tissue allografts can be adapted for other types of allografts, whether organs, hemopoietic cells or other types of cells.

Role of physicians and surgeons in clinical governance

Clinical governance of tissue and cell transplantation requires physicians to be involved in a systematic and wide-ranging approach to improve and maintain quality in transplant recipient care in an environment of transparent responsibility. The processes of ensuring clinical governance have been previously described [1–3] and these provide an important interdisciplinary oversight involving health care professionals to ensure safe, effective, and efficient use of tissue and cell allografts. The roles of the physician in the clinical governance of tissue transplantation have been described by Swanson et al. [1] and have been revised and listed in Table 2.2.

Clinical governance is the responsibility of each individual practicing clinician (surgeons, physicians and other health care professionals, depending on the field of tissue or cell application) but it also provides an opportunity for professional medical societies. Through membership of professional societies, clinicians have opportunities to have a direct effect on the quality and research relating to the allografts they use for patients. Professional societies can influence the type of grafts their members use and the processing which the allografts undergo by working with tissue suppliers and reporting surgical outcome measures and specifying how grafts should be preserved or packaged. Case Study 2.1 illustrates a surgical society in the United Kingdom (UK) that is prospectively contributing to tissue transplantation effectiveness and safety.

Another example is the work by the American Association of Orthopedic Surgeons, which formed a committee in 2002 to contribute to improved allograft safety by working with regulatory and public health

Table 2.2 Responsibilities of surgeons and treating physicians for the clinical governance of cell and tissue transplantation*

Provide advice about the appraisal, provision, medical necessity, and cost effectiveness of new cell and tissue allografts and services.

Collaborate with clinical peers and national professional societies to establish and disseminate guidelines and best practices for the use of allografts supported by evidence-based medicine.

Participate in physician peer review of appropriateness of allograft use by undertaking regular clinical audits, reviewing and monitoring allograft use against measures of best practice, including underuse, overuse, and misuse.

Participate in oversight committees to establish best practices, review clinical audits, and assess the safety, availability, effectiveness, and quality of allografts.

Recognize, investigate and report serious adverse outcomes of allograft use. Undertake counseling of recipients, with appropriate advice where necessary, who have been affected by an adverse event or reaction.

Assist in recalls and look back investigations by notifying and evaluating allograft recipients, if needed.

Promote continuous improvement through analysis of adverse events, errors and near-misses related to allograft handling and use with an interdisciplinary, systems approach in a fair and just environment that does not focus on fear, defensiveness, or blame of individuals.

Promote continuing education to ensure that physicians have the skills, knowledge, and experience necessary for safe and effective transplantation.

Ensure that appropriate procedures are in place for the recognition, appropriate guidance, and corrective action of poor performance.

Promote public and professional support of cell, tissue, and organ donation.

Support and promote research, education, and lifelong learning in all fields related to transplantation.

*These responsibilities are equally applicable to organ transplantation and use of haemopoietic stem cells and those working in the field of assisted reproduction using donated gametes.

organizations following a report of a death due to *Clostridium sordelli* caused by a contaminated fresh femoral condyle [4, 5]. Health care professionals are also involved with the development of European Union-level regulations and working practices relating to vigilance and surveillance, traceability and identification/coding of tissue and cell allografts and other substances of human origin. Clinicians and tissue banking professionals can further exert influence by active dialogue with their regulators.

Clinical effectiveness and clinical audit

Assessing, improving, and maintaining the clinical effectiveness of tissue allografts involve evaluating whether they accomplish their intended

CASE STUDY 2.1

How surgical societies can help with tissue transplant effectiveness and safety

A Surgical Allograft Working Group comprising The British Association for Surgery of the Knee (BASK) and the National Health Service Blood and Transplant Tissue Services (NHSBT) was formed to provide a national forum for professional interaction between the major English provider of tissue allografts (NHSBT) and the major clinical users of tendon, ligament, and meniscal allografts for knee surgery (BASK). The subjects for consideration by this working group are the following:

- To collect and report data on the number of soft tissue allograft implantation procedures conducted in the UK and to maintain a database of outcomes.
- To provide a feedback mechanism for clinical outcome data following soft tissue implantation in the knee in the UK, allowing comparisons to be made of tissue preserved or decontaminated by different methods.
- To prioritize areas for in vitro and clinical research and development aimed at improving the clinical success of soft tissue allografting in the knee.
- To oversee the introduction of new soft tissue allografts, establishing user working groups and reporting clinical outcomes to BASK members.
- To make recommendations to NHSBT Tissue Services on the range and type of soft tissue allografts to be supplied.
- To monitor and report on novel technologies that might improve the success of soft tissue implantation in the knee, keeping BASK members fully informed.
- To monitor and review the safety of soft tissue allografts in the knee, informing BASK members of the risks involved and recommending risk reduction strategies to NHSBT Tissue Services.
- To review the literature in the field, ensuring that BASK members are fully informed of current developments.

In addition, as it becomes appropriate, the Working Group may apply for funding for research and development, and to commission the work when successful.

purpose, are safe, and are used appropriately. Oversight of clinical effectiveness includes assessing whether allograft application produces better outcomes than alternatives, including no surgery at all or the use of a medical device or an autograft. Data are obtained by objective clinical studies and routine reporting of surgical outcomes. The introduction of a new cell or tissue allograft or a new method of use should be scrutinized not only for its clinical effectiveness and safety but also for its cost-effectiveness. For example, evaluation should be made whether an existing allograft used in a new application or whether a new conditioning regimen used before a hemopoietic stem cell transplant produces improved outcomes.

Allograft effectiveness depends not only on the quality of the allograft but also by ensuring that it is used for a clinical indication that has been proven to be effective. Robust peer-reviewed published evidence is fundamental to determine agreed changes in clinical indications for use. Evidence-based medicine involves the application of clinical outcome data to develop clinical practice guidelines as has been applied in other specialty practices over the years [6]. Clinical audit is a form of peer review and is another powerful tool to improve medical practice. Clinical governance requires regular audit to measure individual practitioner's use of allografts against agreed standards and practice guidelines. When practice guidelines are not followed, audits can provide the necessary information to facilitate change.

Education and training

Clinical governance also involves ensuring the initial and continued education and training of physicians and hospital staff. Knowledge about allograft infectious risks, and whether allografts were processed, disinfected, or sterilized, is important in making a choice of the graft type to use and when providing information to patients so they can be aware and give informed consent. A survey in 2006 sponsored by the American Orthopedic Society for Sports Medicine in the United States (USA) showed that there is continued need for surgeons to have accurate information about the grafts they use [7]. Of the surgeons who use allografts, 46% did not know if the allografts they use were sterilized. Most knew very little about the sterilization process used by the tissue supplier, whereas 10% thought unsterilized allografts were not at all safe and 14.6% thought unsterilized allografts were completely safe or nearly so.

Surgeons not only have responsibilities for their own education but a responsibility to educate others, including their patients and other clinical staff. Physicians and surgeons are expected to maintain standards of proficiency and demonstrate ongoing development. This is broader than continued education because it includes competency assessment and improving clinical skills; not merely knowledge acquisition.

Research

It is important for physicians to use tissue and cell allografts based on evidence of safety and effectiveness. Other than with the use of hemopoietic cells, there is currently a relative paucity of controlled clinical trials of the effectiveness and safety of tissue and cell allografts. Many variables in surgical practice have made it difficult to compare the use of grafts. Similarly, there are few studies of how variations in tissue bank practices can result in improved outcomes. These practices may be based on historical precedent rather than being evidence-based. The following chapters in this book include available clinical evidence of the use of tissues and cells, including hemopoietic stem cell therapies and in assisted reproduction. It is incumbent on physicians who use allografts to promote and support studies needed for new transplantation advances in the light of benefits, disadvantages, safety, efficacy, and costs involved.

Oversight, openness, quality improvement

Clinicians should fully participate in interdisciplinary oversight of allograft use, in hospital quality-improvement efforts, and in the open investigation of complaints, errors, accidents, and adverse outcomes of allograft use and near-misses. Clinical governance requires clinicians to accept transparent accountability, teamwork rather than individualism, a systems approach to quality, and a sharing of authority and decision making in improving quality and medical care [8]. Processes open to the scrutiny of others, while respecting individual patient and practitioner confidentiality, are an essential part of continuous quality improvement.

Biovigilance networks

Participation in biovigilance programs is an important part of the clinical governance of transplantation. Biovigilance programs comprise all those opportunities for discovering patients' adverse outcomes associated with implantation of allografts (Table 2.3). A fundamental element of biovigilance is the recognition and reporting of suspected allograft-caused complications by surgeons and physicians or other relevant individuals. Physicians have an ethical obligation to report serious adverse events (and reactions). This is written into opinion 9.032 of the Code of Medical Ethics of the American Medical Association [9]. Reporting must lead to an investigation into the cause and is critically important to allow learning from the root causes of and contributing factors to adverse outcomes and reactions. This ensures improvements in allograft quality and their use. Reporting should allow the timely identification of other recipients of tissue or cells from the same donor, or from the same processing batch, so they can be evaluated as early as possible. Reporting also allows allograft quarantine and recall of tissues or cells in inventory preventing potential recipients from being affected.

Effective biovigilance also requires that reports of complications, such as transmission of disease, reach the tissue banks that process and provide allografts. This is complicated by the global movement of donated organs, tissues, and cells. A single donor may provide several allografts used by many recipients and processing of tissues and cells may result in their integration into composite allografts, medical devices or other tissue-engineered materials. Allografts may be handled or stored by several facilities and may be

Table 2.3 Elements of biovigilance that contribute to allograft safety

Recognition and reporting of suspected allograft-associated adverse outcomes and adverse reactions by the treating physician.

Investigation of adverse outcomes leading to corrective and preventive actions.

National and international biovigilance programs that collate, monitor. and analyze adverse outcomes in recipients.

Use of traceability and coding systems that can link donations with recipients anywhere.

Recalls and look back investigations.

Hospital morbidity and mortality conferences.

Autopsy studies on patients who died after receiving allografts.

Review of health-care facility accident, error and near miss reporting, analysis and quality improvement programs.

Physician audit and peer review of appropriateness of allograft use.

Publication of health-care facility and tissue bank investigations of suspected adverse outcomes.

Qualification of tissue bank suppliers and maintenance of documents listing approved suppliers.

Prospective or retrospective clinical research studies.

Analysis of claims in allograft-related malpractice litigation cases.

distributed widely before final use. Depending on the tissue bank and country of origin, a single type of allograft can carry different names and variations of the donation number and product code as well as words on the label that were designed to provide a unique link to the tissue bank supplier and donor or processing batch. There may be language interpretation issues when tissues and cells traverse international boundaries and uniqueness of identification can only be assured if a unique coding system is used within robust traceability systems. Health care facilities must be able to track from tissue and cell receipt to the recipient or other final destination.

Earlier systems for recognizing adverse outcomes have not been fully effective, which meant that opportunities to recognize, report, investigate and prevent adverse outcomes, particularly regarding transplant-transmitted infections, were missed. The development of regulatory systems in many continents across the world and mandated reporting of adverse outcomes and reactions can help to increase safety. Such reporting would be facilitated by the application of universal coding systems for allograft labeling and record-keeping within traceability systems that can be interpreted and applied in systems used around the world [10, 11]. Ideally, labeling should use a global system.

Need for a biovigilance system

There have been many cases of failed reporting and lack of communication about tissue and organ allograft-transmitted infections by organ procurement organizations, tissue banks, and hospitals [12–14]. In addition there have been gaps in traceability of allografts, and inadequate investigations [12–15]. Consequently some recipients of allografts were unnecessarily infected and others were not identified or evaluated for infection.

Some infectious complications have not been uniformly recognized or reported by transplant surgeons and other physicians caring for recipients. Case Study 2.2 is an example of a sentinel event revealing failures of a biovigilance system along with other deficiencies that led to unnecessary HCV infections of tissue allograft recipients but which subsequently led to corrective actions [13, 14]. Lessons learned from these unfortunate incidents have resulted in improved donor testing, improved communications and improved ability to conduct tissue quarantine and recalls. However, the early recognition and reporting of unexpected outcomes by transplant surgeons and the timely communications to other tissue establishments has remained suboptimal.

Benefits of a biovigilance system

Biovigilance programs involving adverse outcomes of blood transfusion and tissue, cell and organ transplantation can improve patient safety by providing early warning, timely investigation, effective communication and the sharing of data to understand the prevalence and types of adverse outcome. A biovigilance system can provide data for analysis of trends and reduce costs by eliminating errors and inefficiencies, and provide early detection of infectious diseases transmitted after transplantation, including new and re-emerging infectious diseases and other serious adverse outcomes. It can be used to track serious accidents, errors, and process deviations, and quality failures associated with or having the potential for serious adverse outcomes or near-misses. Effective voluntary, centralized biovigilance programs depend on clear and simple confidential reporting by clinicians, hospital personnel, and tissue banks. Reporting must be nonpunitive, nonburdensome, with a standardized data collection system [16, 17]. The importance of a transplantation biovigilance network in which adverse outcomes are reported to a central system and quickly shared with appropriate organizations, and investigated, is further discussed in Chapter 3.

The role of the transplant surgeon in allograft biovigilance programs

Although many components of a biovigilance program do not directly involve transplant surgeons, they and other treating physicians have specific responsibilities [1, 18, 19]. Table 2.4 lists the critical roles of transplant clinicians in improving allograft safety.

CASE STUDY 2.2

Surgeon vigilance in identifying and reporting a postoperative infection due to a virus known to be transmissible by transplantation and poor communication among tissue and organ procurement organizations

Six weeks after repair of an anterior cruciate ligament injury using a donated frozen patellar ligament allograft, the recipient became ill and was diagnosed with hepatitis C virus (HCV) infection [13, 14]. The surgeon reported the HCV infection and an investigation was initiated by tissue bank A that provided the allograft and by public health authorities. The recipient did not receive any blood transfusions and had no other risk factors for HCV exposure and infection.

The patellar ligament allograft had been donated almost two years previously by a deceased donor of four organs and 32 bone, tendon, cornea, vein, and skin allografts that had already been transplanted to other patients. The donor had no HCV risk factors and had been tested and found negative for HCV antibodies. A stored sample of donor blood was tested for HCV RNA and this was found to be positive, thus showing that the donor had an undiagnosed, early seronegative infection when he died.

The subsequent investigation and evaluation of the other recipients in 16 States in the USA and two other countries showed that most recipients did not become infected by HCV. However, HCV infection was found in three organ recipients, a recipient of a frozen saphenous vein allograft, a recipient of a tibialis tendon allograft and three recipients of frozen tendon with bone grafts.

Posttransplant HCV infections had been identified in organ recipients over one year before the contaminated tendons were processed and distributed for use by tissue bank A, but this information was not shared with either tissue bank A or tissue bank B who processed and distributed saphenous vein and tibialis tendon tissue shortly after the original donation. The investigation also discovered an HCV infection in a saphenous vein allograft recipient and two months later an HCV infection in a tibialis tendon allograft recipient had been reported to tissue bank B, but this information was not shared with tissue bank A, the organ procurement agency, or public health authorities. Owing to the findings of this case investigation, tissue donor testing for HCV RNA became a professional standard of the American Association of Tissue Banks and, over 2 years later, it became a federal regulation in the USA. Efforts were initiated nationwide for improved notification and sharing of donor information among tissue banks and organ procurement agencies.

This case illustrated the importance of reporting viral infections in allograft recipients in a timely fashion so the same infection can be prevented in others. It also demonstrates that an investigation can lead to identification of other infected recipients, important process changes in transplantation, and improved safety for future recipients. It also illustrates the adverse effect on recipients when tissue and organ recovery organizations do not communicate effectively.

Table 2.4 The clinician's role in improving the safety of allograft use

Inform patient of risks, benefits and alternatives to allograft use.

Ensure that the risks of an allograft are balanced by the benefits.

Avoid use of unsafe allografts.

Maintain awareness regarding the disease transmission risk of allograft use.

Report all suspected allograft-caused complications.

Cooperate with investigations into suspected adverse outcomes.

Discuss allograft-related complications with peers at hospital morbidity and mortality conferences, and professional meetings.

Cooperate with recall and look back investigations and, when requested, notify and evaluate patients who may have received a contaminated allograft.

Support hospital involvement in allograft safety surveillance programs.

Recognizing and reporting adverse outcomes

Surgeons must maintain awareness of potential adverse clinical outcomes and be willing to help investigate them to determine whether they are complications of the surgery or directly related causally to the tissue or cell allograft. They should discuss and share with their clinical colleagues any case involving an infection or other complication associated with allograft use, particularly at venues such as hospital morbidity and mortality conferences and surgical grand rounds. Surgeons are urged to involve hospital tissue services or another tissue bank physician who is knowledgeable about allografts.

Transplant surgeons and other physicians caring for transplant patients have essential responsibilities for recognizing transplant-transmissible disease, whether infectious, malignant, or another type as discussed in Chapter 4. A history of allograft transplantation should be sought by the physician caring for a patient who has a new diagnosis of any disease that can be transmitted by an allograft. The physician should be particularly suspicious of allograft-transmitted infection when there is unexplained inflammation at the allograft site, laboratory evidence of a new infection, or development of unusual syndromes suggesting disease transmission.

If an infection or other complication is suspected to be associated with allograft use, it should be reported by the physician. In a hospital it should be reported to the hospital tissue storage service and hospital infection control department as soon as possible so it can be investigated and reported to the tissue bank supplier. Reporting adverse outcomes should be a requirement set by hospitals for hospital staff and physicians who have been granted privileges to take care of patients there. In clinics or other facilities it may be necessary to report it directly to the tissue bank and supplier listed on the allograft label. Where there is regulatory oversight it should also be reported as required by regulations. The reporting of an adverse event or reaction triggers an investigation that is essential for correcting errors and accidents and improving safety of tissue use and preventing other recipients of donations from the same donor or same batch being transplanted into other recipients.

Bacterial infections

Although the risk of an allograft-associated bacterial infection is low, the surgeon needs to recognize that grafts can be a source [20]. It is better to be overly suspicious than to miss an infection caused by a bone or tendon allograft. An example of an investigation of a postoperative infection of uncertain cause following allograft use is given in Case Study 2.3. It illustrates how reporting by the surgeon triggers hospital and tissue facility actions in undertaking relevant investigations that ultimately provide useful information for the surgeon and the patient.

A contaminated bone allograft should be suspected when an allograft recipient's infection is deep and when organisms other than those commonly causing wound infections are involved. Not all postoperative bacterial wound infections should be reported as many of these will be a complication of surgery rather than causally related to the graft. Surgeons should consider various factors to determine the likelihood that a postoperative bacterial infection is related to the graft. These include a temporal relationship between the surgical procedure and the onset of the infection, the type of organism, tissue graft processing with minimally processed grafts being a higher risk than highly processed and terminally sterilized grafts, as well as the patient's underlying immune status and medical condition.

Reporting adverse outcomes to patients

Transplant surgeons have roles in the voluntary disclosure of adverse outcomes to patients and should ensure that patients are informed. Professional standards in the USA require hospitals to inform their patients of unanticipated outcomes, especially sentinel events [25]. Several countries and states are enacting disclosure and apology laws pertaining to errors or accidents that may have led to adverse clinical outcomes including those due to a mistake or judgment error.

In the USA, federal legislation (National Medical Error Disclosure Act of 2005) was introduced, but not passed, that called for open disclosure of medical errors to patients, apology, and early compensation. Seven states in the USA have mandated that institutions disclose unanticipated outcomes to patients [26]. It has been predicted that frank and full disclosure will become the norm throughout the USA within a decade and will aid the restoration of the public's trust in the honesty and integrity of the health care system [26]. Opinion 8.121 of the American Medical Association Code

CASE STUDY 2.3

Investigation of a patient who underwent a multi-ligament knee reconstruction and developed a severe operative site infection

After an injury, a 44-year-old female patient underwent a multi-ligament knee reconstruction using frozen irradiated allogeneic anterior tibialis tendon, and posterior tibialis allografts. No pre-implantation cultures were taken at the time of surgery. Postoperatively the patient developed pain and swelling where the grafts were situated, which required hematoma drainage. An infection followed and a variety of low-virulence skin organisms were detected from the wound drainage including diphtheroids, *Acinetobacter baumannii* and coagulase-negative staphylococcus. After antibiotic treatment, residual tissue damage required repair by plastic surgeons but the patient fully recovered without removal of the allografts.

The surgeon did not believe the allografts caused the infection and that it was more likely due to the surgical intervention. However, he did not feel expert in distinguishing between the two potential causes and reported it so it could be investigated.

Possible sources of infection were investigated, which included the operating theatre environment, the arthroscope, the surgical team, the recipient's own skin, or whether the operative wound infection might be due to an allograft donor infection or a failed procedure in the tissue facility such as nonapplication of gamma irradiation to the allograft.

The hospital investigated whether it had any outbreaks of infections from similar organisms in the operating theatre or related surgical areas during the month before and after the operation and it was found that there had been none. There were no signs of failure in the chemo-sterilization procedure used to disinfect the arthroscope.

The allografts were derived from two separate deceased tissue donors. A review of tissue bank records showed that there was no evidence of infection in the tissue donors. There were no reports of infections in any other recipients of tissues derived from these same donors. The tissue bank confirmed that all standard operating procedures had been followed in the procurement and processing of tissue from the implicated donors. A review of pre-processing bacterial testing showed that no bacteria were detected on one of the allografts but the other grew coagulate-negative staphylococcus and *Propionibacterium acnes* but not *Acinetobacter*. As is customary, isolates were not saved on the donation microbiology samples thus DNA sequencing of the staphylococcus from the recipient's wound could not be tested for a match with that detected on the pre-processed allograft. The allograft processing treatments included alcohol disinfection followed by gamma radiation. Records verified that a dose of 25.2–36.4 kGy of gamma radiation was delivered to the allografts a dose validated as an effective sterilization step.

A consulting bacteriology advisor reviewed the data and concluded that the bacterial wound infection's source was endogenous rather than from the allografts or the hospital environment. The conclusion was reported to the surgeon who was then able to report this to the patient.

This case demonstrates the importance of a surgeon's vigilance in reporting a postoperative infection of uncertain cause that enabled a thorough investigation. In this case the allografts were exonerated as a cause but if implicated should have led to corrective actions and improved safety for future recipients of allografts. If the allografts were implicated the surgeon would have been duty-bound to report this to the recipient.

However, the surgeon should not assume that a tissue graft is free of microbial contamination even though the tissue has been packaged in a sealed container, has claims it was sterilized, or has been labeled as sterile. There have been cases of bacterial infections from the use of contaminated tendon allografts during anterior cruciate ligament surgery that were caused by human error when the tissue processor erroneously failed to apply the intended gamma irradiation sterilization step [21]. Infections have also been caused by contaminated tendon, cartilage, and heart valve allografts thought to be free of microbial contamination [22–24]. The contaminant was undetected because final sterility testing by the tissue processor failed. Thus, regardless of the type of tissue allograft used and the sterility assurance claimed, allografts should be considered as a possible cause of posttransplant bacterial infection.

of Medical Ethics recommends that physicians report to their patients any harmful adverse outcomes that are due to error [27]. Western Australia has mandated that serious unanticipated outcomes be disclosed to the patient, preferably by the physician [28, 29]. In the UK, National Health Service policies provide for disclosure so that a patient who has suffered harm as a result of the health care they have received must get an apology [30]. When informing a patient who experienced an allograft complication such as a tissue-transmitted infection, disclosure should include an explanation of the event with an expression of concern, regret, and apology, followed by a projection of future needs for treatment and willingness to assist by including appropriate referral to a specialist as needed for the management of the condition.

Hospital tissue services and clinical governance

The handling of tissue and cell allografts in hospitals requires physician oversight and leadership similar to the requirement for handling of blood components within hospitals. The oversight responsibilities of a hospital tissue service Medical Director and oversight committee are listed in Table 2.5 and have been previously described [1, 18, 19].

Table 2.5 Roles of a hospital tissue services Medical Director and oversight committee

Hospital tissue services medical director	Hospital tissue services oversight committee
Participate in hospital medical staff committees responsible for oversight of tissue and cell allograft use.	Provide oversight of all aspects of tissue and cell transplantation within the hospital to promote a safe, adequate supply of high-quality tissue allografts.
Assist in evaluating qualifications of tissue allograft suppliers.	Review quality of allografts and services, qualifications and certifications of tissue suppliers.
Assist in the investigation and reporting of infectious and other adverse outcomes of allograft use and in taking corrective actions to prevent recurrence	Review reports and investigations of tissue allograft adverse outcomes such as allograft-associated infections.
Participate in auditing of appropriateness of tissue allograft use.	In consultation with the medical staff, establish guidelines for the use of tissue allografts. Establish criteria for auditing the use of tissue allografts and review those not meeting audit criteria for clinical appropriateness.
Assist in recalls and look-back investigations of tissue allografts.	Review recalls and look-back investigations.
Assure compliance with clinical professional standards and governmental regulations.	Review tissue services regulatory and accreditation inspection and compliance reports.
Assist in evaluating suitability of autologous tissue donors including autologous tissue obtained from other hospitals.	Review tissue service quality assessment reports and participate in quality improvement efforts as needed.
Assure that autologous tissue donors with positive infectious disease test results are notified and counseled.	Review tissue service activities including tissue allograft usage trends, outdating, wastage, errors, near-misses and supply shortages.
Provide a link between the hospital tissue service and transplant surgeons and other clinical staff.	Promote tissue transplantation education for the medical staff and hospital employees.
Review and approve exceptional tissue release when there were deviations from written procedures and where release is warranted by clinical situations on a case-by-case basis.	
Review and approve medical-technical procedures	
Assist in the development of policies, processes, and procedures about recipient informed consent.	

There are different models of handling tissue allografts and their receipt and storage in hospitals and there is variation between countries. For example, in the USA, a full supply of allografts is routinely stored by the hospital's tissue service and issued to the operating theater when needed. A hospital tissue service assures that an adequate supply of allografts is obtained from a qualified supplier, inspects incoming allografts, stores allografts and investigates reports of adverse outcomes and reactions. Physicians, including a hospital tissue service Medical Director, are involved with allograft acquisition and storage practices used in the hospital and investigating complications and adverse outcomes. In the UK, the main model involves the direct receipt of allografts from tissue banks and the subsequent short-term storage of grafts in the operating theaters. Depending on the model, there are various levels of clinical and nonclinical hospital staff involvement in the receipt, storage, record-keeping, and other handling of allografts, and autografts, as well as the monitoring of the patient after surgery for the recognition and reporting of adverse outcomes. Some adverse outcomes may be due to the surgery alone or can be due to the allograft if allograft is used. So, for example, an adverse outcome due to infection can result from a patient's own skin flora, for example methicillin-resistant *Staphylococcus aureus* (MRSA). Similarly a hepatitis B transmission from an unrecognized carrier surgeon could occur. Neither of these supposed instances would be due to the allograft. However, a postoperative wound infection due to flora on the allograft or a hepatitis B allograft transmission from the graft or inflammation due to residual chemicals used in graft processing would constitute an adverse reaction to the allograft. When the surgeon and tissue facility Medical Director investigate such outcomes they need to determine whether the complication is due to aspects of surgery or due to the allograft as different corrective and preventative actions would be required in each case.

Oversight responsibility for hospital-based tissue services

In the USA, the Joint Commission, a standards-setting organization for hospitals, requires them to assign responsibility for overseeing the acquisition and storage of tissue allografts and investigation of adverse events throughout the hospital [25]. Complying with these requirements has brought about many positive changes within hospitals nationwide. Handling of tissue allografts within many hospitals had been suboptimal, not centralized, and responsibilities not identified, although some states (i.e., New York and California) require licensure and assignment of responsibility by health care facilities within their borders if they store tissue for transplantation. The Joint Commission does not require that tissue allografts are managed by any specific hospital department or individual, but it does require that hospitals designate oversight responsibility for the organization-wide tissue program operation and identify, by position, persons with responsibility for compliance with accreditation and regulatory requirements. In the UK any organization or department within an organization that stores tissues and cells for human application for more than 24 hours requires a license to do so by the Human Tissue Authority; there are similar requirements which have been introduced into other European Member States through the transposition of the European Commission's Tissue and Cell Directives into national regulations.

In the USA, the site within a hospital that has been most commonly responsible for storing and issuing tissue allografts for transplantation has been the operating room [31]. However, in some hospitals the responsibility for ordering and acquiring tissues and determining that the tissue supplier meets minimum qualification requirements is the purchasing department. In some hospitals, ordering tissue is not centralized and more than one department orders and stores tissue for use in the operating room. Adverse events and reactions after tissue use are not common and hospitals have been uncertain as to how thorough an investigation needs to be and who should conduct it. The focus of responsibility within a hospital for conducting recalls has also sometimes been uncertain and there have been failures in attempts to identify past recipients of allografts [12, 13, 15].

Inspection and acceptance of incoming allografts in hospitals

Inspection of incoming tissue grafts is the responsibility of the hospital tissue services department. Tissue allografts are normally obtained from a tissue supplier and inspected on initial receipt to ensure that the tissue's immediate container is intact and the label is complete, accurate, affixed, and legible before acceptance and placement in storage. In the USA, the Joint Commission requires that hospitals log in all incoming tissues, verify package integrity, and ensure that, when applicable, the transport temperature was controlled and acceptable [25, 32]. Inspection of the shipping container for integrity and for evidence of residual coolant, if applicable, (e.g., wet ice for refrigerated grafts, dry ice for frozen allografts) provides assurance that the required tissue-specific storage environment was maintained during transportation. Upon receipt of tissue allografts at a hospital in the USA, they are stored temporarily or for long periods, most often in areas within the surgical suite or in the blood transfusion service, until used [31].

Expertise that the hospital blood bank/blood transfusion service can offer to serve as a tissue service

A hospital blood bank/blood transfusion service can provide special expertise as a hospital tissue service because the infrastructure that it provides for blood transfusion is very similar to that required for tissues and their transplantation [18, 19, 33–37]. This includes dealing with donated human material, traceability, disease transmission, appropriate use, clinical oversight, storage and monitoring conditions, and investigating adverse reactions among many other skills and functions.

The American Association of Blood Banks (AABB) requires that hospital blood banks/blood transfusion services have a physician responsible for reviewing and approving medical and technical procedures, also known as Standard Operating Procedures (SOPs) [38]. Hospital tissue services should have a Medical Director to liaise with clinicians applying human tissues and cells and who is competent to investigate what may be a complex clinical environment. The blood transfusion service model not only includes oversight by administrative and technical managers and a Medical Director, it also includes oversight by the hospital medical staff in the form of a medical staff committee. This committee could usefully be a template for a medical staff committee with responsibilities (see Table 2.5) to provide oversight of the safety, effectiveness, and appropriateness of allograft use including cycles of auditing.

Tissue supplier qualification and certification

Tissue suppliers should be selected based on their ability to reliably provide high-quality tissues that meet expectations for tissue availability, safety, and effectiveness. The process of qualifying a tissue supplier has been described [1, 18, 19]. Tissue supplier requirements should include registration and evidence of compliance with government regulations with license or accreditation by those regulators according to national or regional law and where appropriate, accreditation by country-specific professional accreditation organizations such as the American Association of Tissue Banks (AATB) and Eye Bank Association of America (EBAA) in the USA [39, 40]. For similar allografts that have special characteristics depending on the supplier, input from clinicians and involvement with the hospital tissue service Medical Director may be important (see Case Study 2.4). A list of approved tissue suppliers should be maintained and updated annually.

Tissue allograft traceability and record-keeping

Hospital tissue services must record all steps concurrently with their performance when handling tissue. Records must provide bi-directional traceability of all tissues from the donor and tissue supplier to the recipients or other final disposition, including the discard of tissue. Case Study 2.5 illustrates the importance of surgeons cooperating with recalls by notifying and evaluating recipients and the importance of hospital record-keeping to enable identification for potentially infected recipients.

Tissue storage

Tissue grafts are stored under various conditions depending on the type of tissue, method of preservation, and packaging. In the USA, hospital tissue services should store tissue allografts according to the AATB standards and

CASE STUDY 2.4

Surgeons wanting new types of tissue allografts that are clinically unproven: the surgeon's role in helping to assess potential providers of tissue allografts

Tissue allografts used in an academic medical center in the USA are acquired by and stored in the hospital blood transfusion service facility. Neurosurgeon A requested the use of a tissue allograft comprising a frozen solution of bits of human amnion and cells from amniotic fluid claimed to be mesenchymal stem cells with the intention to mix this with demineralized cancellous bone allograft for use in cervical spine surgery. Orthopedic surgeon B requested purchase of demineralized cancellous bone allograft supplemented with well-characterized mesenchymal stem cells derived from human adipose tissue. Orthopedic surgeon C requested frozen bone allograft that had most cells removed but retained cells that have markers for mesenchymal stem cells. Of the three potential stem cell allograft products, two were offered by well-known, large not-for-profit tissue banks accredited by the AATB and one was a small for-profit business. None had controlled clinical data that showed effectiveness.

The hospital had an oversight committee responsible to decide whether expensive new surgical equipment and products should be purchased and provided in the operating theater. There was no expertise on this committee to evaluate these requests so a subcommittee was formed to include the potential users of these allografts and the blood transfusion service manager and Medical Director who are responsible for acquiring, storing, and handling tissue allografts.

The tissue storage service Medical Director investigated and reported to the subcommittee facts about the proposed allografts and suppliers. Through this process it was discovered that one of the potential suppliers (the for-profit business selling frozen amnion cells) had not been fully assessed by the hospital to be a qualified vendor, was not accredited by AATB, was not fully registered with the US Food and Drug Administration and was not following good manufacturing practices in their packaging and labeling. This potential supplier had not characterized the cells in their product, had not labeled it properly and their sales staff had made clinical claims unsupported by data. In addition, it was discovered and that the hospital did not have the requirement that their tissue allograft suppliers be AATB accredited. By the process of clinical staff participation in the subcommittee, a potentially dangerous supplier was excluded and a joint conclusion was made to choose only one supplier, to consider use of the requested material as research and to require recipient informed consent before use. In addition, hospital policies were revised and strengthened.

This case demonstrates the importance of a hospital process that involves surgeons in the overview of tissue allograft acquisition and the importance of working together as a team where peer pressure can result in cooperative decision making. In addition, it demonstrates the benefit of storing and handling tissue allografts by the hospital blood transfusion service where a Medical Director can participate as a clinical peer providing objective data for evaluation of new allografts and potential suppliers.

CASE STUDY 2.5

Importance of hospital record-keeping to enable identification of recipients during an allograft recall and surgeon cooperation for evaluation of allograft recipients

Before 1990 HCV had not been discovered and there was no test available for HCV antibodies to be applied to blood, tissue, or organ donors. The new nonspecific test for HCV antibodies, anti-HCV 1.0, first became available in 1990. During that year, two HCV-infected deceased tissue donors were tested and found falsely negative [15]. Many tissue allografts from these two donors were used in patients. In 1992, when the more sensitive anti-HCV 2.0 test became available, stored serum samples from these donors were tested and two were found to be repeatedly reactive and confirmed positive, indicating the presence of HCV infection.

Some unused bone allografts from these two donors were in frozen storage and discarded. Many bone, tendon, and skin allografts had already been used in patients. The tissue bank conducted a look back investigation by notifying hospitals and surgeons who had used these allografts. The surgeons were encouraged to notify their patients and evaluate them for HCV. Recipient notification and blood testing with RNA sequence analysis of HCV from donor and recipients enabled the diagnosis of three recipients proven to have acquired HCV infection through use of frozen bone, ligament, and tendon allografts. Bone that had been irradiated did not transmit HCV.

Not all allograft recipients could be identified because of inadequate hospital record-keeping. Some other recipients were not notified or evaluated because their surgeons did not cooperate.

This case is important because it illustrates a surgeon's responsibility during a look back investigation that can result in the identification of new patients with HCV infections. This can allow their early treatment and implementation of measures to prevent further spread.

This case showed that surgeon participation and good hospital record-keeping are essential for the diagnosis of infected allograft recipients and the reduction of further spread of a potentially lethal virus.

the tissue processor's instructions in the package insert. Compliance with other relevant regulatory standards should be assured in other jurisdictions. Storage records should be retained for a minimum of 10 years but there may be variation in the local or national regulations. Storage procedures should address steps to be taken if the temperature is out of limits or in the event of equipment or power failure, including emergency back-up alternatives in locations that can be monitored on site or remotely.

Tissue autograft collection, storage, and use

The use of a patient's own tissues has advantages and disadvantages over use of allograft tissues obtained from donors. SOPs should address aseptic collection of autografts, microbial testing, packaging, storage, and subsequent issue for use. Procedural recommendations have been published by AATB and the Association of Perioperative Registered Nurses (AORN) [39–41].

Investigating possible allograft-caused serious adverse reactions

Physicians should actively participate in the identification and timely investigation of an infection involving an allograft because it can lead to corrective action that improves safety and can prevent disease transmission to other patients. Investigation should aim to determine whether an infection that seemed to be associated with allograft use was actually caused by a contaminated allograft or had a different cause. For example, in the case of classical Creutzfeldt–Jakob disease (CJD), Maddox et al. [42] estimated that considering the age range of corneal allograft recipients a few cases of CJD might be expected to occur spontaneously in recipients and the fact that they had also received a cornea could be coincidental. During an investigation of an apparent relationship between an adverse outcome and an allograft, it is important to undertake an imputability assessment in which other causative factors, including chance, are considered before deciding that the adverse outcome is actually due to a defective allograft.

When the hospital tissue service is notified of an allograft-related infection, the tissue service Medical Director and hospital infection control or epidemiology service should be notified. All documents pertaining to the investigation should be maintained in an adverse event file. Critical immediate steps should be to sequester and quarantine existing inventory from the same donor, or same processing batch, if known. The tissue supplier should be promptly notified so they, too, can quarantine allografts in inventory, undertake a full investigation, and alert other tissue facilities having received tissue from the same donor or same processing batch.

Investigation of adverse events and reactions requires close cooperation among clinicians. The hospital tissue services Medical Director should discuss the case with the reporting physician to confirm the details of the infection and to learn whether the patient had any risk behaviors or had undergone other medical procedures that could account for the origin of the infection other than from the allograft. The hospital infection control clinicians should be consulted to learn whether there have been outbreaks of the same organism and whether a nosocomial source should be suspected.

If the adverse event involves an infection, is fatal, life threatening, or results in permanent impairment of a body function or a body structure, or necessitates medical or surgical intervention, governmental and public health authorities should be notified as soon as the possibility is identified. Serious adverse outcomes should be reported to a national biovigilance network, if available. A written final report of the investigation identifying any corrective actions should be reviewed by the hospital tissue services Medical Director and hospital infection control clinicians and reported to the surgeon, and the final outcome of the hospital-based investigation must be reported to the relevant public health service and national authority.

Tissue allograft recalls and look back investigations

When a tissue allograft is determined to be contaminated, potentially infectious, or otherwise nonconforming, the other tissues derived from the same deceased donor or processed in the same lot are also suspected to be affected and the tissue bank supplier must notify hospital contacts where the grafts were distributed. The hospital may be instructed to quarantine any unused allografts in inventory and to identify recipients and notify surgeons if the allografts have already been used. Hospitals that re-distributed the recalled grafts are responsible for tracking them further. Surgeons are then advised to contact their patients, inform them and evaluate them. The hospital tissue service Medical Director should be involved in oversight of the recall and be available to assist the surgeon. Recall investigations can be very labor intensive and involve many allografts, surgeons, and potentially infected recipients [43]. From 1997 to 2007, the US Food and Drug Administration issued recalls for 61,607 human tissue allografts, over 59,000 of which were bone and tendon allografts due to improper donor evaluation, contamination, and recipient infections [44]. Case Study 2.6 illustrates the magnitude of a recently published recall effort involving over 4000 tendon and ligament allografts and the surgeon's responsibility to evaluate recipients for infection [43].

Summary

Maintaining and improving the safety and effectiveness of donated allografts require good clinical governance by clinicians. Surgeons and physicians have important direct and oversight roles in recognizing and investigating allograft-associated complications, in participating in clinical audits of allograft use against agreed upon indications, and in establishing appropriate policies and procedures for handling tissue allografts in their health care facility. Participation by clinicians in all aspects of clinical governance is the cornerstone of good practice to optimize transplantation safety and effectiveness.

CASE STUDY 2.6

Surgeon responsibility to report a possible adverse outcome leading an investigation and large scale recalls and evaluation of recipients

Following an anterior cruciate ligament (ACL) reconstruction using a patellar ligament allograft, a patient developed a postoperative infection caused by the unusual bacterium *Elizabethkingia meningoseptica* (formerly *Chryseobacterium meningosepticum*) [43]. Because of uncertainty about the cause the case was reported so an investigation could determine the source of the bacterium. No evidence was found that the contamination was from the hospital environment. The tissue bank had initially received no other reports of infection due to the same organism and found no obvious source in the donor or from the tissue processing. After a second case of infection was reported involving the same unusual organism following ACL repair using an allograft from the same tissue bank, the tissue bank further investigated and discovered that the identical organism had been found in a water drain during routine environmental monitoring of the processing room.

The tissue bank closed the processing facility, improved its microbial monitoring process, and conducted a recall of allografts processed during the same time period in the same facility. The intent of the recall was to withdraw allografts that had not been used and for those that had been implanted, recommend that surgeons notify recipients so they could be evaluated for a similar infection. Over 4000 tendon and ligament allografts had been distributed to over 700 hospitals in the USA, Mexico, and Canada and the surgeons were notified. No further cases of postoperative infection by the same organism were discovered.

This case demonstrated that reporting an unusual infection as a potential adverse outcome can lead to an investigation and corrective and preventive steps, to a large-scale recall, to avoiding further exposure of potentially contaminated allografts, and to evaluating other recipients to determine whether they also became infected.

KEY LEARNING POINTS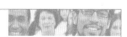

- Clinical governance of tissue and cell transplantation requires that physicians participate in transparent oversight to ensure the effective, safe, efficient, and equitable use of allografts.

- Physicians should audit tissue and cell allograft use against agreed-upon clinical guidelines based on evidence-based medicine to ensure appropriate use.

- By reporting adverse outcomes, the surgeon and other treating physicians improve tissue transplantation safety both within their own hospital and practice and as part of wider national and international biovigilance programs that recognize and investigate allograft-associated complications. This will result in corrective actions and improved safety for patients.

- Physicians in hospitals that acquire, store, and use tissue allografts have oversight responsibilities for their quality, storage, record-keeping, traceability, and for investigating adverse outcomes and conducting recalls. This function is similar to how a hospital handles their blood transfusion services.

References

1. Swanson E, Randell W, Freedman DB. Clinical governance and cell and tissue donation, banking and clinical use, in Warwick RM, Fehily D, Brubaker SA, Eastlund T, eds. Tissue and Cell Donation: An Essential Guide, Wiley-Blackwell, 2009, chapter 13, p243.
2. Scally G, Donaldson LJ. Clinical governance and the drive for quality improvement in the new NHS in England. BMJ 1998;317:61-65.
3. Donaldson LJ, Gray JAM. Clinical governance: a quality duty for health organisations. Qual Hlth Care 1998;7(suppl):37–44.
4. Centers for Disease Control and Prevention. Update: allograft-associated infections – United States, 2002. MMWR 2002;5:201–10.
5. Harner CD, Lo MY. Future of allografts in sports medicine. Clin Sport Med 2009;28:327–40.
6. McMaster P, Rogers D, Kerr M, Spencer A. Getting guidelines to work in practice. Arch Dis Child 2007;92:104–6.
7. American Orthopedic Society for Sports Medicine. 2006 AOSSM Orthopaedic Surgical Procedure Survey on Allografts, http://www.sportsmed.org/tabs/research/downloads/AOSSM06AllograftsSurveyFINALREPORTFINAL.pdf, accessed February 28, 2012; Jost PW, Dy CJ, Robertson CM, Kelly AM. Allograft use in anterior cruciate ligament reconstruction. Hospital for Special Surgery Journal 2011;7:251–256.
8. Perkins R, Pelkowitz A, Seddon M. Quality improvement in New Zealand healthcare. Part 7: clinical governance – an attempt to bring quality into reality. NZ Med J 2006;119:U2259.
9. American Medical Association. Opinion 9.032 – Reporting Adverse Drug or Device Events. Code of Medical Practice. Report: Issued June 1993 based on the report "Reporting Adverse Drug and Medical Device Events." American Medical Association. Chicago, Illinois 60654. USA. http://www.ama-assn.org/ama/pub/physician-resources/medical-ethics/code-medical-ethics/opinion9032.shtml, accessed February 12, 2011.
10. Strong DM, Shinozaki N. Coding and traceability for cells, tissues and organs for transplantation. Cell Tiss Bank 2010;11:305–23.

11. Reynolds M, Warwick RM, Poniatowski S, Trias E. European coding system for tissues and cells: a challenge unmet? Cell Tiss Bank 2010;11:353–64.

12. Simonds RJ, Holmberg SD, Hurwitz RL, et al. Transmission of human immunodeficiency virus type 1 from a seronegative organ and tissue donor. N Engl J Med 1992;326:726–32.

13. Centers for Disease Control and Prevention. Hepatitis C virus transmission from an antibody-negative organ and tissue donor–United States, 2000-2002. Morb Mortal Wkly Rep 2003;52:273–4, 276.

14. Tugwell BD, Patel PR, Williams IT, et al. Transmission of hepatitis C virus to several organ and tissue recipients from an antibody-negative donor. Ann Intern Med 2005;143:648–54.

15. Conrad EU, Gretch DR, Obermeyer KR, et al. Transmission of the hepatitis-C virus by tissue transplantation. J Bone Joint Surg Am 1995;77:214–24.

16. Kaye S, Baddon A, Jones M, Armitage WJ, Fehily D, Warwick RM. A UK scheme for reporting serious adverse events and reactions associated with ocular tissue transplantation. Cell Tiss Bank 2010;11:39–46.

17. Strong DM, Seem D, Taylor G, Parker J, Stewart D, Kuehnert MJ. Development of a transplantation transmission sentinel network to improve safety and traceability of organ and tissues. Cell Tiss Bank 2010;11:335–43.

18. Eisenbrey AB, Eastlund T. Hospital Tissue Management: A Practitioner's Guide. Bethesda MD: AABB, 2008: 1–205.

19. Eastlund T. Tissue and Organ Transplantation and the Hospital Tissue Transplantation Service. Chapter 32. In: Roback JD, editor. AABB Technical Manual. 16th edition. Bethesda, Maryland, USA: AABB Press, 2008: 833–64.

20. Eastlund T. Bacterial infection transmitted by human tissue allograft transplantation. Cell Tiss Bank 2006;7:147–66.

21. Centers for Disease Control and Prevention. Septic arthritis following anterior cruciate ligament reconstruction using tendon allografts – Florida and Louisiana, 2000. MMWR Morb Mortal Wkly Rep 2001; 50:1081–3.

22. Kainer MA, Linden JV, Whaley DN, et al. Clostridium infections associated with musculoskeletal-tissue allografts. N Engl J Med 2004;350:2564–71.

23. Centers for Disease Control and Prevention (CDC). Invasive *Streptococcus pyogenes* after allograft implantation – Colorado, 2003. Morb Mortal Wkly Rep 2003;52: 1174–6.

24. Kuehnert MJ, Clark E, Lockhart SR, Soll DR, Chia J, Jarvis WR. *Candida albicans* endocarditis associated with a contaminated aortic valve allograft: implications for regulation of allograft processing. Clin Infect Dis 1998;27:688–91.

25. Transplant Safety (TS) Chapter, Part III. Transplanting Tissues, The Joint Commission Comprehensive Accreditation Manuals. Oakbrook Terrace, Illinois: The Joint Commission, 2010.

26. Gallagher TH, Studdert D, Levinson W. Disclosing harmful medical errors to patients. N Engl J Med. 2007,356:2713–2729.

27. American Medical Association. Opinion 8.121 – Ethical Responsibility to Study and Prevent Error and Harm (subpart 3). Code of Medical Practice. Report: Issued December 2003 based on the report "Ethical Responsibility to Study and Prevent Error and Harm in the Provision of Health Care," adopted June 2003. American Medical Association. Chicago, Illinois 60654. USA. www.ama-assn.org/ama/pub/physician-resources/medical-ethics/code-medical-ethics.shtml, accessed January 25, 2011.

28. Office of Safety and Quality in Healthcare, Innovation and Health System Reform. WA open disclosure policy: Communication and disclosure requirements for health professionals working in Western Australia. May 2009. Information Series No. 10 (2009). Western Australian Department of Health, East Perth, Western Australia 6004, accessed January 26, 2011, http://www.health.wa.gov.au/circularsnew/attachments/395.pdf.

29. Australian Council for Safety and Quality in Health Care. Open disclosure standard:a national standard for open communication in public and private hospitals following an adverse event in healthcare – 2003 update. Government of West Australia Department of Health. East Perth, Western Australia, http://www.safetyandquality.health.wa.gov.au, accessed February 13, 2011.

30. National Patient Safety Council. Being open when patients are harmed. Safer practice notice Number 10, 2005. U. K. National Health Service, accessed January 26, 2011, www.nrls.npsa.nhs.uk/EasySiteWeb/getresource.axd?AssetID=59991.

31. Kuehnert MJ, Krista L,Yorita KL, Holman RC, Strong DM and the AABB Tissue Task Force. Human tissue oversight in hospitals: a survey of 402 AABB institutional members. Transfusion 2007;47:194–200.

32. Standards for tissue storage and issuance. Accreditation manual for critical access hospitals. 2nd edn. Oakbrook Terrace, Illinois: Joint Commission on Accreditation of Healthcare Organizations, 2003 (updated 2005).

33. Karow A. Should blood transfusion services become organ banks? Transfusion 1975;15:185–6.

34. Meryman HT. The role of blood transfusion services in the development of the regional tissue bank program. Transplant Proc 1976;8:241–244.

35. Murphy AM, Lumley SP, Darg C, Maginnis MJ, McClelland DBL. Bone banking: an extended role of the blood transfusion service. Transfusion Med 1990;1(suppl 1):48.

36. Steckler D, Eastlund T. Tissue banking: the role of the regional blood centre: an American experience in Minnesota. Med Lab Sci 1992;48:147–54.

37. Warwick RM, Eastlund T, Fehily D. Role of the blood transfusion service in tissue banking. Vox Sang 1996:71:71–77.

38. Price TH (ed.) Standards for Blood Banks and Transfusion Services, 27th edn. Bethesda, MD: AABB, 2011.

39. Pearson KA, Brubaker SA (eds) Standards for Tissue Banking. 12th edn. McLean, Virginia, USA: American Association of Tissue Banks, 2008.

40. Anonymous. Medical Standards. Washington, DC: Eye Bank Association of America, 2010.

41. AORN Recommended Practices Committee. Autologous tissue. AORN J 2005;82:871–77.

42. Maddox RA, Belay ED, Curns AT, et al. Creutzfeldt-Jacob disease in recipients of corneal transplants. Cornea 2008;27:851–4.

43. Cartwright EJ, Prabhu RM, Zinderman CE, et al., Food and Drug Administration Tissue Safety Team Investigators. Transmission of *Elizabethkingia meningoseptica* (formerly *Chryseobacterium meningosepticum*) to tissue-allograft recipients: a report of two cases. J Bone Joint Surg Am 2010;92:1501–6.

44. Mroz TE, Joyce MJ, Lieberman IH, Steinmetz MP, Benzel EC, Wang JC. The use of allograft bone in spine surgery: is it safe? Spine J 2009;9:303–8.

3 Development of Vigilance and Surveillance Systems

Scott A. Brubaker[1] and Deirdre Fehily[2]

[1]American Association of Tissue Banks, McLean, VA, USA
[2]National Transplant Centre (CNT), Rome, Italy

Vigilance is an attitude![1]

Dr Luc Noel, World Health Organization
Rome, Italy
June 2007

Introduction

The brief statement that prefaces this chapter is true and unpredictable, and identifies a significant factor that can affect the level of participation in the surveillance and tracking of adverse experiences associated with the use of cell or tissue allografts. It is a fact that formal systems are being developed that will properly detect, report, investigate, assess, monitor, and trend adverse outcomes linked to the therapeutic use of human cells or tissues. These systems are young, even in the most developed countries, and are currently a major focus of activity both for practitioners and regulators. For any such system to work and fulfill its aims, however, there must be willingness to participate at distinct stakeholder levels. Clinicians that use allografts, the cell- and tissue-banking professionals who provide them, key service providers in testing laboratories and irradiation facilities for example, and regulators

---

[1]A meeting about *"Vigilance & Surveillance of HCTT for Human Application in Europe & Globally"* jointly hosted by the World Health Organization and the EU-funded EUSTITE project (European Union Standards and Training in the Inspection of Tissue Establishments).

Tissue and Cell Clinical Use: An Essential Guide, First Edition. Edited by Ruth M. Warwick and Scott A. Brubaker.
© 2012 Blackwell Publishing Ltd. Published 2012 by Blackwell Publishing Ltd.

of these therapeutic products must work together to achieve the goal of an effective "vigilance and surveillance" program. What is the goal? It is to enhance allograft recipient safety using knowledge acquired through collection, analysis, and communication of information from untoward incidents.

During the past 60 years, the donation, processing, and transplantation of human tissues and cells has experienced much growth and matured in many areas: public education about organ and tissue donation; protocols for detection of donors, referral, consent/authorization, screening, and testing; allograft collection and recovery procedures; development of techniques that preserve allografts resulting in the ability to store them and sustain inventories for many years; processing methods that result in technically sophisticated tissue forms and constructs; and the clinical use of these allografts has expanded with this higher rate of availability and variety. During this same period, the circulation of tissues and cells has moved from local, often exclusively within one hospital, to global, with tissues and cells often donated in one country, distributed in large numbers and transplanted to patients located on other continents.

Despite this impressive growth in activity and global impact, vigilance and surveillance of clinical outcomes in recipients are, comparatively, still in their infancy. This chapter explores surveillance schemes in place and new ones that are being developed to fill this gap called "biovigilance." A successful biovigilance system will provide early warning when there is a safety issue; promote rapid exchange of relevant information among stakeholders (across a global network, when indicated); be a basis for evidence-based practice improvement; and, be educational and outcome-driven [1]. In May 2010, the World Health Assembly adopted a resolution [2] that placed vigilance and surveillance of organ, tissue, and cell transplantation indisputably on the World Health Organization (WHO) agenda. Those working at all levels in these fields are expected to embrace these aspects of their work as essential and integral to the care and safety of patients worldwide who need tissue or cell transplants.

Historical experience of adverse clinical outcomes with tissues and cells

There are three general types of adverse outcome related to recipient reactions to allografts. Although considered rare overall, transmission of disease, a toxic or immune reaction, or graft failure can result. The strength of the causal links between these reactions and the application of the tissues or cells may vary and is often referred to as "imputability." Where imputability is low, it is likely that the reaction identified was due to causes other than the tissues or cells transplanted. When imputability is high, it is very likely that the transplanted tissues or cells were the cause of the observed adverse outcome. Disease transmission can occur for the following reasons: micro-organisms including viruses, aerobic and anaerobic bacteria, and fungi/yeasts; parasites; the agent that causes human transmissible spongiform encephalopathy; and, possibly, certain malignancies (see Chapter 4). A toxic reaction to an allograft can be due to sensitivity to reagents (e.g., dimethlysulfoxide used as a cryoprotectant) or drugs (e.g., antibiotics) used during processing of the tissues or cells, and immune complex reactions can occur due to expression of, and reaction to, antigens that are donor-derived (e.g., ABO, RhD, human leukocyte antigen (HLA)) or from non-human animals (e.g., fetal bovine serum used in processing/cryopreservation).

The successful history of therapeutic use of human cells and tissues for transplantation is widely recognized, published, and impressive. However, lessons have been learned from negative experiences as well. Although formal surveillance systems were not in place during the formative years of tissue allograft transplantation, clinicians reported recipient adverse incidents usually through voluntary publications in professional journals. Good examples of this were seen during the 1960s and 1970s when harsh preservation and sterilization techniques were used on human aortic and pulmonary heart valves with hopes of establishing "safe" homograft valve bank inventories [3]. Storage techniques included flash-freezing, freeze-drying, and glutaraldehyde fixation, and sterilization steps included irradiation and treatment with β-propiolactone. Poor clinical results, specifically short-term durability, were experienced so these methods fell out of favor and clinician recommendations against homografts treated using such methods were published in peer-reviewed journals. Cardiothoracic surgeons pioneered development and voluntary participation in an international registry that tracks recipient outcomes while linking them to numerous technical aspects of a specific reconstructive procedure, the Ross (pulmonary autograft or switch) procedure, which uses refrigerated or cryopreserved aortic or pulmonary allograft heart valves. The International Ross Registry was established in 1993. It reports data that track patient demographics and medical history to facilitate identification of patients who would benefit most from this operation [4]; it also trends technical operative considerations of the procedure. Recipient follow-up information is completed 6 months postoperatively and annually thereafter to capture long-term patient outcomes in terms of re-operation, surgical technique, autograft failure, allograft function, and mortality. Although not specifically developed to track efficacy or safety of the allograft used in the procedure, this registry is a wonderful example of a vigilance and surveillance system designed to collect and analyze data used to make improvements to surgical practices that benefit patients worldwide who undergo this procedure. Currently, only the Australian Corneal Graft Registry (ACGR[2]), described later, can claim similar data collection success in the field of tissue transplantation.

---

[2]Acronyms of vigilance programs and projects discussed in this chapter are given in Table 3.1.

Table 3.1 Acronyms of vigilance programs and projects

ACGR	The Australian Corneal Graft Registry.
BIG V&S	The Bologna Initiative for Global V&S led by the World Health Organization (WHO) to take forward the work started in the NOTIFY project (see below).
CTISS	The Canadian Transfusion Transmitted Injuries Surveillance System.
CTOSS	The Canadian Cell, Tissue and Organ Surveillance System.
EUSTITE	An EU-funded project that ran from 2006 to 2009 and developed inspection guidelines for tissue and cell banks and vigilance and surveillance tools and guidance (European Union Standards and Training for the Inspection of Tissue Establishments).
MedWatch	The US Food and Drug Administration (FDA) reporting system for adverse events.
NOTIFY	An initiative launched by the WHO to build a history library of documented types of adverse events and reactions with didactic analysis by international experts (www.notifylibrary.org).
OARRS	The On-line Adverse Reaction Reporting System of the Eye Bank Association of America.
SOHO V&S	An EU-funded project entitled "Vigilance and Surveillance of Substances of Human Origin" promoting a harmonized approach to vigilance and surveillance of tissues and cells in the EU.
S(P)EAR	The vigilance and surveillance system run by the World Marrow Donor Association (WMDA), which includes SEAR (Serious Events and Adverse Effects Registry) for donor reactions, and SPEAR (Serious Product Events and Adverse Effects Registry) for product and recipient incidents.
ttsn	The Transplantation Transmission Sentinel Network (ttsn), a joint vigilance and surveillance initiative launched by three public health agencies in the USA (the Centers for Disease Control, the FDA, and the Health Resources and Services Administration (HRSA), was a prototype internet tracking and reporting system hosted by the United Network for Organ Sharing (UNOS).
TSN	The Transplantation Sentinel Network (TSN) is a national surveillance module for tissue transplants proposed to work in conjunction with a new hemovigilance module (a blood donation and transfusion safety network) being constructed within CDC's National Healthcare Safety Network (NHSN). Together, these modules could be deemed the "US Biovigilance Network Collaborative."

The Serious Events and Adverse Effects Registry (SEAR) vigilance system established by the World Marrow Donor Association is a pioneering global initiative in the field of hematopoietic stem cell transplantation, collecting and sharing information on adverse outcomes in unrelated donors across the global network of bone marrow donor registries [5]. It is the responsibility of the Chief Medical Officer at each donor registry to report any event that leads in the donor to life-threatening disease or death, requires in-patient hospitalization or considerable prolongation of existing hospitalization, or leads to persistent or significant disability/incapacity. Examples are events related to anesthetic, cardiac complications, infective complications, mechanical injury, or hemostasis.

In response to the publication of the European Directives on tissues and cells, the program was enhanced by the addition of the Serious Product Events and Adverse Effects Registry (SPEAR) reporting system. Examples of incidents that are reported include impairment of the quality of the graft (e.g., clots), wrong product infused, damage or loss of graft or part of the graft, serious transportation problems, serious unpredicted transmissible infection risk (e.g., hepatitis B), serious unpredicted non-infection risk (e.g., malignancy), and bacterial infection if the patient becomes unwell.

The need

There is a plethora of published articles about the use of tissue allografts. Most of them address clinical efficacy outcomes when using a specific allograft type. They are usually general reports of the experience of one surgeon or a surgical group, and sometimes successes or failures are correlated with use of certain surgical techniques. Although these reports are very useful, what has not been done on a large scale is to perform organized, controlled studies to determine specific factors that could improve allograft recipient outcomes or that identify and trend causes of adverse reactions. It is accepted that human tissue allografts "work" in the clinical setting; however, details about what works best in relation to specific graft processing methods and donor age are lacking [6]. Chapter 2 describes what can be done on a local basis at a medical facility and this type of control is encouraged, but information collected locally about adverse outcomes could, ideally, feed into a large-scale system to allow recognition of cogent issues on a much broader scale.

Transmissions of disease in the United States (USA) attributable to tissue allografts (see Chapter 4) have been reported in public health agency publications (i.e., Morbidity and Mortality Weekly Report from the Centers for Diseases Control and Prevention) or in professional journals (e.g., *New England Journal of Medicine*, *Annals of Internal Medicine*). However, actively looking for possible adverse reactions in tissue allograft recipients is generally absent today and systems rely on passive reporting.

Except for two long-standing data collection programs involving the use of corneas, no formal data sharing or surveillance programs exist for other tissues or cells. However, efforts are underway to change this and are addressed later in the chapter. The Australian Corneal Graft Registry (ACGR) has been collecting outcome data on cornea transplantation since May 1985 [7], with reports generated every 2 years. Another important collection of vigilance information with a long history is the adverse reaction database hosted by the Eye Bank Association of America (EBAA), established in 1991, and now called the On-line Adverse Reaction Reporting System (OARRS). These are the two premier tissue vigilance systems in the world today. The EBAA has published an OARRS Guidance [8], which outlines triggers for recognition with expectations for reporting primary graft failure or an infection "reasonably likely" to be due to the ocular graft. These data are evaluated annually by a standing committee and reported to a Medical Advisory Board.

Some regulators have pioneered national programs for reporting adverse tissue transplant reactions, building on their experience of pharmacovigilance and hemovigilance. A notable example is the French regulator Agence Française de Sécurité Sanitaire des Produits de Santé (AFSSaPS) which, in early 2004, established a network of vigilance officers in French hospitals to take responsibility for detecting, notifying, and investigating adverse incidents associated with the transplantation of substances of human origin. Theirs is the longest experience of tissue vigilance in Europe and they now collect approximately 100 reports a year, publishing a summary report on their website. It must be assumed that similar numbers of incidents are occurring in other countries where, at least until very recently, no system was in place for collecting or evaluating such reports.

Risk management and vigilance: reporting errors/incidents/near-misses

Some vigilance programs go beyond the communication and management of recipient reactions, requiring the reporting of errors/incidents/near-misses where recipients have not, or not yet, been harmed. In European Union (EU) legislation these are defined as adverse events (as opposed to adverse reactions, where a recipient has been affected) and reporting to regulatory authorities is required if they are considered "serious." The release of large numbers of tissue allografts from donors who had not been correctly selected and where medical histories had been falsified (see Case Study 3.1) is a good example of a serious adverse event followed by major preventive vigilance in the absence of a single recipient reaction. In other cases, the reporting of serious errors, even if the tissues or cells were not distributed for clinical application, can be a source of invaluable information for cell- and tissue-banking professionals, who can take steps to prevent similar occurrences. Serious adverse events can also result in the loss of transplantable material, such as a unique bone marrow donation, highly matched to a specific patient, or the loss of embryos created for a specific couple that followed many failed attempts. Monitoring the causes of such errors can be highly informative for professionals.

It can be difficult to decide whether an adverse event is sufficiently serious to be reported to a regulatory authority. The EUSTITE project [9] proposed

CASE STUDY 3.1

Inadequate donor screening, testing, and records: lack of confirmed transmission of disease

Owing to falsification of donor records including consent that took place over a 2-year period, the largest tissue allograft recall in history occurred in late 2005 and during all of 2006 [27]. Six tissue establishments that processed tissue and distributed it for transplantation had a tissue recovery agreement with a recovery agent who falsified documents and knowingly violated regulations as well as donation and transplantation ethics. Investigations into many donors recovered by personnel at this establishment identified concerns about the validity of donor screening information reported and infectious disease testing. Approximately 28,000 tissue grafts and tissue devices were made available for transplant from donors recovered by this tissue recovery establishment. Eventually, it was determined that approximately: 2200 tissue grafts/devices were not distributed, 15,800 tissue grafts and devices had been implanted, and 8000 tissue grafts/devices were successfully returned or destroyed by end users. However, approximately 700 (2.5%) tissue grafts remained unaccounted for by end users, and the disposition of 1300 (4.6%) tissue devices (i.e., demineralized bone matrix combined with a carrier in the form of a paste, putty, gel, or moldable strips) could not be confirmed by *distributors* and *end users*. Many of these allograft products were considered to be highly processed and, in the exhaustive investigations that ensued, no transmissions of disease to recipients were proven to occur from these donations. The US FDA's Centers for Device Evaluation and Research (CDRH) classified the recall of tissue devices as class III, meaning there was little risk to public health. FDA's Centers for Biological Evaluation and Research (CBER) classified the conventional tissue allografts as a class I recall, equating to a situation in which there is a reasonable probability the product will cause serious adverse health consequences. The tissue banks verified where all grafts were sent; however, internationally, three countries would not release information about the recalled grafts, citing patient confidentiality or their own national privacy laws. There were about 500 tissue grafts unaccounted for in the USA by consignees, and almost 200 tissue grafts and devices unaccounted for internationally. These estimates improved as the recall progressed but exact figures have not been reported. Vigilance in locating all allografts did not prevail, so gaps remain in systems nationally and internationally that affect patient safety. Surveillance for possible transmission of disease was high as lawyers searched for cases using all available forms of advertising; however, so far, no cases have been reported and confirmed to be caused by any of these allografts.

Table 3.2 EU Criteria for the reporting of serious adverse events

Inappropriate tissues/cells have been distributed for clinical use, even if not used.

The event could have implications for other patients or donors because of shared practices, services, supplies, or donors.

The event resulted in a mix-up of gametes or embryos.

The event resulted in loss of any irreplaceable autologous tissues or cells or any highly matched (i.e., recipient-specific) allogeneic tissues or cells. Or,

The event resulted in the loss of a significant quantity of unmatched allogeneic tissues or cells.

criteria for the reporting of serious adverse events to regulatory authorities, which have since been incorporated in the official guidance to EU Member States on annual tissue and cell vigilance reporting to the European Commission. The criteria are shown in Table 3.2.

It is interesting to note an analogous requirement for error reporting in the area of blood banking in the USA. For the past 10 years, the Food and Drug Administration (FDA) has required blood centers and hospital transfusion services to report events associated with testing, storage, or distribution of blood products that deviate from current good manufacturing practices or that affect the safety, purity, or potency of the blood product. Over a 5-year period (2004–2009), an average of less than 9% of hospitals reported blood product deviations. A study revealed that blood bankers did not have clear understanding of what constituted an FDA reportable occurrence; thus the number of reports is likely lower than reality of occurrence [10].

Risk management and vigilance: evaluating emerging hazards

Vigilance aimed at preventing harm to recipients is taken a step further where organizations and authorities develop systems for identifying and communicating new risks to the professional field so that appropriate preventative action can be taken. Such programs usually relate to new disease transmission risks. The WHO plays an essential role in the monitoring and publication of trends in disease transmission and both the USA's Centers for Disease Control and Prevention (CDC) and the European equivalent, the ECDC, actively monitor the spread of disease, and assess the impact and communicate it to the medical community and the public. This activity is new in the EU but has already had significant impact. The ECDC has conducted formal risk assessments on the transmission of Q-fever by transfusion and transplantation after its spread in the Netherlands [11] and evaluates the colonization of Europe by the mosquito vector of West Nile Virus [12] (Figure 3.1), providing useful data to support the development of policy on donor exclusion and testing.

'It can be concluded that the temperate strains of Aedes albopictus are here to stay — and that they will spread. In addition, new populations may become established in other parts of Europe. Surveillance of the introduction and spread of this vector, in particular in areas at risk, is important in order to be prepared for the mosquito's role in the transmission of diseases.'

from Development of *Aedes albopictus*risk maps, ECDC Technical Report, Stockholm, May 2009 [12]

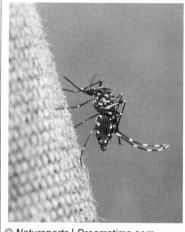

© Natursports | Dreamstime.com

Figure 3.1 *Aedes albopictus.*

Standards and policies for handling adverse outcome reports

Various professional association standards require that tissue or cell establishments must have procedures to handle adverse outcome reports. Since the first edition in 1984, the American Association of Tissue Banks (AATB's) *Standards for Tissue Banking (Standards)* has included requirements to "maintain an adverse reaction file" and to have "recall procedures." As early as 1992, a document was introduced in a technical manual published by the AATB entitled *Protocol for Reporting an Event with the Potential for Disease Transmission* that provided guidance for handling these situations. This was introduced soon after transmission of human immunodeficiency virus (HIV) was realized from allograft tissue and a few tissue grafts from the deceased donation could not be tracked to final disposition by hospitals in the USA [13] (see Case Study 3.2). As a result, in 1993, two related events occurred. First, a new section directed at end users appeared in *Standards* titled *Medical Facility Tissue Storage and Issuance*, which required adverse outcome reporting to the tissue bank and written procedures for responding to allograft recalls. Next, AATB's President, Ted Eastlund, and Executive Director, Jeanne Mowe, successfully influenced a large hospital accreditation group to include similar requirements in their standards for accrediting health care facility "laboratories" (first included by 1996), because hospital clinical laboratories were known to store allograft tissues. This accreditation organization is now called The Joint Commission (on Accreditation of Healthcare Organizations). Similar efforts were directed at the College of American Pathologists (CAP)

CASE STUDY 3.2

Communication gaps, tracking failures

In 1991, an HIV transmission from a frozen (deceased donor) femoral head allograft was discovered to have occurred after use of the graft during hip replacement surgery for an elderly woman. Her surgery had occurred in December 1985 and she now tested positive for HIV-1 antibody without the presence of other medical or behavioral risk factors. The donor was a young, adult male who sustained a gunshot wound to the head during a robbery at a petrol station where he worked. He was an organ and tissue donor and, although two separate blood samples were tested at two different laboratories for each donation event, and plasma dilution (hemodilution) was not an issue, he tested negative for antibodies to HIV (i.e., detection of antibodies to HTLV-III was the testing performed at that time). Although some of the organ donor recipients experienced episodes of immune deficiency soon after transplantation, a link to the donor was not suspected. Within weeks, three organ recipients seroconverted to positive for HIV antibody, but risk in two was attributed to receipt of blood transfusions before 1985 from untested blood donors. The third organ recipient met established criteria and was reported to the state health department as an AIDS case, but no formal system was in place to link these events to the common donor. None of this information was communicated to the tissue bank or the eye bank involved in recovering tissue from the same donor. Fifty-three tissue grafts were made available for transplantation, of which two tissue grafts were not implanted and 46 allograft tissues were implanted (including both corneas). In the course of the investigations that followed, it was confirmed that seven recipients of organs or tissues from this donor tested positive for HIV-1; four organ recipients and three recipients of minimally processed "fresh frozen" tissue grafts. Five tissue grafts (more than 9% of all tissue grafts) remained unaccounted for by hospitals that received them. This was a case where communication gaps occurred among transplantation professionals and tissue allograft tracking failures by health care facilities were evident [13].

and they, too, soon included tissue handling requirements in their Transfusion Medicine Checklist used for inspection/accreditation, and later in their Reproductive Medicine Checklist.

In the USA, more tissue allograft recalls and adverse events occurred in the late 1990s and during the early years of the twenty-first century (see Case Study 3.3). During investigations and recall efforts, it was clearly apparent that tissue grafts were routinely stored in departments other than the clinical laboratory at health care facilities. This prompted The Joint Commission in 2005 to include tissue-handling standards in each of five *Comprehensive Accreditation Manuals* for hospitals, ambulatory care (centers), critical

CASE STUDY 3.3

Communication gaps, tracking failures (again)

A male donor in his forties with a history of hypertension and heavy alcohol use died of an intracranial hemorrhage in October 2000. He had an undetected hepatitis C viremia and, although his blood sample tested negative for antibodies to hepatitis C virus (anti-HCV), his tissues and organs infected several recipients [28]. In this case, 91 tissues and organs were made available for transplantation from the donor and 40 patients received transplants within 22 months of donation. The index case that identified a recipient became infected with HCV from the donor occurred 1½ years after donation; she received a tissue graft (tendon with bone). Although two recipients (one tissue, one organ) had been diagnosed with HCV within 4 and 6 months after transplantation, linking this infection to the donor did not occur. Many tissue grafts were processed after these recipients were recognized as contracting new HCV infections; however, communication to other stakeholders involved did not occur and tissue allografts were distributed. This could have been avoided. Ultimately, HCV transmission occurred in eight recipients: three of three organ recipients, one of two saphenous vein recipients, one of three tendon recipients, and three of three recipients of tendon with bone. Recipients were located in 16 states in the USA and two other countries. Viral isolates were genetically related to those of the donor so there was no question of viral origin in these recipients who tested positive. This case demonstrates a continuing lack of communication among transplant centers, organ procurement organizations, and tissue banks, and it additionally identified limitations of viral antibody testing. Questions remain, however. Can this lack of recognition of a donor-derived infection, and failed communication among stakeholders, still occur today?

access hospitals, office-based surgery, as well as laboratories. These standards and their descriptive expectations, listed as "elements of performance," describe the need for procedures to be maintained for tissue oversight responsibility, tissue supplier qualification, tissue receipt/storage/preparation/tracking/recalls, and investigating and reporting recipient adverse events. These requirements are now found in The Joint Commission's *Transplant Safety Chapter*, which also includes requirements related to organ donation and transplantation. Officials at the AATB continue to collaborate with The Joint Commission to update these standards as necessary.

During this period, use of tissue allografts grew rapidly in North America and the appearance of tissue distributors (intermediary agents) began to grow as well. As a response in 1996, the AATB developed a section in *Standards* specific for tissue distribution intermediaries. It included requirements for this entity to have procedures that address tracking, recalls, and reports of adverse outcomes. These developments over the course of more than 15 years have been critical in filling major gaps. There is now nationwide awareness and emphasis on safe tissue handling by distributors and the clinician/end-user. Clear expectations exist which require investigation and reporting of an adverse outcome without delay.

Some other professional standards that require procedures for investigating adverse events and reactions include the EBAA's *Medical Standards* (at G1.000) since 1990, and the Canadian Standards Association's *General Requirements* in Z900.1-03 (at Clause 19) since 2003. The European Association of Tissue Banks' Standards and the FACT/JACIE Standards for hematopoietic stem cell facilities also require such systems to be in place. The Council of Europe's *Guide to Safety and Quality of Organs, Tissues and Cells* [14] recommends that all serious adverse events and reactions such as identified transmission of disease should be reported in a timely manner to public health authorities, processing institutions and, where relevant, to the donor's personal physician (with the donor's consent), as well as physicians involved in transplantation or implantation of the organ/tissue/cell. An EU-funded project called European Quality Systems in Tissue Banking (EQSTB) produced a guideline for tissue banks and a specific audit guide, both of which highlighted the need to ensure that robust systems are in place to report and investigate adverse incidents.

Tissue and cell reporting requirements of authorities

In its *Aide Memoire* issued in 2007 for National Health Authorities on *Access to Safe and Effective Cells and Tissues for Transplantation* [15], the WHO called on health authorities to provide national oversight of these activities with surveillance and vigilance, including transplantation-transmitted disease. This was reinforced in 2010 when the World Health Assembly adopted resolution WHA63.22 [16], which reiterates the importance of post-transplantation surveillance systems in ensuring appropriate levels of safety and quality for patients being treated with substances of human origin.

The development of adverse outcome reporting systems by regulatory authorities at the local or national level has often been stimulated by high-profile incidents that questioned the safety of tissue or cell allografts. This was the case in the USA when the states of New York and Florida implemented requirements for tissue banks in 1993. In New York, these laws were codified at Title 10 New York Codes, Rules and Regulations (NYCRR) in Part 52 and require licensure of tissue banks and transplant centers. Adverse outcome reporting and records requirements are included, and there is required reporting by tissue banks within seven calendar days if an "error" or "accident" was reported that involved a distributed allograft. Each licensed establishment must also submit an annual activity report that provides a denominator so prevalence of adverse reporting can be estimated. Although Florida's Agency for Health Care Administration is not involved in the investigation, an adverse reaction must be reported to them by the tissue bank within one working day of receipt of the notice from a physician or a hospital.

The US FDA promulgated regulations that became effective in 2005 that continue to use MedWatch [17] for reporting suspected adverse reactions caused by cell or tissue allograft products. These regulations require cell and tissue establishments to investigate and report adverse reactions to FDA when a reported reaction is fatal, life threatening, results in permanent impairment of a body function or permanent damage to a body structure, or necessitates medical or surgical intervention, including hospitalization. If any report of communicable disease transmission is suspected to be reasonably associated with the allograft after an investigation has been performed, it must be reported. This is the same system the agency uses for other FDA-regulated products such as drugs, biologics, medical devices, cosmetics, and dietary supplements. When association is reasonably attributed, reporting within 15 days, and an update every 15 days thereafter, is expected. Otherwise, the MedWatch system can also be used on a voluntary basis by end-users or patients. Additionally, a tissue establishment must investigate all deviations related to a cell/tissue product they distributed that violated "core" requirements. All follow-up actions that have been or will be taken in response to the occurrence of the deviation (e.g., a recall) must be communicated to FDA within 45 days of the occurrence [18].

In Canada, Heath Canada's Cell, Tissue and Organ regulations are different in that reporting within 24 hours of receipt of an initial adverse reaction report is required (regardless of suspicion or results of an investigation) and updates are expected every 15 days thereafter.

Article 11 of EU Directive 2004/23/EC requires Member State regulators (known as "competent authorities") to implement systems for reporting, investigating, registering, and communicating information about serious adverse incidents. The Directives go beyond many vigilance systems by requiring serious incidents to be reported to the regulator, even if a patient has not been harmed. The definitions differentiate between cases where harm to a recipient or a living donor has occurred and cases where an adverse incident has occurred that might have, or might still, cause harm.

Serious Adverse Reaction: (SAR) an unintended response, including a communicable disease, in the donor or in the recipient associated with the procurement or human application of tissues and cells that is fatal, life-threatening, disabling, incapacitating or which results in, or prolongs, hospitalisation or morbidity.

Serious Adverse Event: (SAE) any untoward occurrence associated with the procurement, testing, processing, storage and distribution of tissues and cells that might lead to the transmission of a communicable disease, to death or life-threatening, disabling or incapacitating conditions for patients or which might result in, or prolong, hospitalisation or morbidity.

These definitions are mirrored in EU legislation for blood and blood products and for organs (Directive 2010/53/EU). The tissue and cell directives place the "tissue establishment" at the center of the vigilance system, requiring them to provide information to procurement organizations and to clinical users on how to report and investigate. Directive 2006/86/EC provides more detail on reporting and investigation requirements, and includes standard vigilance data sets to be included in individual reports and in an annual report to be provided by each Member State to the European Commission.

Tissue and cell vigilance and surveillance systems in development

European Union Standards and Training in the Inspection of Tissue Establishments (EUSTITE)

One of the principal objectives of the EUSTITE project was to support EU competent authorities in the implementation of the requirements of EU legislation for vigilance of tissues and cells. As described previously, the project developed a set of agreed criteria for the reporting of serious adverse events (SAEs). It also developed severity and imputability tools to facilitate a common approach to the evaluation of serious adverse reactions (SARs), which are now incorporated in the guidance provided by the European Commission to Member States for the completion of their annual vigilance reports. An impact assessment tool was proposed to support tissue establishments and regulators in the evaluation of the broader impact of any specific incident, taking into account not only impact on a specific patient but also on the transplant system or the donation system, where negative media coverage, for instance, might result in the loss of public confidence in the system. The project provided guidance on the management and communication of SAREs (includes both serious adverse reactions and events) within individual Member States and when they have implications across borders.

The EUSTITE tools and guidance were piloted over a 1-year period in 20 EU countries. Participating vigilance officers applied the tools to all cases reported to them and provided the details to the project of each case. In total, 306 incidents were reported during the year, almost equally distributed between SARs and SAEs. The exercise demonstrated the value of consolidated data collection in a region like Europe where individual national case numbers would be very small. The reported cases involved all kinds of tissues and cells, including corneas, hematopoietic stem cells, gametes and embryos, and bone, and the events reported had occurred at all stages from procurement to distribution.

After the publication of the pilot report, a series of Vigilance Recommendations were developed and provided to the European Commission [9]. These addressed areas that needed further clarification and development (particularly in the field of assisted reproduction and in cases of illegal and fraudulent activity). The recommendations are being taken forward in a further EU-funded project known as SOHO V&S (Vigilance and Surveillance of Substances of Human Origin, www.sohovs.org), which will develop detailed guidance and training on investigation of SARE. The project is led by several EU regulators but also has the collaboration of many regulators and professional societies within and outside the EU, in recognition of the need for a global approach to vigilance of tissues and cells.

Cell, tissue, and organ surveillance system

In Canada, similar systems are actively being explored and developed. The Public Health Agency of Canada (PHAC) is working collaboratively with Health Canada to develop a cell, tissue, and organ surveillance system (CTOSS) [19]. The aim is to establish an expected frequency of adverse events and to assess the feasibility of implementing a prospective surveillance system. Pilot projects in a few provinces include retrospective chart reviews of musculoskeletal and ocular tissue transplant recipients. There is also consideration for linkage with Canada's national hemovigilance system, the Transfusion Transmitted Injuries Surveillance System (TTISS).

Transplantation Sentinel Network

Soon after the turn of the twenty-first century, public health authorities in the USA identified gaps in patient safety and focused on the need to improve communication between institutions that recover, process, distribute, and implant allografts. This was underscored by the potential for one donor to affect up to seven recipients of organs and an average of nearly 50 tissue allograft recipients. It was also recognized that many organ donors, approximately 37% in one survey [20], are donors of tissue. In addition, allograft tissue processing (also known as "manufacturing") has evolved and minimizes the risk for many tissues; however, for lightly processed tissues, risk of contamination from recovery remains, and for all tissues could be introduced during processing. In 2005, three public health agencies in the USA (CDC, FDA, and Health Resources and Services Administration (HRSA)) convened a workshop [21] to discuss strategies for improving safety of patients related to donor-transmitted infections. Further development of current systems and establishment of a new network to promote rapid recognition, reporting, cooperation, investigation, and stakeholder communication were agreed priorities. Subsequently, a cooperative agreement was awarded by CDC to the United Network for Organ Sharing (UNOS), resulting in development of the Transplantation Transmission Sentinel Network (ttsn) [22, 23]. The ttsn prototype was a secure, online database for cross-referencing and registering organ and tissue donors, transplanted allografts, and recipient adverse reactions. The prototype demonstrated the potential to improve communication avenues across all stakeholders in the event of a suspected adverse reaction. In 2008, a limited pilot project was undertaken where participants tested the system. Improvement areas were identified and, although the project's government funding ended, specifications needed to build a system emerged from the experience. The CDC gathered more input for operation of a national Transplantation Sentinel Network (TSN) [24] and more recently (in early 2011) a request for information [25] was issued in hopes of soliciting ideas for a public–private partnership from interested stakeholders about a plan for developing a national biovigilance network. The "TSN" could be developed as a surveillance module in conjunction with a new hemovigilance module (a blood donation and transfusion safety network) being constructed within CDC's National Healthcare Safety Network (NHSN). Together, these could be deemed the "US Biovigilance Network Collaborative." Responses to the request for information about a public–private partnership for biovigilance remain to be evaluated, and identifying funding avenues will be a significant hurdle. Concerns about biovigilance for organs, tissues, and cells, or lack thereof, were previously identified and reported in 2009 by an advisory committee to the Secretary of Health and Human Services but these gaps remain to be filled [26].

AATB's role in the USA

In 2008, the AATB formed a multi-agency task force with a mission to fill some gaps identified from surveys performed for the ttsn project. This task force is developing a Guidance Document titled "Identifying, Reporting, and Investigating Tissue Recipient Adverse Reactions." Its aim is to promote professional inter-communication, establish vigilance, and improve surveillance in the proper recognition, reporting, and investigation of possible tissue allograft-caused adverse reactions. Primary stakeholders include end-user clinicians and the clinicians who later provide medical care to tissue allograft recipients, public health authorities, and tissue-banking professionals. One section will provide clinicians with necessary tools to recognize, report, and assist with the investigation of a possible allograft-caused disease transmission or graft failure (see descriptions of criteria in Box 3.1). Tissue establishments handling these reports will be given a template containing

Box 3.1 AATB Proposal

The essential role of the clinician in detecting tissue recipient reaction triggers

To facilitate proper recognition and investigation of a possible transmission of disease caused by an allograft, guidelines have been suggested based on experience with investigations in the USA [29, 30]. *Recognition criteria include clinical events as well as laboratory test results and other medically relevant findings.* It is important to select criteria that are manageable and have reasonable sensitivity, because reporting of common community-acquired infections that occur postoperatively (flu, colds, etc.) is not desired. When reviewing past reports of allograft-caused infections from the literature, allograft removal has not been a factor that would capture cases so this is not used as an indicator. Recipient symptoms were recognized between 2 and 113 days postoperatively and patients were generally re-admitted within 30 days of surgery. When disease transmission was proved to occur from a tissue allograft, unexpected organisms were cultured from the surgical site or wound. If this occurs, clinicians should suspect tissue allograft transplanted at this site as the possible source. A 6-month period was selected, instead of 1 year for recognition of a bacterial or fungal infection, because this is evidence-based using information from investigations of confirmed disease transmission from tissue. Criteria for suspected parasitic or viral disease transmission is 1 year after surgery because of the potential for delays in recognition of a recipient's symptoms or test results. Suspected cases involving a human transmissible spongiform encephalopathy have no timeline limitation. The following criteria provide guidelines (recognition triggers) that should be followed by clinicians when identifying a possible allograft-caused reaction.

Bacterial or fungal
Signs of inflammation or infection (e.g., pain, swelling, purulent discharge, lymphadenopathy) from or near an operative site within 6 months of implantation associated *with at least one of the following*:

- fever;
- positive culture or gram stain from within the operative site or from purulent drainage (not a superficial swab culture); or
- positive blood culture (consideration of other patient sources for the bacteremia must be investigated).

Parasitic or viral
Signs and symptoms consistent with an unexpected viral agent or parasitic disease (e.g., fever, rash, lymphadenopathy, hepatitis, or possible neurological

symptoms/encephalitis; and/or confirmed infectious disease test result (e.g., serologic, molecular) within 1 year after implantation.

Hypersensitivity or toxicity
Signs, symptoms, or clinical evidence suggestive of graft rejection or other failure, or a recipient reaction suggestive of an immune response to a foreign stimulus, that occurs within days or weeks of the transplant.

Malignancy
Signs and symptoms consistent with a new malignancy at an unexpected body site within 18 months after implantation. Molecular studies of malignancy in the recipient and any archived samples from the donor may be needed to confirm or exclude suspicion.

Human transmissible spongiform encephalopathy
Any period after transplant should be considered.

- Creutzfeldt–Jakob disease (CJD): signs and symptoms consistent with a combination of: progressive dementia; typical electroencephalogram (EEG) (generalized triphasic periodic complexes at approximately one per second); and at least two of the following: myoclonus; visual impairment or cerebellar signs; pyramidal or extrapyramidal signs; or, akinetic mutism.
- Variant CJD: signs and symptoms consistent with a combination of persistent painful sensory symptoms and/or psychiatric symptoms at clinical presentation; dementia and development 34 months after illness onset of ataxia and at least one of the following three neurologic signs: myoclonus, chorea, or dystonia; a normal or an abnormal EEG, but not the diagnostic EEG changes often seen in classic CJD; and duration of illness of over 6 months.
- Or, any positive test result for protease-resistant prion protein (PrP).

expectations for performing a proper investigation and this will satisfy requirements to maintain AATB accreditation. This guidance will also contain reporting requirements and parameters to be used for closing an investigation based on all information acquired. Harmonization with terms and processes used by EUSTITE is a goal. When the guidance is finalized, formal public support from professional associations of clinicians will be sought and mass distribution of the document is planned along with educational presentations at major, relevant meetings. The initial focus is to develop systems that will properly handle reports of SARs involving allograft tissue recipients and future projects may include guidelines for dealing with SAEs.

Project Notify and the Bologna Initiative for Global Vigilance and Surveillance

In the context of worldwide circulation of tissues and cells, the benefits of sharing vigilance information globally are obvious. Serious adverse events and reactions occur rarely but each one represents a learning opportunity that should be communicated widely so that effective and timely corrective and preventive actions can be taken to protect donors and patients. The WHO has collaborated with the EU project SOHO V&S and the Italian National Transplant Centre to coordinate the collation of a historic library of event and reactions types, by human substance type, with references to the relevant documents or publications where the incidents are recorded. A broad international group of experts in tissue and cell banking, organ, tissue, and cell transplantation, assisted reproduction, disease transmission, and the regulation of these fields collaborated to collect and insert the cases of which they were aware and provided additional information related to the initial alerting signals and the means of confirmation of imputability, from their own experience. A meeting was held in Bologna to review the work and plan the way forward in February 2011 (report available at www.organsandtissues.net).

Several outcomes of the Notify project and the Bologna meeting have taken forward the work of building tools to support effective vigilance and surveillance under the banner of the Bologna Initiative for Global Vigilance and Surveillance (BIG V&S). The valuable catalogue of information gathered through the Notify project has now been transferred to a public, searchable database on a dedicated website (www.notifylibrary.org). Experts from across the globe continue to add new cases and to provide analysis of new information the cases provide. On the same website, didactic documents relating to each major category of adverse reaction or event (infection, malignancy, process or clinical errors, genetic transmissions, and reactions in donors), written by the Notify expert groups are available. The group continues to communicate and is working on standardizing terminology for vigilance to improve international communication.

Universal coding to promote biovigilance

Tissue or cell grafts are commonly identified by a code assigned by the tissue establishment. To log in or track the allograft, a person involved with handling the graft upon receipt for storage or when used for a patient must transcribe the identification numbers and/or letters that contain the code to a logbook or enter it into a database, and eventually enter it into the patient's medical record. Long alphanumeric identifiers of various configurations exist for these identification codes, which greatly increases the chance for making clerical mistakes, leading to gaps in tracking. This is a concern related to patient safety, especially if there is an adverse reaction or a tissue allograft recall. End-user compliance with steps involved with tracking allografts is critical and they are the most diverse of all the stakeholders involved in biovigilance efforts. Making it easier to handle and track cell and tissue allografts should be a priority; thus, a universal coding and labeling system should be used on a global scale because allografts often travel across regional and national borders. Experience with recall events and international distribution begs for a global universal coding system to facilitate tracking. So the development of any biovigilance system needs to consider how this can be accomplished using unique coding and labeling systems that are already established and used for similar medical products of human origin (i.e., blood and blood components). Tissue vigilance and surveillance systems should harmonize terminology so there is an ability to collect global information that can be evaluated to identify potential trends, improve products and services, and aid overall goals for patient safety related to biovigilance.

Conclusion (and hope)

The aptitude of the professionals involved who affect the success of biovigilance systems is not lacking, so the hope is that positive attitudes prevail and stakeholders understand their roles and comply. Clinicians should be committed to monitoring their patients who are recipients of tissue or cell allografts, be vigilant in reporting when there is a qualified suspicion of an adverse reaction caused by the allograft, and remain actively involved in the subsequent investigation by the allograft supplier through to closure of the case file. Cell- and tissue-banking professionals providing allografts should also be vigilant in three general areas for which only they can be responsible. They should (1) have active surveillance programs directed at recipients of their allografts who are considered to pose the highest risk, (2) thoroughly investigate without delay all reports received of adverse reactions when there is suspicion they were caused by an allograft, and (3) share any corrective and preventive actions implemented as a result of these investigations so knowledge improvement on a global scale can be realized. Three expectations of regulators are equally important to the management of a successful biovigilance program. As public health protectors, regulating bodies or competent authorities should (1) promulgate policy (legal basis) that enhances participation by clinicians and cell- and tissue-banking professionals in a formal biovigilance network, (2) ensure that participation is not punitive-driven because it is, in the end, based on principles of voluntary engagement, and (3) provide initial, and ensure ongoing, financial support for biovigilance programs because public health and consumer protection is their oversight responsibility. A combination of regulatory and professional cooperative efforts seems to be the best formula for success. Where adverse outcomes occur in the context of international distribution, compliance with systems and regulations that exist where a serious adverse reaction or event occurred should be required by all entities involved, but the regional or national systems from where the allograft was sourced cannot be ignored. Respect for each other's concerns and expectations should be mutual.

The expectations of roles described here should be viewed as obligations, not only to the recipients of these life-saving or life-enhancing allografts, but also to the tissue and cell donors and the myriad of people associated with the donation process. Clinicians, cell- and tissue-banking professionals, and their regulators all play critical roles in the stewardship of these human-derived gifts. The programs described in this chapter must be a priority and continue or we have failed this important part of our safety mission. Desire to succeed must foster positive attitudes towards biovigilance.

KEY LEARNING POINTS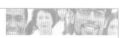

- Formal systems are being developed to properly detect, report, investigate, assess, monitor, and trend adverse outcomes linked to the therapeutic use of human cells or tissues but, for any such system to work and fulfill its aims, there must be willingness to participate at distinct stakeholder levels.

- Although considered rare overall, there are three general types of adverse outcome related to recipient reactions to allografts: transmission of disease, a toxic or immune reaction, or graft failure. The strength of the causal links between these reactions and the application of the tissues or cells may vary and is often referred to as "imputability."

- Enhancement of allograft recipient safety can be accomplished using knowledge acquired through collection, analysis, and communication of information from untoward incidents but, without knowledge of these incidents, safety is not fully addressed.

- A successful biovigilance system should be a combination of regulatory and professional cooperative efforts that provide early warning when there is a safety issue by promoting rapid exchange of relevant information among stakeholders (across a global network, when indicated), being a basis for evidence-based practice improvement, and being educational and outcome-driven.

- Clinicians should (1) have active surveillance programs directed at recipients of their allografts determined to pose the highest risk, (2) thoroughly investigate without delay all reports received of adverse reactions when there is suspicion it was caused by an allograft, and (3) share any corrective and preventive actions implemented as a result of these investigations so knowledge improvement on a global scale can be realized.

- As public health protectors, regulating bodies or competent authorities should (1) promulgate policy (legal basis) that enhances participation by clinicians and cell- and tissue-banking professionals in a formal biovigilance network, (2) ensure that participation is not punitive-driven because participation is, in the end, based on principles of voluntary engagement, and (3) provide initial, and ensure ongoing, financial support for biovigilance programs because public health and consumer protection is their oversight responsibility.

References

1. Williams AE. Biovigilance in the United States: efforts to bridge a critical gap in patient safety and donor health. Meeting of the Advisory Committee on Blood Safety and Availability, April 30, 2009.
2. Eighth Plenary Meeting of the Sixty-Third World Health Assembly, May 21, 2010, A63/VR/ 8. WHA63.22. Annex 8. WHO Guiding Principles on Human Cell, Tissue and Organ Transplantation, Guiding Principle 10. http://apps.who.int/gb/ebwha/pdf_files/WHA63-REC1/WHA63_REC1-en.pdf (accessed July 2, 2011).
3. Hopkins RA. Cardiac Reconstructions with Allograft Tissues, Springer Science + Business Media, 2005.
4. http://ihimf.pyrontechnologies.com/pdfs/281%20-%20The%20Ross%20Procedure%20-%20Current%20Registry%20Results.pdf (accessed July 2, 2011).
5. SEAR summary from 2003 to 2010. http://www.worldmarrow.org/index.php?id=493 (accessed July 22, 2011).
6. Sikka RS, Narvy SJ, Vangsness CT Jr. Anterior cruciate ligament allograft surgery: underreporting of graft source, graft processing, and donor age. Am J Sports Med 2011;39:649–55.
7. http://hdl.handle.net/2328/1002 (accessed July 2, 2011).
8. http://www.restoresight.org/files/oarsguidance809.pdf (accessed 02 July 2011).
9. Fehily D, Sullivan S, Noel L, et al. Improving vigilance and surveillance for tissues and cells in the European Union: EUSTITE, SOHOV&S and Project NOTIFY. Organs Tissues & Cells 2012;15(2).

10. Lam R, Bryant BJ. Knowledge of food and drug administration reportable deviations. Transfusion 2011;51:1619–23.

11. ECDC Risk Assessment on Q-fever. http://ecdc.europa.eu/en/press/news/Lists/News/ECDC_DispForm.aspx?List=32e43ee8%2De230%2D4424%2Da783%2D857 42124029a&ID=367 (accessed July 22, 2011).

12. http://ecdc.europa.eu/en/publications/Publications/0905_TER_Development_of_Aedes_Albopictus_Risk_Maps.pdf (accessed July 22, 2011).

13. Simonds RJ, Holmberg SD, Hurwitz RL, et al. Transmission of human immunodeficiency virus type 1 from a seronegative organ and tissue donor. N Engl J Med 1992;326:726–32.

14. Council of Europe. Guide to Safety and Quality of Organs, Tissues and Cells, 4th edition, 2010.

15. World Health Organization (2007). Access to Safe and Effective Cells and Tissues for Transplantation, Aide Memoire, http://www.who.int/transplantation/AM-HCTTServices.pdf (accessed July 2, 2011).

16. World Health Organization (2010). Sixty-third world health assembly, Resolution WHA63.22, Agenda item 11.21, Human organ and tissue transplantation, May 21, 2010, http://apps.who.int/gb/ebwha/pdf_files/WHA63/A63_R22-en.pdf (accessed July 2, 2011).

17. MedWatch: The FDA Safety Information and Adverse Event Reporting Program http://www.fda.gov/Safety/MedWatch/default.htm (accessed July 2, 2011).

18. US Department of Health and Human Services, Food and Drug Administration, Current Good Tissue Practice for Human Cell, Tissue, and Cellular and Tissue-Based Product Establishments; Inspection and Enforcement; Final Rule, November 24, 2004. http://frwebgate.access.gpo.gov/cgi-bin/getdoc.cgi?dbname=2004_register&docid=fr24no04-9.pdf (accessed July 2, 2011).

19. Summative Evaluation of the Blood Safety Contribution Program – Final Report, Component 3000: Cells, Tissues and Organs Surveillance System (CTOSS), Public Health Agency of Canada, http://www.phac-aspc.gc.ca/about_apropos/reports/2008-09/blood-sang/2f-eng.php (accessed July 2, 2011).

20. Brubaker S. AATB-accredited OPOs: recovery-related survey report, October 2006.

21. http://www.aatb.org/files/BOOTS%20-%20ORGAN%20AND%20TISSUE%20Workshop%202005%20final%20report.pdf (accessed July 2, 2011).

22. http://www.aatb.org/files/TTSN%20Description%20AATB%20-%20January%20 2007.pdf (accessed July 2, 2011).

23. http://www.aatb.org/files/TTSN%20-%20Year%20Two%20Annual%20 Update%20Report%20Revised%202008.pdf (accessed July 2, 2011).

24. http://edocket.access.gpo.gov/2009/E9-22658.htm, accessed July 2, 2011.

25. Request for Information (RFI) to Identify and Obtain Relevant Information from Public or Private Entities with an Interest in Biovigilance, A Federal Register Notice by the Health and Human Services Department on 25 April 2011, http://www.cdc.gov/niosh/ocas/pdfs/sec/ames/fr042511-185.pdf, accessed July 2, 2011.

26. Biovigilance in the United States: Efforts to Bridge a Critical Gap in Patient Safety and Donor Health, Public Health Service (PHS) Biovigilance Task Group, April 2009, http://www.hhs.gov/ash/bloodsafety/biovigilance/ash_to_acbsa_oct_2009.pdf.pdf (accessed July 2, 2011).

27. FDA orders Biomedical Tissue Services, Ltd., to cease manufacturing and to retain existing inventories of human cells, tissues and cellular and tissue-based

products (HCT/Ps), February 3, 2006. http://www.fda.gov/NewsEvents/Newsroom/PressAnnouncements/2006/ucm108589.htm (accessed July 2, 2011).

28. Tugwell BD, Patel PR, Williams IT, et al. Transmission of hepatitis C virus to several organ and tissue recipients from an antibody-negative donor. Ann Intern Med 2005;143:648–54.

29. Organ and Tissue Safety Workshop (2007) Advances and Challenges, Record of the Proceedings, June 5–6, 2007, Reston, VA, USA.

30. American Association of Tissue Banks. Identifying, Reporting and Investigating Tissue Recipient Adverse Reactions, draft Guidance Document, 2011.

4 Diseases Transmitted by Transplantation of Tissue and Cell Allografts

Ted Eastlund[1] and Ruth M. Warwick[2]
[1]University of New Mexico, Albuquerque, NM, USA
[2]University of Bristol, Bristol, UK

Introduction

Transplant surgeons and other treating physicians need to know about the risk and natural history of diseases that are transmissible through the transplantation or application of human organ, tissue, and cell allografts. By being aware of transmissible diseases and when and how these usually appear after transplantation, clinicians will be able to recognize them and discern whether the disease is allograft-associated. A timely diagnosis of a transmitted disease allows institution of early therapy and an assessment of whether the disease is possibly contagious so that measures to prevent spread to others can be initiated.

Preventing the spread of an allograft-associated transmissible disease to others can be achieved by prompt reporting of the disease to the hospital, the tissue bank, and relevant public health authorities so timely investigation about the cause can allow quarantine of implicated material in inventory and prevent further use of allografts from the same donor or same batch of processed tissue or cells. This will also allow the identification and evaluation of others who may have already received allografts from the same donor or same batch. A cooperative investigation by the hospital, tissue bank, and public health authorities is a critically important process that can lead to corrective actions that improve the safety of transplantation for future patients. Thus, awareness and reporting of postoperative diseases by the transplant surgeon and other treating physicians is very important. This chapter addresses diseases transmitted by transplantation, with emphasis on

Tissue and Cell Clinical Use: An Essential Guide, First Edition. Edited by Ruth M. Warwick and Scott A. Brubaker.
© 2012 Blackwell Publishing Ltd. Published 2012 by Blackwell Publishing Ltd.

tissue allografts, and when and how they become recognizable along with measures taken for their prevention.

Allograft viability and safety

Processed bone allografts are the most frequently transplanted human material in the world and the most used in the USA. Over one to two million processed bone allografts are used annually compared with over 20 million blood components used each year in the USA. In comparison, organ and cell transplants, including hematopoietic stem cells (HSCs), sperm, and ova, number in the tens of thousands each year.

The risk of transmitting disease to recipients of organ, tissue, and cell allografts is less with allografts that are nonviable and which have been processed to contain few cells (Table 4.1). The most commonly used bone allografts are those that have most of the cells and lipids removed, are exposed to disinfectants, and often demineralized and sterilized. For a large portion of bone allografts, processing also includes freeze-drying. The success of bone and tendon allograft use does not depend on cellular viability for effectiveness but on filling defects, providing support and strength and a scaffold of non-cellular matrix for the ingrowth and incorporation of the patient's own cells. Because of this, they can be vigorously disinfected and even sterilized. None of the reported cases of viral, bacterial, or fungal transmissions were due to this type of processed bone allografts [1, 2].

The clinical success of transplantation of other tissues, such as corneal allografts, depends on their cellular viability and continued metabolic activity and these types of allograft cannot undergo sterilization steps. Unprocessed frozen bone (e.g., femoral heads) containing marrow and lipids, tendons and ligaments with unprocessed bone ends, viable cartilage, refrigerated and frozen unprocessed skin are also in common use. Cryopreservation with dimethyl sulfoxide or glycerol as a cryoprotectant is the long-term storage method usually used for heart valves, semen, vessels, HSCs, and sometimes for skin and cartilage allografts to maintain cellular viability. The cases of tissue allograft-transmitted disease due to viruses, bacteria, and fungi involve these relatively unprocessed frozen, refrigerated, or fresh tissues that may contain large numbers of cells that are viable. A rare exception to this generalization is Creutzfeldt–Jakob disease (CJD), which is caused by prion proteins that are resistant to the usual disinfectants and which have been transmitted by freeze-dried dura mater allografts [3–8].

An accurate estimate of the incidence of disease transmission from tissue allografts is not available because of the lack of controlled studies; but the risk is low. As a whole, blood-borne viral disease transmission risk from tissue allografts is presumed to be greater than from blood transfusion but

Table 4.1 Allograft viability and risk of disease transmission

	Viable allografts	Allografts not containing viable cells*
Description	Fresh refrigerated cartilage	Frozen lyophilized bone, tendon
	Cryopreserved meniscus	Frozen frozen/lyophilized ligament, fascia
	Cryopreserved heart valve	Frozen sterilized costal cartilage
	Fresh/refrigerated cornea	Lyophilized dura mater
	Fresh/refrigerated/cryopreserved Skin	Acellular dermal matrix
	Hematopoietic stem cells	Frozen lyophilized pericardium
	Organs	Frozen ear ossicles
	Fresh/refrigerated/cryopreserved Vessels	
	Semen and oocyte	
	Blood cells	
Characteristics	Contains many viable cells	Nonviable, mostly matrix
	Cellular metabolism preserved	Mostly processed acellular
Matrix	May be antibiotic treated	May be chemically disinfected
	Cannot be sterilized	May be sterilized
	Has the potential to transmit neoplastic, metabolic, genetic, immunological infectious diseases	

*These allografts are processed with most cells removed, exposed to antibiotics, alcohol, and other disinfectants, and often sterilized. Depending on the degree of processing, some viable cells may remain.

less than from organ transplants or hematopoietic stem cell transplantation (HSCT) [9].

Many cases of serious and even fatal infections and malignancies are transmitted through organ transplantation each year in the USA [10]. Even though worldwide organ transplants number only in the tens of thousands each year, the magnitude of the morbidity and mortality from transmitted disease dwarfs that seen with blood transfusions and tissue transplantation. Some of the reasons for this are that the organ is unprocessed, not disinfected and contains large numbers of viable cells that are transplanted to a patient who is deliberately immune suppressed to prevent rejection of the new organ.

In addition, organ allografts from donors who carry more risk for disease transmission are acceptable when there may be no other deceased, brain-dead organ donor available and the recipient may urgently need a life-saving transplant to survive. Use of organ donors with encephalitis and other neurologic conditions of unknown cause has resulted in transmissions of fatal viral and amoebic infections [11–16]. In contrast, most tissue allografts and blood transfusion components can be obtained, screened, and stored to be safely available for emergencies and for scheduled surgery. Many of these types of blood component or tissue allograft are life enhancing more than life saving. There are exceptions in that blood transfusion availability can facilitate life saving surgery or chemotherapy and similarly heart valve and skin allografts can be life saving. It follows that a greater level of safety can be expected for blood transfusion and for tissue allografts than can currently be tolerated for organ transplants with such a short supply. This means that professional standards and government directives and regulatory requirements should be as stringent for tissue donors and tissue allografts as they are for blood donors and transfusions [17] especially when tissues may not be processed.

Infectious diseases transmitted by organ, tissue, and HSCs

Surgeons and other clinical staff are often aware of the most common infectious diseases transmitted by blood transfusion but are generally less aware of disease transmission by tissue, organ, and HSCT. Table 4.2 shows the spectrum of infectious diseases reported to have been transmitted from tissue, organs, and hematopoietic cells and compares these with similar transmissions by blood transfusion. Several of the same fatal and nonfatal infections have been transmitted by all these types of substance of human origin, but many infections have been reported with only one, two, or three types of allograft. The large number of transmitted diseases observed with some allografts but not others should alert clinicians to their potential transmission by hitherto uninvolved allografts.

Bacterial and fungal infections transmitted by tissue allografts

In the past, most attention given to disease transmission through tissue and cell allografts has focused on the blood-borne transmissible viruses human immunodeficiency virus (HIV), hepatitis B virus (HBV), hepatitis C virus (HCV), and human T-cell lymphotropic virus (HTLV). There were occasional cases of bacterial and fungal contamination of bone, cornea, skin, heart valve, tendon, pericardial, and cartilage allografts that caused occasional infections in patients [1, 2]. The threat from bacterial and fungal contamination to recipients has been thought to be minimal but several recently reported nonfatal cases, and two fatal cases, have again drawn attention to bacterial [24–27] and fungal [28, 29] contamination as an important problem. Table 4.3

Table 4.2 Infectious diseases transmitted by transfusion and organ, tissue and HSCT

Blood transfusion	Tissue allograft	Organ allograft	Hematopoietic stem cell allografts
HBV, HCV, HTLV-I	HBV, HCV, HTLV-I	HBV, HCV, HTLV-I	HBV, HCV, HTLV-I
HIV	HIV	HIV	HIV
CMV, EBV	CMV, EBV	CMV, EBV	CMV, EBV
Bacteria	Bacteria	Bacteria	Bacteria
Variant CJD	Classic CJD		—
Malaria	—	Malaria	Malaria
Parvovirus	—	Parvovirus	Parvovirus
Toxoplasmosis	—	Toxoplasmosis	Toxoplasmosis
Dengue [18]		Dengue [19]	Dengue [20]
—	Fungi	Fungi	Fungi
West Nile virus	—	West Nile virus	—
Trypanosoma cruzi (Chagas disease)	—	*Trypanosoma cruzi* (Chagas disease)	—
Filariae (*W. bancrofti*)	—	Filariae (*W. bancrofti*)	—
Leishmaniasis	—	Leishmaniasis	—
Syphilis		Syphilis	
	Tuberculosis, Non-tuberculous mycobacteria [21]	Tuberculosis	—
—	Rabies	Rabies	—
—	Herpes simplex	Herpes simplex	—
Babesiosis		Human papilloma virus (from hand transplant) [22]	Scrub typhus (*Orientia tsutsugamushi*)
Colorado tick fever (virus)	—	Lymphocytic choriomeningitis virus	Brucellosis
Tick-borne encephalitis (virus)	—	Human herpes virus-8 [23]	—
Hepatitis E virus	—	Adenovirus	
Rocky Mountain spotted fever (*Rickettsia rickettsia*)	—	*Balamuthia mandrillaris* (amoeba)	
		Strongyloidiasis	
		Schistosomiasis	

Table 4.3 Infectious disease transmission and the type of tissue allografts

Organism	Type of tissue allograft						
Bacteria	Fresh cornea	Fresh skin	Fresh cartilage	Frozen tendon	Frozen bone	Frozen pericardium	Cryopreserved heart valve
Mycobacterium	Frozen bone	Cryopreserved heart valve	Refrigerated artery				
Fungi	Fresh cornea	Cryopreserved heart valve					
HIV*	Frozen bone	Frozen tendon					
Hepatitis C	Frozen bone	Frozen tendon	Cryopreserved saphenous vein	Refrigerated artery			
Hepatitis B	Fresh cornea	Cryopreserved heart valve					
Rabies	Fresh cornea	Fresh artery					
Creutzfeldt–Jakob disease	Freeze-dried dura mater	Fresh cornea					
Epstein–Barr virus	Fresh nerve						
Cytomegalovirus	Fresh skin						
Herpes simplex	Fresh cornea						
Human T-cell lymphotropic virus, type I (HTLV-I)	Frozen bone						

*In 1986 recipient HIV seroconversion followed the use of allograft skin, processing not specified, for a burned patient from a donor whose HIV test result was not checked before transplantation but was subsequently found to be positive. However, there was no further investigation of the incident and no Western Blot confirmatory testing performed, so proof of transmission cannot be considered unequivocal [33].

CASE STUDY 4.1

Fatal *Clostridium* sepsis due to use of a contaminated allograft

A 23-year-old man received part of a fresh, refrigerated femoral condyle allograft used in reconstruction of knee cartilage and three days later died of *Clostridium sordellii* sepsis due to contamination of the allograft by the same bacterium [24, 25]. An investigation uncovered 14 other cases of allograft-associated *Clostridium* sp. infection from refrigerated tendons, femoral condyles, or menisci provided by the same tissue bank. Many had not been reported to the tissue bank [26]. Contributing factors leading to contamination of so many allografts included that the antibiotics used in processing were not effective against this organism, post-processing culturing was not sensitive enough, and complaints from hospitals were not investigated well and corrective actions were not developed or implemented.

Prevention of disease transmission is an important role of surgeons and their teams. Systematic reporting of adverse outcomes, by clinicians, both to the supplying tissue banks and to regulatory authorities, can give early warning which can highlight new and emerging threats. Such reporting can prevent other patients from receiving tissues that might also carry a risk of transmitting infection to the recipient, either from an implicated donor or from the same processing batch. Such reports can highlight procedural deficiencies in the tissue bank which, if not corrected, could place further recipients at risk. This type or reporting is an essential component to tissue and cell vigilance and surveillance. These types of investigation could not take place unless:

- tissue banks and hospitals where clinicians apply allografts have excellent communication between users of allografts and their supplying tissue banks;
- there are effective procedures for bi-directional traceability to and from the recipient and the donor, and organizations have the ability to undertake comprehensive allograft tracking;
- allograft labeling with agreed upon coding of the donor identification and of the allografts facilitates linkage between all organs and tissues from a single donor;
- reporting disease transmission from allograft use is undertaken at local, national, and international levels as allografts are often distributed very widely across borders; and
- clinicians and their teams are educated to be aware of and to recognize potential risks of infection or other diseases that can be associated with allografts.

CASE STUDY 4.2

Severe group A streptococcal knee infection from contaminated tendon allograft

A 17-year-old male received a hemi-patellar tendon allograft during repair of an anterior cruciate ligament injury. One day later he had pain, redness, fever and rigors [27]. Six days later, the allograft was removed and a fasciotomy of the thigh was needed. Group A *Streptococcus pyogenes* grew from the wound and excised tissues. Fevers persisted for another seven days and the wound again grew *S. pyogenes*, requiring hospitalization and another course of antibiotics. Initial information suggested that the allograft donor died of a medication overdose and an autopsy supported that diagnosis. After the transplant surgeon reported the serious infection after using an allograft from this donor, a more careful investigation into the cause of death of the donor demonstrated the following.

1. The donor had been misdiagnosed by the emergency room physician, the autopsy pathologist and, ultimately, the tissue bank medical director. The cause of death was revised to be streptococcal sepsis and toxic shock-like syndrome with back pain, vomiting, fever, rash, and hypotension;
2. Group A *Streptococcus pyogenes* was recovered from pre-processing cultures of other tissues obtained from the same donor, from autopsy-stored tissues, and from postmortem donor blood. Group A *Streptococcus pyogenes* from the donor was proven to be the same as that found in the patient, using bacterial gene sequence analysis;
3. Investigation showed that the effectiveness of tissue processing steps at the supplying tissue bank had not been properly validated; and,
4. Antibiotics used in processing were ineffective in eradicating the contaminant.

   The surgeon must be aware that:

1. infections in their allograft recipient may arise from a donor and may have implications for other recipients;
2. communication with other transplant surgeons, tissue banks and transplant infectious disease experts is necessary so that, in the event of a possible transplant transmitted infection, appropriate action can be taken for the index case as well as for other recipients and potential recipients; and
3. surgeons and tissue banks must have policies and procedures in place to ensure both can appropriately investigate and act on the relevance of an infection in an allograft recipient and the importance of rapid communication with the supplying tissue bank.

depicts the diseases transmitted by tissue transplantation and the type of tissue allografts that have been implicated. Note that, except for CJD transmission by dura, all the cases involved unprocessed fresh, refrigerated, or frozen unprocessed allografts.

Testing of allografts for bacterial and fungal contamination before implantation

Sampling of the allograft or transport solution for bacterial culture immediately before implantation is a practice that is performed during most organ transplantations. Some physicians have also recommended culturing the tissue allograft immediately before implantation because of the worry that the allograft could be contaminated.

However, a positive result from pre-implantation sampling can often be a low-virulence contaminant acquired from the operating room environment during collection. A positive result can also be of limited or no importance when the isolate is a low-virulence bacterium ordinarily found in the operating theatre environment, or on the patient's skin, or when only a small quantity of bacteria is found. These low virulence organisms are often contaminants and pose little threat to recipients who routinely receive prophylactic antibiotics and antibiotic irrigation solutions intraoperatively during surgery.

Hou et al. [30] confirmed that pre-implantation testing can give positive results for bacteria that do not cause infections in patients. With the routine performance of pre-implantation cultures of thawed frozen bone allografts, they found that 22 (1.6%) of 1353 implanted allografts had a positive swab culture. Only four of these 22 patients (18.2%) developed infection. However, the bacteria found in wound cultures of the infected recipients were different from those found by the swab culture of thawed allografts except in one case. In this last case the wound culture grew *Candida* and the allograft swab grew a yeast-like organism. Further testing was not performed to determine whether these coincidental findings of yeast occurred by chance or represented a contaminated allograft.

Pre-implantation testing can give false-positive results creating serious but unneeded concern for patient safety and superfluous investigations and additional antibiotics given to the patient. Mermel et al. [31] found *Comomonas acidovorans* on four bone allografts when sampled immediately before implantation in four patients. Later, it was discovered that reports of bacterial growth were falsely positive and due to contamination of a water bath sonicator used in the microbiology laboratory to prepare tissue samples and not actually a contamination of the graft itself.

When the sampling is performed immediately before use, it takes days for the results to be available and the test result has limited clinical use. Rarely, it may retrospectively aid in determining the source of a postoperative infection. Aho et al. [32] reported deep bacterial infections in two of 63 patients receiving frozen unprocessed large bone allografts. *Pseudomonas aeruginosa* and *Staphylococcus epidermidis* were identified from pre-implantation sampling immediately before surgery and later from the recipient site of infection. Both allografts had negative cultures at the time of recovery from the donor and before frozen storage. Although the bacteria could have been acquired from the operating theatre environment, the negative recovery cultures could have been falsely negative due to sampling and testing limitations and the allograft could have been contaminated before frozen storage.

Pre-implantation microbial testing of bone and other tissue allografts can provide important information for improving the safety of allograft use and further studies are warranted. For example, studies are important when implementing new processes and procedures, when starting a new tissue bank, when investigating adverse microbial events in transplant recipients, and whenever the safety of the allograft needs investigation. However, because over a million bone, tendon, and other tissue allografts are used annually in the USA, and tissue allograft recipients are not usually as immune-compromised as organ and HSCT recipients, routing pre-implantation testing is not recommended by most tissue banks and tissue banking professional organizations.

Viral infections transmitted by tissue allografts

Tissue transplantation has resulted in donor-to-recipient transmission of HIV [34–37], hepatitis B [38, 39] and hepatitis C [40–44] viruses, human T-cell lymphotropic virus [45], rabies [11, 46–48], *Herpes simplex* [49, 50], Epstein-Barr virus (EBV) [51], and cytomegalovirus [52]. Some of these have occurred in the past decade and because they were eventually recognized, reported, and investigated, lessons have been learned that have improved safety for future recipients. There have been nine cases of HIV transmission through bone transplantation, all of which were from untested donors or from donors tested during the first year when insensitive testing was first available [34–36]. Cases of HCV transmission to multiple organ and tissue recipients in 2000 and 2002 from a common donor have brought about necessary improvements in communication between organ and tissue allograft organizations, triggered the implementation of donor blood testing for HCV nucleic acids (HCV NAT), and emphasized the importance of good record keeping. A case of donor-to-recipient *Herpes simplex* transmission by cornea transplantation brought attention to herpes viruses such as cytomegalovirus (CMV), EBV, and *Herpes simplex* that infect most individuals at an early age and remain latent for years afterwards. The infection can appear in recipients of tissues and organs either as a reactivation of an old infection or as a new infection transmitted from the donor of the allograft [49, 50]. A case of rabies transmission by an arterial allograft in 2004 demonstrated the difficulty of accurately diagnosing rabies in donors and the infectious risk of using an artery from a high-risk donor for an organ recipient. It also demonstrated that, in the USA, arterial tissue allografts procured during organ recovery are not subjected to the same professional standards and government directives and regulations as vascular tissues from deceased tissue donors [11]. Recently, an HCV-positive organ-associated arterial allograft was erroneously chosen from storage instead of an HCV-negative artery and used during organ transplantation causing an unnecessary HCV infection. This case brought about a change in the practice of deliberately storing HCV-positive vessels with HCV-negative vessels for possible use in HCV-positive organ recipients [44].

CJD after tissue transplantation

Sporadic (also known as classical) CJD is a transmissible spongiform encephalopathy with rapidly progressive fatal dementia caused by abnormal prion proteins. It occurs sporadically at a worldwide rate of 0.5–2 cases each year per million population. It has been transmitted by intracerebral electrodes used during neurosurgery, by use of growth hormone derived from human pituitaries, and by the use of cornea and dura mater allografts. There have been approximately 196 cases of CJD transmitted from contaminated dura mater allografts worldwide, most of which took place in Japan and were associated with pooled processed dura mater [6, 7]. No confirmed cases of CJD transmission by organ transplants or HSCT have been reported.

The CJD incubation period after transplants of Lyodura® brand dura mater is very long, with over 130 Japanese cases developing an average of 11.8 years (median 12.4 years, range 1.2–24.8 years) after use of dura mater allograft which had been supplied from a single manufacturer in Germany [6, 7].

Two patients who died of CJD received cornea allografts from donors with CJD 18 months and 30 years earlier [3, 4]. The initial symptoms that developed after transplantation of dura and corneas were ataxia, dysarthria, memory loss, personality change, myoclonus, nystagmus, and decreased ability to speak followed by rapidly progressive dementia.

The CJD cases from contaminated Lyodura brand dura allografts occurred due to pooling of dura from many donors during processing and from inadequate donor screening by the German company. Almost all of the implicated Lyodura allografts were transplanted in Japan between 1978 and 1993, with most between 1983 and 1987. Cases of Lyodura-associated CJD also occurred in several other countries, including the USA, Spain, and New Zealand. Consequently the clinical use of dura allograft nearly ceased. Many patients died unnecessarily because Lyodura continued in use long after it was clearly implicated as being the cause. Neurosurgeons were not warned early enough, the manufacturing company and hospitals did not conduct a timely recall, a distributor continued to sell Lyodura, and the national government where most was used failed to issue directives and warnings to cease use of Lyodura in a timely fashion [7, 8].

Recently, there was the first of two reports of presumed transmission of CJD from dura mater allograft with the name brand Tutoplast®, processed by a different company in Germany [53]. Dura allografts from this company had not been implicated in CJD transmission previously. Another case occurred in Canada in a patient 11 years after receiving a Tutoplast allograft in 1993 but it has not been proven that CJD was caused by the allograft [54, 55]. Results from the investigation of the donor and other recipients of tissue from the same donor, if conducted, have not been published. Maddox et al. [56] have emphasized that rare diseases such as CJD that occur sporadically in an older population can be expected to occur also by chance in older recipients of corneas and other allografts.

Some cases of CJD from dura mater involved donors who had clinical signs of CJD. These donors would not be accepted today. The two cases of CJD from corneal allografts involved clearly symptomatic donors and today's professional standards and government directives and regulations would require exclusion of these donors.

Because there is no effective therapy, CJD is always fatal, and the causative prions are resistant to many common disinfectants and sterilants, prevention is most important. Several donor selection precautions are now in place to reduce the risk.

New variant CJD (vCJD) was first described in 1996 in the UK and is believed to have resulted from consumption of cattle products contaminated with prions responsible for bovine spongiform encephalopathy. After many studies showing that classical CJD does not seem to be transmissible by blood transfusions, there have been a few cases of vCJD transmitted by blood transfusion and possibly by fractionated plasma products in the UK. So far no cases of vCJD have been reported from tissue, organ, or HSCT or gametes. Although there is currently no test for vCJD that can be applied to blood samples, there have been suggestions that deceased donors could be tested for vCJD using non-blood analytes. A pilot study using tonsil tissue from deceased doors as the analyte has been undertaken [57].

Recognizing post-transplantation infections that were transmitted by the tissue allograft

Variable and sometimes long incubation periods and microbial and infection latency creates the need for prolonged vigilance by the tissue allograft transplant surgeon and other clinicians caring for patients. Unlike bacterial infection, which can present as a severe local infection days to weeks after surgery, some other allograft-associated infections can remain asymptomatic and not become apparent until long after surgery because of latency periods between the inoculation of the organism and the onset of symptoms or the ability to test and detect the infection. This varies with the exposure dose, the type of organism, the test sensitivity, and recipient factors (Table 4.4). Physicians should suspect allograft-transmitted HIV, or hepatitis B or C viral

Table 4.4 Neoplastic diseases of donor origin transmitted by organ, tissue, and HSCT

Tissue allografts	Organ allografts	Hematopoietic stem cell allografts
Papillary adenocarcinoma (from cornea)	Post-transplant lymphoproliferative disorders	Post-transplant lymphoproliferative disorders
Glioma (from cornea)	Non-Hodgkin's lymphoma	Non-Hodgkin's lymphoma
	Renal cell carcinoma	Acute myelogenous leukemia
	Choriocarcinoma	Acute lymphocytic leukemia
	Melanoma	Chronic myelogenous leukemia
	Sarcoma	Chronic lymphocytic leukemia
	Astrocytoma	
	Glioblastoma multiforme	
	Medulloblastoma	
	Pancreas adenocarcinoma	
	Colon adenocarcinoma	
	Prostate adenocarcinoma	
	Breast adenocarcinoma	
	Lung adenocarcinoma	
	Lung small-cell carcinoma	
	Lung bronchioloalveolar carcinoma	
	Hepatocellular carcinoma	
	Ovarian carcinoma	
	IgA myeloma	
	Multiple myeloma	
	Urothelial carcinoma	
	Undifferentiated small-cell neuroendocrine carcinoma	

infection, if the patient has no risk factors or other likely cause and was transplanted up to a few months before its clinical onset. Although transmitted viral infections can be clinically silent, many will cause an acute viral syndrome. Fever, rash, enlarged nodes, and diarrhea in two patients developed three weeks after receipt of HIV-contaminated frozen femoral head and frozen patellar tendon allografts [34, 35]. Symptomatic HCV infection developed six weeks after implantation of a contaminated tendon allograft [42,

43]. Both HCV and HBV can cause chronic infections that are silent until chronic liver disease and liver failure develop many years later.

Classic CJD has been transmitted by contaminated dura allograft. Symptoms of classic CJD developed at a median time of 12.4 years after use of freeze-dried dura mater and one case presented after 24.8 years [6]. CJD was transmitted in 1974 when a patient received a corneal allograft from a donor who died of autopsy proven CJD [3]. The graft was implanted 18 months before the patient presented with an 8-month illness resulting in death. One other cornea recipient developed CJD 30 years after a transplant [4].

Fungal contamination of a heart valve allograft caused a severe febrile illness with fungemia that developed 17 days after surgery but was cured with antifungal therapy [28]. The white cell count was normal. Infected heart and heart valve allografts can also remain asymptomatic for months. A heart transplant recipient developed *Aspergillus fumigatus* endocarditis from an infected organ donor but had no symptoms or fever for over five months [58]. In an unpublished case, a patient who died from fungal infection after implantation of a contaminated human heart valve allograft did not develop symptoms of infection until five months later (T. Eastlund, unpublished observation). This patient's hospitalizations were related to septic mycotic emboli causing stroke followed by osteomyelitis of the spine.

The use of human rib allografts for spine surgery that were contaminated with *Mycobacterium tuberculosis* led to chronic tubercular wound infections in several patients but, in one, it caused disseminated tuberculosis that was not clinically apparent until two months later [59]. Mycobacterial infections in cardiovascular grafts have been reviewed [60]. Khanna and Munro reported a case of fatal miliary tuberculosis developing eight months after receiving a human heart valve allograft and concluded that the infection arose from the transplanted valve [61]. Anyanwu et al. reported several cases of miliary tuberculosis that developed from a few weeks to 12 months after surgical implantation of contaminated human heart valve allografts [62]. Non-tuberculous mycobacterium has been transmitted by use of a refrigerated arterial allograft. A pre-implant culture of the allograft grew *Mycobacterium hominis,* and an *M. hominis* wound infection with hematoma rupture developed after surgery [61].

Most confirmed cases of bacterial infections transmitted by contaminated corneal allografts occurred 3–32 days after surgery with a median of seven days [63]. *Candida* infections from contaminated corneal allografts can also become symptomatic early but many do not until after several weeks after surgery [64].

Transmission of infectious disease through organ transplantation

Infectious diseases transmitted by organ transplantation have been reported more often and with more types of microorganism than those transmitted by tissue transplantation (Table 4.2).

CMV and EBV commonly cause infections after organ and HSCT and they most often occur due to reactivation of endogenous latent virus. In some seronegative recipients they can be due to new donor-derived infections. The common blood-borne viruses such as HIV, HBV, HCV, and HTLV have been transmitted by organs, HSCs, blood transfusion, and tissues. Blood transfusions, organs, and HSCTs have transmitted malaria [65–68], parvovirus [69, 70], toxoplasmosis [71–76] and dengue [18–20]. Rabies has been transmitted by organ transplantation [12, 13]. An interesting case involved transmission of human papilloma virus infection and warts from hand transplant surgery has also been reported [22].

Syphilis and parasites such as leishmania, microfilariae, and *Trypanosoma cruzi* [77, 78] have been transmitted by organs [77] and blood transfusion but not by tissue, HSCs, or gametes.

Several other organisms cause serious infectious disease in the USA but have only recently been identified as being capable of transmission through organ transplantation. For example, lymphocytic choriomeningitis virus (LCMV) is known for its disastrous teratogenic effects in newborns. The deadly result of its infection was recently shown to follow its transmission by organ transplantation [79].

Subsequently, a new LCMV-related arenavirus was discovered to cause fatal infections in three recipients of organs after transmission from a single donor [80]. Transmission of this arenavirus by transfusion, tissue, or cell transplantation or gamete use has not been demonstrated. Another of the many disquieting examples of transmission is *Chlamydia pneumoniae*, a serious cause of pneumonia in humans and recently reported as probably transmitted through lung transplantation and to contribute to complications such as bronchiolitis obliterans syndrome [81].

This occurs frequently but rarely result in transmission of infection. There is likely under-recognition of bacterial transmission because transient fevers without a documented cause and infections caused by common bacteria may not be recognized as donor-derived. Several donor-to-recipient transmissions of tuberculosis through organ transplantation have been reported [82, 83]. A diagnosis can be difficult and its onset may be delayed by months.

Fungal disease transmissions by organ transplantation, including aspergillosis and *Candida*, are associated with significant morbidity [58]. Transmissions of coccidiomycosis, endemic in parts of the USA, demonstrate the difficulty in differentiating active and potentially infectious disease from quiescent disease in prospective donors [84].

Donor-derived parasitic infections have been a significant cause of morbidity and mortality in organ recipients and may be difficult to diagnose [76]. Transmissions of the trypanosome causing Chagas' disease [78], leishmaniasis [85], strongyloidiasis [86], and the amoeba *Balamuthia mandrillaris* have recently been reported [15, 16]. The transmission of *Balamuthia* demonstrated that prospective organ donors with neurologic conditions, such as unexplained encephalitis, can harbor infectious transmissible disease and should be excluded from donation [16].

Transmission of infectious disease through HSCT

Except for cases of CMV and EBV, donor-to-recipient transmission of infections during HSCT occurs rarely. Infectious disease transmission by both HSCT and tissue allografts occurs much less frequently that by organ transplantation. There have been rare cases of transmission of HIV [87], HCV [88], HBV [89, 90], HTLV-I [92], parvovirus [91], dengue [20], scrub typhus [93], brucellosis [94], and the parasites toxoplasmosis [95] and malaria [96, 97] through HSCT (Table 4.2). Stem cells can become contaminated during processing and infusion of bacterially contaminated stem cells has caused acute reactions and bacteremia [98–100].

Transmission of neoplastic diseases through organ, tissue, and HSCT

Table 4.4 lists reported transmissions of malignancies by organs, tissues, and HSCs. So far, there have been no reports of donor-derived malignancies transmitted by blood transfusion and only two through tissue allografts, both from cornea donors. There is a very low possibility of transmitting malignancies from use of tissue allografts for immunocompetent recipients even if the allograft contains viable cells but the possibility should be kept in mind. There have been two cases of accidental transplantation of patient-derived malignancies into the hands of surgeons through needle stick injury [101, 102]. This demonstrates that viable fresh malignant cells may be able to be transplanted across the immunological barrier into immune competent persons. Animal studies have shown that lymphoma can be transmitted through the transplantation of frozen and cryopreserved ovarian tissue into healthy recipient mice [103]. Despite this, tissue allografts that have been processed or frozen likely have a low number of viable cells and the risk of transmitting malignancy can be practically excluded.

Malignancy transmitted by organ transplantation

There have, however, been many more reports of malignancies transmitted from organ donors during organ transplantation than from other forms of transplantation [104]. This may be due to the large reservoir of fresh viable malignant cells that can be present in an organ and the severe immunosuppression due to drugs administered to the organ recipient to prevent organ rejection. The risk of malignancy transmission by organ transplantation is a serious one and prevention is difficult or to be certain that an organ donor is free of an undiagnosed malignancy. In some cases a donor malignancy had metastasized to the donor's brain and caused death from intracerebral

Table 4.5 Transmission of autoimmune, alloimmune, genetic, and metabolic diseases through organ and HSCT

HSCT	Organ transplant
Graft versus host disease, acute and chronic	Graft versus host disease, acute
PLS (RBC alloantibodies: acute hemolysis)	PLS (RBC alloantibodies: acute hemolysis)
Idiopathic autoimmune thrombocytopenia	PLS (acute thrombocytopenia)
Sarcoidosis	Sarcoidosis
Vitiligo	Vitiligo
Atopy, atopic dermatitis	Severe peanut allergy
Alopecia areata	Factor VIII deficiency (hemophilia A)
Autoimmune thyroid disease: autoimmune thyroiditis, thyrotoxicosis	Factor XI deficiency
Coeliac disease	Factor XII deficiency
Type 1 diabetes mellitus	
Gaucher's disease	
G6PDH deficiency	
IgA deficiency	
Myasthenia gravis	
Anti-phospholipid syndrome	
Anti-pancreatic antibodies	
Cyclic neutropenia	

hemorrhage, which may have hidden the small underlying metastatic brain tumor. This may be of increasing importance as older donors are being considered owing to organ shortages.

Renal cell carcinoma is reported most frequently but malignant melanoma and choriocarcinoma occur frequently [104]. Malignancies transmitted through organ transplantation (Table 4.5) include carcinomas, lymphomas, and melanomas from various sites. An unusual case of donor-derived malignancy involved a man who received a kidney transplant and later developed metastatic ovarian carcinoma [105]. Proving that a malignancy was transmitted by organ transplantation requires a histological comparison between the tumor in the recipient and the donor, and often karyotyping, fluorescent in situ hybridization, or other molecular methods to demonstrate a gender match between donor and recipient, or DNA nucleic acid sequencing to exclude pattern mismatches. Early diagnosis and demonstrating that the malignancy is unequivocally of donor origin is important because it determines therapy; if of donor origin, a reduction in immunosuppressive medication and possible explantation of the graft is of immediate importance. To be effective, both of these interventions need timely recognition and diagnosis.

Malignancies transmitted by organ transplantation have been first diagnosed either very quickly, as early as one day after surgery or first recognized as long as more than a year after surgery. In some, transmitted malignancies have been limited to the transplanted organ and in others they have been first diagnosed after widespread metastasis.

Malignancy transmitted by tissue allografts

Two cases of tumors transmitted by corneal transplantation were reported, one many decades ago in Japan and another in 1990 in the USA [106, 107]. Both came from corneal transplants obtained from donors harboring known malignancies. One corneal donor who died in 1990 of disseminated poorly differentiated adenocarcinoma had known choroidal masses in the eye when the corneal allograft was removed for use in another patient. However, despite the transplantation of corneas from donors with malignancies, studies have suggested that the incidence of cancer in cornea recipients is no different from the general population [108]. There have not been any cases reported of malignancy transmission after use of skin, heart valve, or the most commonly used allografts, bone and tendon. Some bone allografts, such as femoral heads that are obtained as a discard during hip arthroplasty, are stored frozen and used without processing. Even though cells can survive long-term storage at −80°C in bone [109–111] and may contain malignant cells [112–114], no cases of bone allograft transmission of malignancy have been found.

Histologic studies of donated frozen femoral heads have shown that some femoral heads from patients with no known malignancies contain malignant cells. Sugihara et al. [112] reported that femoral heads from many patients with no known malignancy contain malignant cells. In a separate study, Zwitser et al. [113] studied femoral heads donated by patients with no history of malignancy and found low grade lymphoma cells in six of 504 donor femoral heads. Long-term follow-up of these six donors found that one developed a B-cell lymphoma in an inguinal lymph node and one developed chronic lymphocytic leukemia. Sugihara found malignant lymphoma in two of 137 femoral heads. Palmer et al. [114] examined 1146 donated femoral heads and found well-differentiated lymphocytic lymphoma cells in two and a low-grade chondrosarcoma in one. Despite these findings, there have been no reports that femoral heads transmit malignancies. The low prevalence of femoral heads containing malignant cells and the small inoculum along with the immunocompetency of the bone graft recipient probably account for the lack of malignancy transmission.

With rare exceptions, prospective donors who have active malignancies, lymphomas, or leukemias are excluded from donating blood, tissues, and organs. Prospective donors who have primary malignancies of the brain without spread are considered eligible to be a source of organs and often, depending on the tissue bank and country, as a source of tissue allograft. Many tissue banks will accept deceased tissue donors who have a remote history of malignancy but donor eligibility policies vary widely. Those that accept donors with a history of malignancy require curative therapy and may require at least three to five years of a disease-free status.

Transmission of malignancies by HSCT
Hematologic malignancies, but not solid tumors, have been transmitted by HSCT [104, 115]. Acute and chronic leukemias and non-Hodgkin's lymphoma have been transmitted. The leukemias can be transmitted directly from the donor or can arise *de novo* from circulating donor cells years later [104].

Post-transplant lymphoproliferative disease
Post-transplantation lymphoproliferative disease (PTLD) is both an infectious disease caused by a common oncogenic virus, the EBV, and is a malignant disease similar to non-Hodgkin's lymphoma. PTLD complicates organ transplants and HSCT but not tissue transplants or blood transfusions. The organ graft is a common site for PTLD especially during the first year after transplantation but it regularly occurs at other sites throughout the body. Mortality rates of 5–55% have been observed [116]. Most of the PTLD after HSCT are donor cell derived while most PTLD following solid organs are recipient derived [104]. Transmission through transplantation to immune suppressed recipients results in *de novo* infection of recipient B-lymphocytes by EBV of donor origin. Early diagnosis allows early treatment and a better prognosis [117]. Therefore awareness of its clinical presentation is important. PTLD has developed as early as 15 days after transplantation, commonly appears within one year but may occur years later [117].

The most common systemic symptoms are fever, fatigue, sore throat, hepatic or splenic enlargement, poor appetite, and weight loss. Treatment of PTLD includes discontinuing immunosuppression, removal of the affected organ or lymph nodes (excisional therapy), antiviral therapy, anti-human CD20 antibody (rituximab) infusion, and EBV-targeted T-lymphocyte infusions.

Transmission of immunologic diseases of donor origin through organ and HSCT

Graft-versus-host disease
Graft-versus-host disease (GVHD) is a well-known complication of blood transfusion [118], organ transplantation [119, 120] and HSCT [121]. GVHD is due to donor-derived lymphocytes contained in the donated allograft.

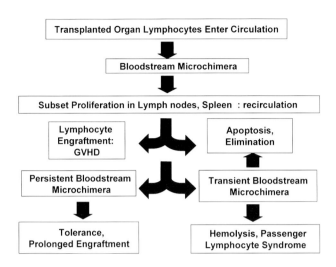

Figure 4.1 Fate of donor lymphocytes transplanted with an organ and passenger lymphocyte syndrome (PLS).

Instead of gradually being eliminated in the recipient, donor lymphocytes can continue to circulate and engraft, though this is usually a transient phenomena (Figure 4.1).

After leaving the transplanted organ and recirculating as a lymphocyte chimeric state, donor lymphocytes can become established in tissue to cause cytotoxic injury and GVHD or can proliferate and produce antibody against the recipient's red cells and cause hemolysis. This cause of hemolysis is called the passenger lymphocyte syndrome (PLS).

Donor-derived lymphocytes can exert cytotoxic destructive effects against recipient's cells and tissues especially the patient's liver, skin, intestine, and marrow, causing GVHD. Clinical manifestations include severe diarrhea, hepatitis with jaundice, and an extensive red rash. GVHD is a risk of organ and HSCT but is not expected after use of tissue allografts or gametes owing to their absolute or relative lack of viable lymphocytes.

GVHD after organ transplantation and blood transfusion appears rarely, usually in its acute form, and is poorly responsive to any treatment with most affected patients dying in less than 21 days. Blood transfusion or organ transplantation associated GVHD results in marrow hypoplasia with pancytopenia because the marrow is another target of donor-derived lymphocytes and as a consequence, fatal infection and bleeding are not unusual. In contrast, the marrow in HSCT-related GVHD is not necessarily hypoplastic because the engrafted marrow is of donor origin and is not a target.

In HSC transplants both acute and chronic GVHD are common. They are treated and managed more successfully but are still accompanied by serious morbidity and mortality. HSCT not only delivers donor-derived lymphocytes directed against normal recipient cells and tissues resulting in GVHD, but the engrafted donor lymphocytes also exert a very important and beneficial anti-leukemia and anti-tumor effect. This is a key element in the success of HSCT in treating malignant diseases.

Passenger lymphocyte syndrome: "graft-versus-host" hemolytic anemia

PLS with hemolytic anemia has complicated organ and HSCT. After transplantation of an organ, donor lymphocytes contained in the organ (passenger lymphocytes) leave the organ, pass through the patient's lymph nodes and spleen, and recirculate (Figure 4.2).

Because organ and HSC recipients receive immune suppressive drugs and the allograft is histocompatible, donor-derived lymphocytes are not readily

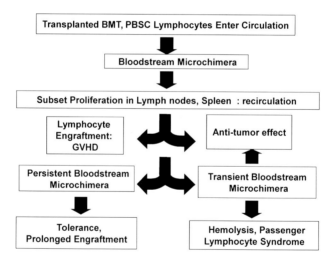

Figure 4.2 Fate of lymphocytes after bone marrow transplant (BMT) or peripheral blood stem cells (PBSCs) leading to passenger lymphocyte syndrome (PLS). As the bone marrow or PBSC engraft, donor lymphocytes proliferate and circulate. Persistent circulation of donor and recipient lymphocytes (microchimaera) predicts prolonged tolerance and acceptance of the hematopoietic graft. Circulating donor cytotoxic lymphocytes are responsible for an anti-tumor effect, enabling a cure for the underlying malignancy for which the transplant was given. Transient proliferation of donor lymphocytes can cause PLS in which there is transient antibody-mediated hemolysis of recipient RBC due to sensitized donor lymphocytes producing antibodies against recipient RBC antigens that are identical to RBC antigens to which the donor was previously exposed while alive.

eliminated from the circulation. Their persistence can affect the immune function of the patient and be both beneficial by modulating tolerance with prolonged graft acceptance and function, and harmful by mounting an antibody response against the recipient [122]. Donor-derived lymphocytes can mount a humoral response, resulting in red cell antibodies directed against the patient's unmatched blood group antigens and causing hemolytic anemia [123]. Hemolysis due to transient donor-derived antibodies is a complication of organ transplantation and bone marrow or peripheral blood stem cells transplants, but generally not when cord blood is used. Presumably, this is because cord blood lymphocytes are less capable than adult lymphocytes of mounting an immune response, do not strongly produce isohemagglutinins, anti-A or anti-B, and have not been sensitized or exposed to foreign antigens before birth.

Hemolytic anemia due to donor-derived antibodies depends on previous sensitization of the organ or HSCT donor to a blood cell antigen absent in the donor but present in the recipient. This is more likely with donors having minor ABO incompatibility with the recipient, e.g., donor blood group O with circulating anti-A and anti-B and the recipient is blood group A [122]. Others at risk include recipients of organ and stem cell transplants from donors with antibodies to minor red blood cell (RBC) antigens such as rhesus (Rh), Kidd, and Duffy [124–127]. Hemolytic anemia due to PLS has occurred with liver, lung, heart, kidney, pancreas, and intestine transplants, occurring more frequently after transplantation of organs with large amounts of donor lymphoid tissue such as with liver or combined heart-lung transplants. When there is minor ABO incompatibility between organ donors and liver or lung transplant recipients, hemolysis of some degree is seen in most patients.

In most cases hemolysis due to donor ABO antibodies develops within two weeks of the transplant and is mild and self-limited being treated by use of red cell transfusions of organ donor blood type. Antibodies are usually present for one to three weeks after the transplant but circulating donor-derived antibodies have been observed for over one year. In contrast, hemolysis and organ donor-derived anti-D usually develop later and persist for months in organ recipients [123, 124].

Organ and HSCT donors usually have their blood typed for ABO and screened for RBC antibodies. Transplant surgeons should be aware of the possibility of PLS whenever RBC antibodies incompatible with the recipient are encountered preoperatively or when the donor has a history of autoimmune thrombocytopenia, is a female with a child born with hemolytic disease of the newborn or thrombocytopenia (neonatal alloimmune thrombocytopenia), or is a donor with any other autoimmune disease associated with autoantibodies that theoretically can be transiently transferred by passenger lymphocytes after transplantation.

Passenger lymphocyte syndrome: "graft-versus-host" thrombocytopenia in recipients of organs and HSCs

Though occurring infrequently, passenger lymphocytes can also produce platelet antibodies and cause thrombocytopenia [128] in organ and HSC recipients. As a form of PLS there have been cases of severe antibody-mediated thrombocytopenia with transient bleeding that developed rapidly after transplanting organs from donors with idiopathic (autoimmune) thrombocytopenia purpura (ITP) [129, 130].

There have been other cases of ITP after liver transplantation but these represent new cases of ITP, rather than PLS, developing an average of 53 months after transplantation. These cases did not have donors with thrombocytopenia or known ITP and the thrombocytopenia was probably due to transplant-related altered immunity instead of PLS [131].

Transmission of autoimmune thrombocytopenia by bone marrow transplantation

ITP of donor origin may have been transferred to recipients with donor cells capable of engrafting and proliferating in the marrow graft producing platelet autoantibodies having specificities identical to those of the donor [132–134].

Transmission of metabolic and genetic diseases of donor origin by organ and HSCT

Organ transplants carry the risk of transmitting non-infectious, non-malignant diseases such as autoimmune, metabolic, and genetic diseases of donor origin (Table 4.6). Rare cases have been reported of acquired hemophilia A in a liver recipient due to donor-derived factor VIII antibodies, unrecognized before transplantation, and separate cases of factor XI and factor XII deficiencies transmitted by liver transplantation [135–137]. Vitiligo has been transmitted by way of combined liver-kidney transplant [138].

Severe allergies have been carried from the donor to the recipient by organ transplantation. Liver and lung transplant recipients have had allergic and anaphylactic reactions to peanuts with no personal history of a previous allergy but it was later established that the peanut allergy was transferred by the transplanted organ from donors who had serious peanut allergies and died from anaphylactic reactions to peanuts [139–142].

Interestingly there is also a case report of a patient who had peanut allergy cured inadvertently when a bone marrow transplant was performed for another reason [143]. Hematopoietic stem cell transplantation results in an engrafted donor marrow and donor immune system which can, like organ transplantation result in transmitting inherited conditions, deficiencies or diseases in the recipient that were previously present in the donor. Examples of these diseases include the antiphospholipid syndrome [144], Gaucher's disease [145], celiac disease [146], glucose-6-phosphatase deficiency [147], diabetes [148], myasthenia gravis [149, 150], autoimmune thyroiditis and other thyroid disease [151–153], and possible sarcoidosis [154]. A patient can become immunoglobulin-A (IgA)-deficient after a transplant of a marrow from an IgA-deficient donor while others with IgA-deficiency have been unexpectedly cured by marrow transplants from a normal donor [155–157]. Marrow transplantation has transferred atopy, allergen-specific IgE and asthma, and allergen-specific, IgE-mediated hypersensitivity reactions [158–162]. Other case reports have demonstrated that marrow transplantation from normal donors can cure allergic disease such as latex allergy and atopic dermatitis [163–165]. Serious cyclic neutropenia has been accidentally transferred to several patients by marrow transplantation [166]. Hemoglobin S trait has been transmitted by cord blood transplantation [167] and bone marrow transplant has transmitted vitiligo [168].

Disease transmission and complications due to assisted reproduction using donated sperm and ova

This section addresses transmission of infectious disease, harmful immune reactions and genetic diseases unintentionally inherited from sperm or ovum donations. Table 4.6 depicts the diseases transmitted by sperm, ova, and embryos using assisted reproduction technologies. Although gametes, organs, and HSC are viable, metabolically active and capable of sustaining malignant cell growth, malignancy transmission from the donor to the recipient is mainly a feature of organ and HSC transplantation to immuno-suppressed patients, not through gamete use by immunocompetent persons (Tables 4.4 and 4.6). Genetic, inherited diseases are readily transmitted by donated gametes, organs, and HSC; whereas, neoplastic, metabolic and immune diseases are transmitted more readily through organ and HSC transplantation (Tables 4.5 and 4.6).

Complications of assisted reproduction

Assisted reproduction has become a common practice and carries with it complications associated with transmitting disease from the gamete donor to the recipient as well as complications due to the technical procedures themselves. Technical complications arise from ovulation induction, ova retrieval, laparoscopy, anesthesia, laboratory processing of gametes, the techniques used for in vitro fertilization and embryo transfer, intracytoplasmic sperm injection, gamete intrafallopian transfer, and zygote intrafallopian transfer, and even the less complicated intrauterine insemination using washed sperm.

Table 4.6 Diseases transmitted by assisted reproduction technology

Semen		Ovum	Embryo	Gestational carrier
Infection	Metabolic, genetic	Metabolic, genetic	Infection	Antibody-mediated
HIV	Hypertrophic cardiomyopathy	Cystic fibrosis	Hepatitis B virus	Hemolytic disease of the newborn
Hepatitis B virus	Severe congenital neutropenia			Neonatal alloimmune thrombocytopenia
Herpes simplex virus, type 2	Fragile X syndrome			
Chlamydia trachomatis	Autosomal dominant polycystic kidney disease			
Ureaplasma urealyticum	Atopy: eczema, allergies Autosomal			
Gonorrhea				
Bacteremia, sepsis from intra-uterine insemination procedure				

HIV transmission

Many HIV infections in women were caused by sperm donations from HIV-infected men obtained at a time when a blood test for HIV antibodies was not yet in use and donor criteria did not exclude men who had sex with other men [169–173]. In the landmark report by Stewart et al. [169], four of eight recipients of donated sperm became infected with HIV from cryopreserved semen donated by a paid asymptomatic HIV carrier. One woman had generalized, persistent lymphadenopathy whereas the other three were symptom-free three years later and their three children were healthy and not infected. These early reports led to the practice of requiring that sperm donations be cryopreserved and that the donor is retested three months later to eliminate the possibility of accepting sperm donations during the seronegative period of early infection. Later, when a long immunosilent case of HIV infection was found, retesting after six months instead of three months became a requirement.

Many of these reports showed that not all recipients of sperm from HIV-positive men became infected with HIV. Because of this, when couples want to have children and the father is HIV-positive, many have resorted to in vitro washing and manipulation of the sperm to eliminate or reduce its infectivity. There have been thousands of inseminations of sperm from an HIV-positive partner where the sperm was washed and prepared in vitro before use by intrauterine injection or intracytoplasmic sperm injection. Neither the female gestational partner nor the newborn child became infected [174].

HBV transmission

In the 1980s it was not standard practice by all semen banks and fertility clinics to test donors for HBsAg. Berry et al. [175] reported a case of acute HBV infection in a woman after insemination by a donor who was subsequently found to be a carrier of HBV. HBsAg was demonstrated in his blood and semen donations. Another study detailed an outbreak of HBV infections in recipients of embryos processed at a single laboratory. In an earlier era when pooled human serum was used as an embryo culture medium during in vitro fertilization (IVF) in the laboratory, the sera became contaminated with HBsAg and gametes and embryos became contaminated. The use of these embryos caused HBV infection in many women [176].

Transmitted bacterial infections

Fiumara [177] reported a case of gonorrhea infection due to the use of contaminated fresh sperm for insemination. Two days after donation and use of the fresh sperm in a physician's office, the donor became symptomatic and gonorrhea was diagnosed and treated by another physician. He did not notify the inseminating physician. Two days after insemination, the husband and wife had sex and two to three days after this the husband developed urinary frequency, dysuria, and urethral purulence. This was diagnosed as an acute gonorrhea infection and treated. At the same time, six days after insemination, the asymptomatic wife was seen to have cervical redness and some purulence in the cervical os leading to a diagnosis of gonorrhea. This case demonstrated the importance of testing semen donations for gonorrhea, that donated sperm can transmit infection, and cause secondary spread to others and that donors should report an infection that develops soon after donating. It also demonstrates that these infections can be asymptomatic in women while being acutely symptomatic in men.

It is not unusual to find *Trichomonas vaginalis*, group B streptococcus, and genital mycoplasmas in the semen of healthy men [178]. Hill et al. [179] detected *Ureaplasma urealyticum* in 39% and *Mycoplasma hominis* in 12% of semen samples from infertile men. Transmission of mycoplasma and chlamydia infection through insemination has been documented [180–182].

Genital herpes virus can be isolated from semen in asymptomatic men, and a case of transmission through sperm donation was documented in a seronegative woman by restriction enzyme analysis of the HSV-2 isolates obtained from the donor's semen and from the recipient's cervix [183]. During intrauterine insemination bacteria can be introduced into the fallopian tubes and pelvic peritoneum causing pelvic infection. Sacks et al. [184] documented a case of *Escherichia coli* septicemia related to an intrauterine insemination. The pathogenic bacteria can originate from contaminated sperm or the vagina bacterial flora. Stone et al. [185] reported in one case that the bacteria in the pelvis were the same as found in the sperm before intrauterine insemination. Caprino et al. [186] reported a case of *Enterococcus faecalis* bacteremia after nine attempts at insemination with subsequent infective endocarditis and mitral valve regurgitation in the recipient, needing surgical repair. The same organism was found in vaginal cultures.

Transmission of inherited diseases

Certain forms of hypertrophic cardiomyopathy (HCM) are genetically transmitted and can cause heart failure at a young age and sudden death due to arrhythmia. Maron et al. [187] reported several cases of acquiring inherited cardiomyopathy from a single semen donor. The donor was asymptomatic with no known heart disease and donated sperm over a two-year period resulting in 22 offspring by insemination of unrelated recipients, as well as two offspring he conceived with his wife. The donor was later shown to be affected by a novel beta-myosin heavy-chain mutation that caused HCM, after an offspring was clinically diagnosed with this disease. Of the 24 offspring, nine were genetically affected. One died at age two years owing to progressive heart failure with marked hypertrophy, and two were still alive with extreme left ventricular hypertrophy at age 15 years.

Another genetic disease transmitted by sperm is fragile X syndrome. A girl with the fragile X premutation obtained the premutation allele from donated sperm and has clinical characteristics of fragile X syndrome including emotional problems and neuropsychological difficulties presenting as learning disabilities and is at high risk for ovarian failure [188]. Several cases of severe congenital neutropenia have been confirmed as being inherited from a sperm donor [189, 190]. This mode of transmission was discovered because all of the patients were, by chance, cared for by the same hematologist and that physician pursued the family history which led to the diagnosis.

Transmission of the cystic fibrosis gene has been documented through ova donation and in this case cystic fibrosis was diagnosed soon after birth. The ovum donor was chosen carefully but no history of inherited disease was apparent or disclosed at the time of donation and the result of routine donor testing for the cystic fibrosis gene was also not disclosed to the parents. Two months after their child was born, the ova provider notified the parents that the donor had a positive test for being a cystic fibrosis carrier [191, 192]. In another unfortunate case, semen was obtained from a donor with a family history of kidney disease but this history was not disclosed to the family. At age six the offspring developed autosomal dominant polycystic kidney disease [192, 193].

Diseases from the mother or other gestational carrier

During gestation the fetus is at risk of transplacentally transmitted diseases arising from the mother or surrogate gestational carrier. These may be infectious, malignant, or immune in nature. Immunohematologic disorders such as hemolytic disease of the newborn arise owing to antigenic disparity between the mother and fetus. Accurate diagnosis and treatment can be complicated because parental red cell antigens are unknown when IVF and anonymous gamete donors are used. Conditions suspected to be complication of assisted reproduction should be reported and investigated and corrective actions initiated to prevent the same from occurring in others. If embryos are selected based on histocompatibility, the reduced histocompatibility barrier can create a theoretic risk of transplacental spread of metastatic malignancy to the fetus should the mother develop a malignancy during pregnancy. Malignancies wholly arising in the mother have spread to the fetus. As reviewed by Alexander et al. [194], malignant melanoma is reported most frequently but others including breast and lung carcinoma, leukemia and lymphoma have been involved [195]. Choriocarcinoma, an intrauterine malignancy arising within the placenta, has frequently metastasized to the mother and occasionally to both the mother and the fetus [196].

Hemolytic disease of the newborn and fetus facilitated by donated ova

There have been several reported cases of hemolytic disease of the newborn and fetus due to transplacental transfer of maternal antibodies to fetal ABO and Rh red-cell antigens inherited by the fetus through ova donation [197–201].

These cases were often discovered by the immunohematology reference laboratory when anomalous antigen typings of newborn and parental red cells were found during testing of immune hemolytic anemia in a newborn. Consequently a more detailed investigation into the maternal pregnancy history revealed that assisted reproduction had taken place using donated ova, a fact that the mother's physician had not provided and that the reluctant mother had concealed.

Neonatal alloimmune thrombocytopenia due to use of surrogate carriers or donated ova

Anti-platelet antibodies and neonatal alloimmune thrombocytopenia developed due to exposure in utero to incompatible platelet antigens inherited

CASE STUDY 4.3

Gene mutation transmitted by sperm donation causing heart disease in offspring

A 23-year-old healthy male with no history of heart disease donated sperm 95 times over a two-year period, resulting in 22 known offspring [196]. Several years later after he had two children of his own, he was notified that one of the 22 offspring of his sperm donations developed an inheritable heart disease with a novel beta-myosin heavy-chain mutation and hypertrophic cardiomyopathy (HCM). His paternal grandmother died of a "heart attack" at age 54 and both parents had histories of prosthetic heart valve placement. He was evaluated and found to have left ventricular hypertrophy and fibrosis and a positive test for the gene mutation. A lookback investigation of the offspring was initiated. Of the 22 children from at least 13 families, 16 were tested for the mutation, and eight were positive. One of the two children conceived with his wife was also positive. Of the nine mutation-positive children ranging in ages from two to 16 years and who were mutation-positive, two males were age 15 and had evidence of HCM with severe left ventricular hypertrophy, one with exertional chest pain and fatigue and the other with presyncope and palpitations. One 15-year-old received an implanted cardioverter-defibrillator for prevention of sudden death, a recognized complication of young athletic males with HCM. One young child died at age 2.5 years of intractable heart failure due to obstructive HCM while waiting for a heart transplant. He was tested for the gene mutation retrospectively from a stored blood sample and found positive.

This case demonstrated the following:

1. how undiagnosed genetic carriage of HCM by voluntary sperm donation can result in untreatable heart failure, chronic illness, and risk for sudden death in offspring.
2. the importance of physicians and patients to report unexpected illnesses and complications so implicated donors can be identified and evaluated;
3. the sperm bank medical director's professional responsibility and duty to warn, including the notification and evaluation of all the other sperm recipients.

through donated ova [202]. Four infants were born severely thrombocytopenic owing to platelet-specific human platelet antigen (HPA)-1a antigen incompatibility and transplacental passage of maternal platelet antibody to the fetus during gestation. There were two with intracranial hemorrhage and another with fetal death in utero. Three cases involved incompatible antibody production by HPA-1a-negative surrogate gestational carriers and the fourth was an HPA-1a-negative mother implanted with an embryo involving donor egg and husband sperm.

Importance of risk awareness by the organ, tissue, and cell transplant surgeons and other treating physicians

Transplant transmitted infections, malignancies, and other diseases can become apparent at any time after the transplant or implant procedure. Most arise at characteristic subsequent time periods but there are no careful published observations about latency times to clinical presentation for various allografts. However, some transmitted diseases such as CJD have demonstrated latency periods measurable in decades rather than weeks or months. Thus it is apparent that lifelong vigilance by the treating physician and the patient is required.

Because a recipient will see many physicians during their lifetime after the transplant, the transplant surgeon is just one of many important participants important in the recognition, diagnosis and treatment of allograft transmitted diseases. Recipients and their families must be aware of the possibility, albeit remote, of allograft transmitted disease and the transplant surgeon and treating physicians should have processes in their departments and clinics to detect such possibilities associated with transplant procedures. Recipients and their families must also be aware that the patient has been transplanted with a substance of human origin, which, by its nature, has a very small but distinct risk of disease transmission and that their future treating physicians must be made aware of their history of receiving an allograft with its associated risks and latency periods.

KEY LEARNING POINTS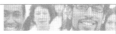

- The risk of transmitting infections and malignances through tissue transplantation is very low but real.
- The risk of transmitting diseases through organ transplantation and HSCs is higher and the spectrum of transmitted diseases is wider.
- Transplant surgeons and other treating physicians and recipients need to be aware of the disease transmission risks from receiving substances of human origin: tissue, cell, blood, and organ allografts.
- Early recognition and reporting can trigger an investigation, improve medical care, and aid the early institution of therapy and prevention of spread of the same disease to others.

References

1. Eastlund T, Strong DM. Infectious disease transmission through tissue transplantation. In: Phillips GO, ed. Advances in Tissue Banking. Vol 7. Singapore: World Scientific Publishing Co, 2003:51–131.
2. Eastlund T. Bacterial infection transmitted by human tissue allograft transplantation. Cell Tissue Bank 2006;7:147–66.
3. Duffy P, Wolf J, Collins G, DeVoe AG, Streeten B, Cowen D. Possible person-to-person transmission of Creutzfeldt–Jakob disease. N Engl J Med 1974;290:692–3.
4. Heckmann JG, Lang CJ, Petruch F, Druschky A, Erb C, Brown P et al. Transmission of Creutzfeldt–Jakob disease via a corneal transplant. J Neurol Neurosurg Psychiatry 1997;63:388–90.
5. Brown P, Brandel JP, Preese M, Sato T. Iatrogenic Creutzfeldt-Jakob disease. The waning of era. Neurology 2006;67:389–93.
6. Centers for Disease Control and Prevention. Update: Creutzfeldt-Jakob Disease Associated with Cadaveric Dura Mater Grafts – Japan, 1978–2008. MMWR 2008;57:1152–54.
7. Hamaguchi T, Noguchi-Shinohara M, Nozaki I, Nakamura Y, Sato TT, Kitamoto T, Mizusawa M, Yamada M. The risk of iatrogenic Creutzfeldt-Jakob disease through medical and surgical procedures. Neuropathology 2009;29:625–631.
8. Tanaka S, Fukushima M. Size of Creutzfeldt-Jakob Disease Epidemic Associated with Cadaveric Dura Transplantation. Neuroepidemiology 2010;34:232–7.
9. Zou S, Dodd RY, Stramer SL, Strong DM; Tissue Safety Study Group. Probability of viremia with HBV, HCV, HIV, and HTLV among tissue donors in the United States. N Engl J Med. 2004;351:751–9.
10. Ison MG, Hager J, Blumberg E, Burdick J, Carney K, Cutler J et al. Donor-derived disease transmission events in the United States: data reviewed by the OPTN/UNOS disease transmission advisory committee. Am J Transplant 2009;9(8):1929–35.
11. Ison MG, Nalesnik MA An update on donor-derived disease transmission in organ transplantation. Am J Transplant 2011;11:1123–30.
12. Srinivasan A, Burton EC, Kuehnert MJ, et al. Rabies in Transplant Recipients Investigation Team: transmission of rabies virus from an organ donor to four transplant recipients. N Engl J Med 2005;352:1103–11.
13. Hellenbrand W, Meyer C, Rasch G, Steffens I, Ammon A. Cases of rabies in Germany following organ transplantation. Euro Surveill 2005;10:2917. http://www.eurosurveillance.org/ViewArticle.aspx?ArticleId=2917
14. Fischer SA, Graham MB, Kuehnert MJ et al. Transmission of lymphocytic choriomeningitis virus by organ transplantation. N Engl J Med 2006;354:2235–49.
15. Kusne S. Regarding unexpected severe and life-threatening donor-transmitted viral infections and use of high-risk behavior donors. Liver Transplant 2008;14:1564–68.
16. Centers for Disease Control. *Balamuthia mandrillaris* transmitted through organ transplantation – Mississippi, 2009. MMWR 2010;59:1165–70.
17. Fehily D, Warwick RM. Safe tissue grafts. Should achieve same standards as for blood transfusion. Brit Med J. 1997;314:1141–2.
18. Tambyah PA, Koay ES, Poon ML, Lin RV, Ong BK. Dengue hemorrhagic fever transmitted by blood transfusion. N Engl J Med 2008; 359:1526–1527.

19. Tan FL, Loh DL, Prabhakaran K, Tambyah PA, Yap HK. Dengue haemorrhagic fever after living donor renal transplantation. Nephrol Dial Transplant 2005;20: 447–8.
20. Rigau-Pérez JG, Vorndam AV, Clark GG. The dengue and dengue hemorrhagic fever epidemic in Puerto Rico, 1994–1995. Am J Trop Med Hyg. 2001;64: 67–74.
21. Marini H, Merle V, Frébourg N, Godier S, Bastit D, Benadiba L, Menguy E, Quesney M, Plissonnier D, Czernichow P. Mycoplasma hominis wound infection after a vascular allograft. J Infect. 2008;57:272–4.
22. Bonatti H, Brandacher G, Margreiter R, Schneeberger S. Infectious complications in three double hand recipients: experience from a single center. Transplant Proc. 2009 41:517–20.
23. Dudderidge TJ, Khalifa M, Jeffery R, Amlot P, Al-Akraa M, Sweny P. Donor-derived human herpes virus 8-related Kaposi's sarcoma in renal allograft ureter. Transpl Infect Dis. 2008;10:221–6.
24. Centers for Disease Control. Notice to readers: Unexplained deaths following knee surgery-Minnesota, November 2001. MMWR 2001;50:1080.
25. Centers for Disease Control. Update: allograft-associated bacterial infections – United States, 2002. MMWR 2002;51:207–10.
26. Kainer MA, Linden JV, Whaley DN, Holmes HT, Jarvis WR, Jernigan DB, Archibald LK. Clostridium infections associated with musculoskeletal-tissue allografts. N Engl J Med 2004;350:2564–71.
27. Lee EH, Ferguson D, Jernigan D, Greenwald M, Cote T, Bos JE, Guarner J, Zaki S, Schuchat A, Beall B, Srinivasan A. Invasive group-A streptococcal infection in an allograft recipient. A case report. J Bone Joint Surg (Am). 2007;89:2044–7.
28. Kuehnert MJ, Clark E, Lockhart SR, Soll DR, Chia J, Jarvis WR. Candida albicans endocarditis associated with a contaminated aortic valve allograft: implications for regulation of allograft processing. Clin Infect Dis 1998;27:688–91.
29. Eastlund T. Unpublished observation.
30. Hou CH, Yang RS, Hou SM. Hospital-based allogenic bone bank: 10-year experience. J Hosp Infect. 2005;59:41–5.
31. Mermel LA, Josephson SL, Giorgio C. A pseudo-epidemic involving bone allografts. Infect Control Hosp Epidemiol 1994;15:757–8.
32. Aho AJ, Hirn M, Aro HT, Heikkila JT, Meurman O. Bone bank service in Finland. Experience of bacteriologic, serologic and clinical results of the Turku Bone Bank 1972–1995. Acta Orthop Scand. 1998;69:559–65.
33. Clarke JA. HIV transmission and skin grafts. Lancet 1987;i:983.
34. Centers for Disease Control and Prevention. Transmission of HIV through bone transplantation: case report and public health recommendations. MMWR 1988; 37:597–9.
35. Simonds RJ, Holmberg SD, Hurwitz RL, Coleman TR, Bottenfield S, Conley LJ, et al. Transmission of human immunodeficiency virus type 1 from a seronegative organ and tissue donor. N Engl J Med 1992;326:726–32.
36. Schratt HE, Regel D, Kiesewetter B, Tscherne H HIV Infektion durch kaltekonservierte Knochentransplantate. (HIV infection caused by cold preserved bone transplants). Unfallchirurg 1996;9:679–84.
37. Li C-M, Ho Y-R, Liu Y-C. Transmission of human immunodeficiency virus through bone transplantation: a case report. J Formos Med Assoc 2001;100:350–1.

38. Hoft RH, Pflugfelder SC, Forster RK, Ullman S, Polack FM, Schiff ER. Clinical evidence for hepatitis B transmission resulting from corneal transplantation. Cornea 1997;16:132–37.

39. Morris A, Strickett MG, Barratt-Boyes BG. Use of aortic valve allografts from hepatitis B surface antigen-positive donors. Ann Thorac Surg 1990;49:802–5.

40. Eggen BM, Nordbø SA. Transmission of HCV by organ transplantation. N Engl J Med 1992;326:411; author reply 412–3.

41. Conrad EU, Gretch DR, Obermeyer KR, et al. Transmission of the hepatitis-C virus by tissue transplantation. J Bone Joint Surg Am 1995;77:214–24.

42. Centers for Disease Control and Prevention. Hepatitis C virus transmission from an antibody-negative organ and tissue donor–United States, 2000–2002. MMWR Morb Mortal Wkly Rep. 2003;52:273–4, 276.

43. Tugwell BD, Patel PR, Williams IT, et al. Transmission of hepatitis C virus to several organ and tissue recipients from an antibody-negative donor. Ann Intern Med 2005;143:648–54.

44. Centers for Disease Control. Potential transmission of viral hepatitis through use of stored blood vessels as conduits in organ transplantation – Pennsylvania, 2009. MMWR 2011;60:172–4.

45. Sanzén L, Carlsson A. Transmission of human T-cell lymphotrophic virus type 1 by a deep-frozen bone allograft. Acta Orthop Scand 1997;68:72–4.

46. Houff SA, Burton RC, Wilson RW, et al. Human-to-human transmission of rabies virus by corneal transplant. N Engl J Med 1979;300:603–4.

47. Javadi MA, Fayaz A, Mirdehghan SA, Ainollahi B. Transmission of rabies by corneal graft. Cornea 1996;15:431–3.

48. Srinivasan A, Burton EC, Kuehnert MJ, et al. Rabies in Transplant Recipients Investigation Team: Transmission of rabies virus from an organ donor to four transplant recipients. N Engl J Med 2005;352:1103–11.

49. Robert PY, Adenis JP, Denis F, Alain S, Ranger-Rogez S. Herpes simplex virus DNA in corneal transplants: prospective study of 38 recipients. J Med Virol. 2003;71:69–74.

50. Cleator GM, Klapper PE, Dennett C, et al. Corneal donor infection by herpes simplex virus: herpes simplex virus DNA in donor corneas. Cornea 1994;13:294–304.

51. Larsen M, Habermann TM, Bishop AT, Shin AY, Spinner RJ. Epstein-Barr virus infection as a complication of transplantation of a nerve allograft from a living related donor. Case report. J Neurosurg 2007;106:924–8.

52. Kealey GP, Aguiar J, Lewis RW 2nd, Rosenquist MD, Strauss RG, Bale JF Jr. Cadaver skin allografts and transmission of human cytomegalovirus to burn patients. J Am Coll Surg 1996;182:201–5.

53. Hannah EL, Belay ED, Gambetti P, et al. Creutzfeldt-Jakob disease after receipt of a previously unimplicated brand of dura mater graft. Neurology 2001;56:1080–83.

54. Tutoplast Dura graft; possible association with Creutzfeldt-Jakob disease. Public Health Agency of Canada: Canadian Adverse Reaction Newsletter. 2004;14(3).

55. 2007 Update CJD in Canada. CJD in a recipient of Tutoplast Dura. Public Health Agency of Canada. September 2003.

56. Maddox RA, Belay ED, Curns AT, Zou WQ, Nowicki S, Lembach RG, Geschwind MD, Haman A, Shinozaki N, Nakamura Y, Borer MJ, Schonberger LB. Creutzfeldt-Jakob disease in recipients of corneal transplants. Cornea 2008;27:851–4.

57. Warwick RM, Armitage WJ, Chandrasekar A, Mallinson G, Poniatowski S, Clarkson A. (2010). A pilot to examine the logistical and feasibility issues in testing deceased tissue donors for vCJD using tonsil as the analyte. Cell Tissue Bank 2012;13:53–61.

58. Keating MR, Guerrero MA, Daly RC, Walker RC, Davies SF. Transmission of invasive aspergillosis from a subclinically infected donor to three different organ transplant recipients. Chest 1996;109:1119–24.

59. James JIP. Tuberculosis transmitted by banked bone. J Bone Joint Surg Br 1953;35B:578.

60. Warwick RM, Magee JG, Leeming JP, et al. Mycobacteria and allograft heart valve banking: an international survey. J Hosp Infect 2008;68:255–61.

61. Khanna SK, Munro JL. Homograft aortic valve replacement: Seven years' experience with antibiotic treated valves. Thorax 1981;36:330–7.

62. Anyanwu CH, Nassau E, Yacoub M. Miliary tuberculosis following homograft valve replacement. Thorax 1976;31:101–6.

63. Hassan SS, Wilhelmus KR, Dahl P, et al. Infectious disease risk factors of corneal graft donors. Arch Ophthalmol 2008;126:235–9.

64. Schotveld JH, Raijmakers AJ, Henry Y, Zaal MJ. Donor-to-host transmitted Candida endophthalmitis after penetrating keratoplasty. Cornea 2005;24:887–9.

65. Chiche L, Lesage A, Duhamel C et al. Posttransplant malaria: first case of transmission of Plasmodium falciparum from a white multiorgan donor to four recipients. Transplantation 2003;75:166–8.

66. Fischer L, Sterneck M, Claus M, et al. Transmission of malaria tertiana by multiorgan donation. Clin Transplant 1999;13:491–5.

67. Einollahi B. *Plasmodium falciparum* infection transmitted by living kidney donation: a case report from Iran. Ann Transplant 2008;13:75–8.

68. O'Donnell J, Goldman JM, Wagner K, Ehinger G, Martin N, Leahy M, Kariuki N, Dokal I, Roberts I. Donor-derived Plasmodium vivax infection following volunteer unrelated bone marrow transplantation. Bone Marrow Transplant 1998;21:313–4.

69. Yango A Jr, Morrissey P, Gohh R, Wahbeh A. Donor-transmitted parvovirus infection in a kidney transplant recipient presenting as pancytopenia and allograft dysfunction. Transpl Infect Dis. 2002;4:163–6.

70. Heegaard ED, Laub Petersen B. Parvovirus B19 transmitted by bone marrow. Br J Haematol 2000;111:659–61.

71. Mayes JT, O'Connor BJ, Avery R, et al: Transmission of *Toxoplasma gondii* infection by liver transplantation. Clin Infect Dis 1995;21:511–5.

72. Barcan LA, Dallurzo ML, Clara LO, et al: Toxoplasma gondii pneumonia in liver transplantation: survival after a severe case of reactivation. Transpl Infect Dis 2002;4:93–6.

73. Anthuber M, Sudhoff F, Schuetz A, Kemkes BM. Donor-transmitted infections in heart transplantation – HIV, CMV, and toxoplasmosis. Transplant Proc. 1991; 23:2634–5.

74. Campbell AL, Goldberg CL, Magid MS, et al: First case of toxoplasmosis following small bowel transplantation and systematic review of tissue-invasive toxoplasmosis following noncardiac solid organ transplantation. Transplantation 2006;81: 408–17.

75. Martín-Dávila P, Fortún J, López-Vélez R, et al. Transmission of tropical and geographically restricted infections during solid-organ transplantation. Clin Microbiol Rev 2008;21:60–96.

76. Kotton CN, Lattes R. Parasitic infections in solid organ transplant recipients. Am J Transplant 2009;9 (Suppl 4):S234–51.

77. Cortes NJ, Afzali B, MacLean D, et al. Transmission of syphilis by solid organ transplantation. Am J Transplant 2006;6:2497–9.

78. Centers for Disease Control. Chagas disease after organ transplantation. Los Angeles, California, 2006. MMWR 2006;55:798–800.

79. Fischer SA, Graham MB, Kuehnert MJ et al. Transmission of lymphocytic choriomeningitis virus by organ transplantation. N Engl J Med 2006;354: 2235–49.

80. Palacios G, Druce J, Du L et al. A new arenavirus in a cluster of fatal transplant-associated diseases. N Engl J Med 2008;358:991–8.

81. Kotsimbos TC, Snell GI, Levvey B, et al. *Chlamydia pneumoniae* serology in donors and recipients and the risk of bronchiolitis obliterans syndrome after lung transplantation. Transplantation 2005;79:269–75.

82. Edathodu J, Alrajhi A, Halim M, Althawadi S. Multi-recipient donor-transmitted tuberculosis. Int J Tuberc Lung Dis 2010;14:1493–5.

83. Centers for Disease Control. Transplantation-transmitted tuberculosis – Oklahoma and Texas, 2007. MMWR 2008;57(13):333–6.

84. Proia L, Miller R. Endemic fungal infections in solid organ transplant recipients. Am J Transplant. 2009;9 (Suppl 4):S199–207.

85. Antinori S, Cascio A, Parravicini C, Bianchi R, Corbellino M. Leishmaniasis among organ transplant recipients. Lancet Infect. Dis 2008;8:191–9.

86. Rodriguez-Hernandez MJ, Ruiz-Perez-Pipaon M, Cañas E, Bernal C, Gavilan F. *Strongyloides stercoralis* hyperinfection transmitted by liver allograft in a transplant recipient. Am J Transplant 2009;9:2637–40.

87. Furlini G, Re MC, Bandini G, Albertazzi L, La Placa M. Antibody response to human immunodeficiency virus after infected bone marrow transplant. Eur J Clin Microbiol Infect Dis 1988;7:664–6.

88. Shuhart MC, Myerson D, Childs BH, et al. Marrow transplantation from hepatitis C virus seropositive donors: transmission rate and clinical course. Blood 1994;84:3229–35.

89. Locasciulli A, Alberti A, Bandini G, et al. Allogeneic bone marrow transplantation from HBsAg+ donors: a multicenter study from the Gruppo Italiano Trapianto di Midollo Osseo (GITMO). Blood 1995;86:3236–40.

90. Tedder RS, Zuckerman MA, Goldstone AH, et al. Hepatitis B transmission from contaminated cryopreservation tank. Lancet 1995;346:137–40.

91. Heegaard ED, Laub Petersen B. Parvovirus B19 transmitted by bone marrow. Br J Haematol 2000;11:659–61.

92. Kikuchi H, Ohtsuka E, Ono K, et al. Allogeneic bone marrow transplantation-related transmission of human T lymphotropic virus type I (HTLV-I). Bone Marrow Transplant 2000;26:1235–7.

93. Kang SJ, Park KH, Jung SI, et al. Scrub typhus induced by peripheral blood stem cell transplantation in the immunocompromised patient: diagnostic usefulness of nested polymerase chain reaction. Transfusion 2010;50:467–70.

94. Ertem M, Kürekçi AE, Aysev D, Unal E, Ikincioğulları A. Brucellosis transmitted by bone marrow transplantation. Bone Marrow Transplant 2000;26: 225–6.

95. Jurges E, Young Y, Eltumi M, et al. Transmission of toxoplasmosis by bone marrow transplant associated with Campath-1G. Bone Marrow Transplant 1992;9:65–6.

96. Dharamasena F, Gordon-Smith E. Transmission of malaria by bone marrow transplantation. Transplantation 1986;42:228.

97. O'Donnell J, Goldman JM, Wagner K et al. Donor-derived *Plasmodium vivax* infection following volunteer unrelated bone marrow transplantation. Bone Marrow Transplant 1998;21:313–4.

98. Stroncek DF, Fautsch SK, Lasky LC, Hurd DD, Ramsay NK, McCullough J. Adverse reactions in patients transfused with cryopreserved marrow. Transfusion 1991;31:521–6.

99. Lazarus HM, Magalhaes-Silverman M, Fox RM, Creger RJ, Jacobs M. Contamination during in vitro processing of bone marrow for transplantation: clinical significance. Bone Marrow Transplant 1991;7:241–6.

100. Webb IJ, Coral FS, Andersen JW, et al. Sources and sequelae of bacterial contamination of hematopoietic stem cell components: implications for the safety of hematotherapy and graft engineering. Transfusion 1996;36:782–8.

101. Gartner HV, Seidl C, Luckenbach C, et al. Genetic analysis of a sarcoma accidentally transplanted from a patient to a surgeon. N Engl J Med 1996;335:1494–7.

102. Gugel EA, Sanders ME. Needle-stick transmission of human colonic adenocarcinoma. N Engl J Med 1986;315:1487.

103. Shaw JM, Bowles J, Koopman P, Wood EC, Trounson AO. Fresh and cryopreserved ovarian tissue samples from donors with lymphoma transmit the cancer to graft recipients. Hum Reprod 1996;11:1668–73.

104. Gandhi MJ, Strong DM. Donor derived malignancy following transplantation: a review. Cell Tissue Bank 2007;8:267–86.

105. Lipshutz GS, Mihara N, Wong R, Wallace WD, Allen-Auerbach M, Dorigo O, Rao PN, Pham PC, Pham PT. Death from metastatic donor-derived ovarian cancer in a male kidney transplant recipient. Am J Transplant 2009;9:1253.

106. Hata B. The development of glioma in the eye to which the cornea of a patient, who suffered from glioma, was transplanted. Acta Soc Ophthalmol Jap 1939;43: 1763–7.

107. McGeorge AJ, Vote BJ, Elliot DA, Polkinghorne PJ. Papillary adenocarcinoma of the iris transmitted by corneal transplantation. Arch Ophthalmol 2002;120: 1379–83.

108. Salame N, Viel JF, Arveux P, Delbosc B. Cancer transmission through corneal transplantation. Cornea 2001;20:680–2.

109. Heyligers IC, Klein-Nulend J. Detection of living cells in non-processed but deep-frozen bone allografts. Cell Tissue Bank 2005;6:25–31.

110. Simpson D, Kakarala G, Hampson K, Steele N, Ashton B. Viable cells survive in fresh frozen human bone allografts. Acta Orthop 2007;78:26–30.

111. Weyts FA, Bos PK, Dinjens WN, et al. Living cells in 1 of 2 frozen femoral heads. Acta Orthop Scand 2003; 74: 661–4.

112. Sugihara S, van Ginkel AD, Jiya TU, van Royen BJ, van Diest PJ, Wuisman PIJM. Histopathology of retrieved allografts of the femoral head. J Bone Joint Surg Br 1999;81B:336–41.

113. Zwitser EW, de Gast A, Basie MJ, van Kemenade FJ, van Royen BJ. B-cell lymphoma in retrieved femoral heads: a long term follow up. BMC Musculoskelet Disord 2009;10:53.

114. Palmer SH, Gibbons CL, Athanasou NA. The pathology of bone allograft. J Bone Joint Surg Br 1999; 81:333–5.

115. Niederwieser D, Appelbaum FR, Gastl G et al. Inadvertent transmission of a donor's acute myeloid leukemia in bone marrow transplantation for chronic myelocytic leukemia. N Engl J Med 1990;322:1794–6.

116. Bakker NA, van Imhoff GW, Verschuuren EA, van Son WJ. Presentation and early detection of post-transplant lymphoproliferative disorder after solid organ transplantation. Transplant Int 2007;20:207–18.

117. Khedmat H, Taheri S. Early onset post transplantation lymphoproliferative disorders: analysis of international data from 5 studies. Ann Transplant 2009; 14:74–7.

118. Rühl H, Bein G, Sachs UJ. Transfusion-associated graft-versus-host disease. Transfus Med Rev 2009;23:62–71.

119. Smith DM, Agura ED, Ausloos K, Ring WS, Domiati-Saad R, Klintmalm GB. Graft-vs-host disease as a complication of lung transplantation. J Heart Lung Transplant 2006;25:1175–7.

120. Weinstein A, Dexter D, KuKuruga DL, Philosophe B, Hess J, Klassen D. Acute graft-versus-host disease in pancreas transplantation: a comparison of two case presentations and a review of the literature. Transplantation. 2006;82:127–31.

121. Siegal D, Xu W, Sutherland R, et al. Graft-versus-host disease following marrow transplantation for aplastic anemia: different impact of two GVHD prevention strategies. Bone Marrow Transplant 2008;42:51–6.

122. Triulzi DJ, Nalesnik MA. Microchimerism, GVHD, and tolerance in solid organ transplantation. Transfusion 2001;41:419–26.

123. Ramsey G. Red cell antibodies arising from solid organ transplants. Transfusion 1991;31:76-86.

124. Ainsworth CD, Crowther MA, Treleaven D, Evanovitch D, Webert KE, Blajchman MA. Severe hemolytic anemia post-renal transplantation produced by donor anti-D passenger lymphocytes: case report and literature review. Transfus Med Rev 2009;23:155–9.

125. Cserti-Gazdewich CM, Waddell TK, Singer LG, et al. Passenger lymphocyte syndrome with or without immune hemolytic anemia in all Rh-positive recipients of lungs from rhesus alloimmunized donors: three new cases and a review of the literature. Transfus Med Rev 2009;23:134–45.

126. Leo A, Mytilineos J, Voso MT, et al. Passenger lymphocyte syndrome with severe hemolytic anemia due to an anti-Jk(a) after allogeneic PBPC transplantation. Transfusion 2000;40:632–6.

127. Hareuveni M, Merchav H, Austerlitz N, Rahimi-Levene N, Ben-Tal O. Donor anti-Jk(a) causing hemolysis in a liver transplant recipient. Transfusion 2002;42: 363–7.

128. West KA, Anderson DR, McAlister VC, et al. Alloimmune thrombocytopenia after organ transplantation. N Engl J Med 1999;341:1504–7.

129. Friend PJ, McCarthy LJ, Filo RS, et al. Transmission of idiopathic (autoimmune) thrombocytopenic purpura by liver transplantation. N Engl J Med 1990;323: 807–11.

130. de la Torre AN, Fisher A, Wilson DJ, Harrison J, Koneru B. A case report of donor to recipient transmission of severe thrombocytopenia purpura. Transplantation 2004;77:1473–4.

131. Taylor RM, Bockenstedt P, Su GL, Marrero JA, Pellitier SM, Fontana RJ. Immune thrombocytopenic purpura following liver transplantation: A case series and review of the literature. Liver Transplant 2006;12:781–91.

132. Minchinton RM, Waters AH, Kendra J, Barrett AJ. Autoimmune thrombocytopenia acquired from an allogeneic bone-marrow graft. Lancet 1982;ii:627–9.

133. Waters AH. Autoimmune thrombocytopenia acquired from allogeneic bone-marrow graft: compensated thrombocytopenia in bone marrow donor and recipient. Lancet 1983;ii:1430.

134. Cahn JY, Chabot J, Esperou H, Flesch M, Plouvier E, Herve P. Autoimmune-like thrombocytopenia after bone marrow transplantation. Blood 1989;74: 2771.

135. Hisatake GM, Chen TW, Renz JF, et al. Acquired hemophilia A after a liver transplantation: a case report. Liver Transplant 2003;9:523–6.

136. Clarkson K, Rosenfeld B, Fair J, Klein A, Bell W. Factor XI deficiency acquired by liver transplantation. Ann Intern Med 1991;115:877–9.

137. Osborn NK, Ustundag Y, Zent CS, Wiesner RH, Rosen CB, Narayanan Menon KV. Factor XII deficiency acquired by orthotopic liver transplantation: case report and review of the literature. Am J Transplant 2006;6:1743–5.

138. Bradley V, Kemp EH, Dickinson C, Key T, Gibbs P, Clatworthy MR. Vitiligo following a 141 combined liver-kidney transplant. Nephrol Dial Transplant 2009;24: 686–8.

139. Phan TG, Strasser SI, Koorey D, et al. Passive transfer of nut allergy after liver transplantation. Arch Intern Med 2003;163:237–9.

140. Legendre C, Caillat-Zucman S, Samuel D, et al. Transfer of symptomatic peanut allergy to the recipient of a combined liver-and-kidney transplant. N Engl J Med 1997;337:822–4.

141. Trotter JF, Everson GT, Bock SA, Wachs M, Bak T, Kam I. Transference of peanut allergy through liver transplantation. Liver Transplant 2001;7:1088–9.

142. Khalid I, Zoratti E, Stagner L, Betensley AD, Nemeh H, Allenspach L. Transfer of peanut allergy from the donor to a lung transplant recipient. J Heart Lung Transplant 2008;27:1162–4.

143. Hourihane JO, Rhodes HL, Jones AM, Veys P, Connett GJ. Resolution of peanut allergy following bone marrow transplantation for primary immunodeficiency. Allergy 2005;60:536–7.

144. Ritchie DS, Sainani A, D'Souza A, Grigg AP. Passive donor-to-recipient transfer of antiphospholipid syndrome following allogeneic stem-cell transplantation. Am J Hematol 2005;79:299–302.

145. Gratwohl A, Corny P, Speck B. 1979. Bone marrow transplantation from a donor with Gaucher's disease. Transplantation 28:266.

146. Bargetzi M, Schönberger A, Tichelli A et al. Celiac disease transmitted by allogeneic non-T cell-depleted bone marrow transplantation. Bone Marrow Transplant 1997;20:607–9.

147. Orlandi E, Varettoni M, Bergamaschi G, Lazzarino M. First episode of acute hemolysis due to G6PD deficiency in a middle-aged woman and transmission of the enzymatic defect through bone marrow transplant. Haematologica 2004;89: ECR04.

148. Lampeter EF, McCann SR, Kolb H. Transfer of diabetes type 1 by bone-marrow transplantation. Lancet 1998;351: 568–9.

149. Smith CI, Aarli JA, Bieberfeld P et al. Myasthenia gravis after bone-marrow transplantation. Evidence for a donor origin. N Engl J Med 1983;309:1565–8.

150. Smith CIE, Aarli JA, Biberfeld P, et al. Myasthenia gravis after bone-marrow transplantation. N Engl J Med 1983;309:1565–8.

151. Thomson JA, Wilson RM, Franklin IM. Transmission of thyrotoxicosis of autoimmune type by sibling allogeneic bone marrow transplant. Eur J Endocrinol 1995;133:564–6.

152. Kishimoto Y, Yamamoto Y, Ito T et al. Transfer of autoimmune thyroiditis and resolution of palmoplantar pustular psoriasis following allogeneic bone marrow transplantation. Bone Marrow Transplant 1997;19:1041–3.

153. Aldouri MA, Ruggier R, Epstein O, Prentice HG. 1990. Adoptive transfer of hyperthyroidism and autoimmune thyroiditis following allogeneic bone marrow transplantation for chronic myeloid leukaemia. British Journal of Haematology 74: 118-119.

154. Heyll A, Meckenstock G, Aul C et al. Possible transmission of sarcoidosis via allogeneic bone marrow transplantation. Bone Marrow Transplant 1994;14: 161–4.

155. Hammarstrom L, Lonnqvist B, Ringden O, Smith CIE, Wiebe T. Transfer of IgA deficiency to a bone-marrow-grafted patient with aplastic anaemia. Lancet 1985;1:778.

156. Rogers RL, Javed TA, Ross RE, Virella G, Stuart RK, Frei-Lahr D. Transfusion management of an IgA deficient patient with anti-IgA and incidental correction of IgA deficiency after allogeneic bone marrow transplantation. Am J Hematol 1998;57:326–30.

157. Kurobane K, Riches PG, Sheldon J, Jones S, Hobbs JR. Incidental correction of severe IgA deficiency by displacement bone marrow transplantation. Bone Marrow Transplant 1991;7:494.

158. Tucker J, Barnetson RSC. Atopy after bone marrow transplantation. Br Med J 1986;290:116–7.

159. Bellou A, Kanny G, Fremont S, Moneret-Vautrin DA. Transfer of atopy following bone marrow transplantation. Ann Allergy Asthma Immunol 1997;78: 513–6.

160. Walker SA, Riches PG, Wild G, et al. Total and allergen-specific IgE in relation to allergic response pattern following bone marrow transplantation. Clin Exp Immunol 1986;66:633–9.

161. Agosti JM, Sprenger JD, Lum LG, et al. Transfer of allergen-specific IgE-mediated hypersensitivity with allogeneic bone marrow transplantation. N Engl J Med 1988;319:1623–8.

162. Hallstrand TS, Sprenger JD, Agosti JM, Longton GM, Witherspoon RP, Henderson WR Jr. Long-term acquisition of allergen-specific IgE and asthma following allogeneic bone marrow transplantation from allergic donors. Blood 2004;104: 3086–90.

163. Wahn V, Laws HJ, Bode CP, Burdach SE. Cure of latex allergy by bone marrow transplantation. Eur J Pediatr 1999;158:88.

164. Koharazawa H, Kanamori H, Takabayashi M, et al. Resolution of atopic dermatitis following allogeneic bone marrow transplantation for chronic myelogenous leukemia. Bone Marrow Transplant 2005;35:1223–4.

165. Khan F, Hallstrand TS, Geddes MN, Henderson WR Jr, Storek J. Is allergic disease curable or transferable with allogeneic hematopoietic cell transplantation? Blood 2009;113:279–90.

166. Krance RA, Spruce WE, Forman SJ, et al. Human cyclic neutropenia transferred by allogeneic bone marrow grafting. Blood 1982;60:1263–6.

167. Ruiz-Argüelles GJ, Reyes-Núñez V, Garcés-Eisele J, et al. Acquired hemoglobin S trait in an adult patient with secondary acute myelogenous leukemia allografted with matched unrelated umbilical cord blood cells using a non-ablative conditioning regimen. Haematology 2005;8:492–6.

168. Alajlan A, Alfadley A, Pedersen KT. 2002. Transfer of vitiligo after allogenic bone marrow transplantation. J Am Acad Dermatol 46: 606–10.

169. Stewart GJ, Tyler JP, Cunningham AL, et al. Transmission of human T-cell lymphotropic virus type III (HTLV-III) by artificial insemination by donor. Lancet 1985;2:581–5.

170. Chiasson MA, Stoneburner RL, Joseph SC. Human immunodeficiency virus transmission through artificial insemination. J Acquir Immune Defic Syndr 1990;3:69–72.

171. Araneta MR, Mascola L, Eller A, O'Neil L, Ginsberg MM, Bursaw M, Marik J, Friedman S, Sims CA, Rekart ML, et al. HIV transmission through donor artificial insemination. JAMA 1995;273:854–8.

172. Wortley PM, Hammett TA, Fleming PL. Donor insemination and human immunodeficiency virus transmission. Obstet Gynecol 1998;91:515–8.

173. Ross RS, Elgas M, Roggendorf M. HIV-1 transmission through artificial insemination. Lancet 1998;351:1812–3.

174. Vitorino RL, Grynstejn BG, de Andrade CA, et al. Systematic review of the effectiveness and safety of assisted reproduction techniques in couples serodiscordant for human immunodeficiency virus where the man is positive. Fertil Steril 2011;13:1684–90.

175. Berry WR, Gottesfeld RL, Alter HJ, Vierling JM. Transmission of hepatitis B virus by artificial insemination. JAMA 1987;257:1079–81.

176. van Os HC, Drogendijk AC, Fetter WP, Heijtink RA, Zeilmaker GH. The influence of contamination of culture medium with hepatitis B virus on the outcome of in vitro fertilization pregnancies. Am J Obstet Gynecol 1991;165:152–9.

177. Fiumara NJ. Transmission of gonorrhoea by artificial insemination. Br J Vener Dis 1972;48:308–9.

178. Peeling R, Embree J. Screening for sexually transmitted infection pathogens in semen samples. Can J Infect Dis Med Microbiol 2005;16:73–6.

179. Hill AC, Tucker MJ, Whittingham DG, Craft I. Mycoplasmas and in vitro fertilization. Fertil Steril 1987;47:652–5.

180. Barwin BN. Transmission of *Ureaplasma urealyticum* by artificial insemination by donor. Fertil Steril 1984;41:326–7.

181. Broder S, Sims C, Rothman C. Frequency of postinsemination infections as reported by donor semen recipients. Fertil Steril 2007;88:711–3.

182. Nagel TC, Tagatz GE, Campbell BF. Transmission of *Chlamydia trachomatis* by artificial insemination. Fertil Steril 1986;46:959–60.

183. Moore DE, Ashley RL, Zarutskie PW, Coombs RW, Soules MR, Corey L. Transmission of genital herpes by donor insemination. JAMA 1989;261:3441–3.

184. Sacks PC, Simon JA. Infectious complications of intrauterine insemination: a case report and literature review. Int J Fertil 1991;36:331–9.

185. Stone SC, de la Maza LM, Peterson EM. Recovery of microorganisms from the pelvic cavity after intracervical or intrauterine artificial insemination. Fertil Steril 1986;46:61–5.

186. Caprino E, Cortesi G, Villani R, Caccia ME, Lauria F, Nava S. Infectious endocarditis following artificial insemination. A clinical case report and review of the literature (Italian). Minerva Cardioangiol 1994;42:493–6.

187. Maron BJ, Lesser JR, Schiller NB, Harris KM, Brown C, Rehm HL. Implications of hypertrophic cardiomyopathy transmitted by sperm donation. JAMA 2009;302:1681–4.

188. Wirojanan J, Angkustsiri K, Tassone F, Gane LW, Hagerman RJ. A girl with fragile X premutation from sperm donation. Am J Med Genet A 2008;146:888–92.

189. Boxer LA. Severe congenital neutropenia: genetics and pathogenesis. Trans Am Clin Climatol Assoc 2006;117:13–31.

190. Boxer LA, Stein S, Buckley D, Bolyard AA, Dale DC. Strong evidence for autosomal dominant inheritance of severe congenital neutropenia associated with ELA2 mutations. J Pediatr 2006;148:633–6.

191. Paretta v Medical Offices for Human Reproduction, 760 NYS 2d 639 (2003). Recorded in Paretta v. Medical Offices for Human Reproduction d/b/a Center for Human Reproduction, et al., 2003 N.Y.

192. Daar JF, Brzyski RG. Genetic screening of sperm and oocyte donors: ethical and policy implications (editorial). JAMA 2009;302:1702–4.

193. Bauman JH. Discovering Donors: Legal Rights to Access Information About Anonymous Sperm Donors Given to Children of Artificial Insemination in Johnson v. Superior Court of Los Angeles County. Golden Gate University Law Review. 2001;31:193–218. http://digitalcommons.law.ggu.edu/ggulrev/vol31/iss2/4 (Accessed March 6, 2011).

194. Alexander A, Samlowski WE, Grossman D, et al. Metastatic melanoma in pregnancy: risk of transplacental metastases in the infant. J Clin Oncol 2003;21:2179–86.

195. Liu J, Guo L. Intraplacental choriocarcinoma in a term placenta with both maternal and infantile metastases: a case report and review of the literature. Gynecol Oncol 2006;103:1147–51.

196. McNally OM, Tran M, Fortune D, Quinn MA. Successful treatment of mother and baby with metastatic choriocarcinoma. Int J Gynecol Cancer 2002;12:394–8.

197. Mitchell S, James A. Severe hemolytic disease from rhesus anti-C antibodies in a surrogate pregnancy after oocyte donation. A case report. J Reprod Med 1999;44:388–90.

198. Freund GG, Finke C, Kirkley SA. Anomalous ABO inheritance explained by ovum transplantation. Transfusion 1995;35:61–2.

199. Patel RK, Nicolaides K, Mijovic A. Severe hemolytic disease of the fetus following in vitro fertilization with anonymously donated oocytes. Transfusion 2003;43:119–20.

200. Mair DC, Scofield TL HDN in a mother undergoing in vitro fertilization with donor ova. Transfusion 2003;43:288–9.
201. Zuppa AA, Cardiello V, Lai M, Cataldi L, D'Andrea V, Romagnoli C. ABO hemolytic disease of the fetus and newborn: an iatrogenic complication of heterologous assisted reproductive technology-induced pregnancy. Transfusion 2010;50: 2102–4.
202. Curtis BR, Bussel JB, Manco-Johnson MJ, Aster RH, McFarland JG. Fetal and neonatal alloimmune thrombocytopenia in pregnancies involving in vitro fertilization: A report of four cases. Am J Obstet Gynecol 2005;192:543–7.

5   Use of Vascular Allografts

P. Dominic F. Dodd[1] and Jeffery Dattilo[2]

[1]Sheffield Vascular Institute, Sheffield, UK
[2]Vanderbilt University Medical Center, Nashville, TN, USA

Introduction

The development of vascular allografts has closely followed the development of vascular surgery itself. Since the start of the twentieth century, the search for the optimal vascular graft has seen the use of allografts rise and fall. Although the commonest cause of arterial occlusive disease is atherosclerosis, blood vessels are also affected by aneurysmal disease, infection, trauma, iatrogenic injury, and involvement in malignancy affecting adjacent tissues. Before the twentieth century, vascular treatment was limited to cauterization of bleeding or ligation of aneurysmal arteries [1]. The introduction of general anesthesia made prolonged and complex surgery feasible and opened the way for a massive surge in the diversity and complexity of surgical interventions possible.

Surgeons are sometimes required to repair or replace a major blood vessel and to achieve this will use an autograft or allograft vascular conduit. The development of vascular allograft use reflects the need to find suitable alternatives to a patient's own vessels. A significant contribution to this development involved pioneering work using allografts and xenografts [2] demonstrating the feasibility of vascular reconstruction, most notably by Alexis Carrel and Claude Guthrie at the beginning of the twentieth century [3, 4].

This chapter discusses the role of allografts in vascular reconstruction over the last century and the current and likely future application of these tissues. Currently, vascular allografts are used to replace or repair large and

Tissue and Cell Clinical Use: An Essential Guide, First Edition. Edited by Ruth M. Warwick and Scott A. Brubaker.
© 2012 Blackwell Publishing Ltd. Published 2012 by Blackwell Publishing Ltd.

medium-sized arteries or veins. They are used in cardiovascular, reconstructive, and solid-organ transplantation surgery.

The human body's largest vessels are the aorta and vena cava. The aorta arises from the left ventricle of the heart and gives rise to branches leading to the whole of the systemic circulation. The aorta typically has a diameter of 25–30 mm in the thorax and gradually reduces in diameter to 12–18 mm where it terminates in the abdomen in the iliac arteries, which are 6–9 mm in diameter. The major cerebral, upper limb, and splanchnic vessels are typically 5–8 mm in diameter, whereas the medium-sized vessels of the thigh, the deep and superficial femoral arteries, are also 5–8 mm in diameter. Corresponding veins are typically 10–20% larger. The major arteries deliver oxygenated blood at flow rates of up to 20 liters per minute at a pressure of up to 200 mmHg. Arterial replacement conduits need, therefore, to be mechanically resilient, but also must be non-thrombogenic and biocompatible.

The disease process most commonly affecting arteries in the population of the developed world is atherosclerosis. This is a progressive condition starting in late teens with the formation of fatty streaks, advancing with time to form cholesterol-laden plaques that can ultimately lead to arterial occlusion, amputation, and/or end-organ damage. The specialty of vascular surgery has evolved to diagnose and manage the effects of these conditions.

Vascular surgery

The use of allografts in vascular surgery spans the past 100 years. Throughout this time, enthusiasm for allografts has waxed and waned as developments in allograft processing have competed with the availability of improved prosthetic vascular grafts. Most recently, development of endovascular stent-grafts has reduced reliance on conventional grafts to replace diseased arteries and it is likely that this trend in minimization will continue in the future, pending long-term clinical results.

Vascular grafts are most often used as conduits to repair or replace diseased arteries or veins. In essence, the conduit should allow the passage of blood without restriction to flow or activation of the coagulation, inflammation or immune pathways. At the time of writing there is still a lack of this type of graft. Such is the burden of atherosclerosis in the developed world that most activity in vascular biology research has focused on understanding the processes responsible for this condition. There has been a relative paucity of research into the development of the ideal conduit. Tissue-engineering solutions are currently the most attractive but complex remedies to provide durable biocompatible grafts. Conventional options meanwhile are relied upon with only modest success for long-term outcomes.

Table 5.1 Features of an ideal vascular conduit

Vascular conduit biocompatibility
Tensile strength
Resistance to suture pullout (see Plate 5.1)
High radial burst pressure
Compliance
Durability
Inert
Non-toxic
Immunologically compatible
Non-thrombogenicity
Resistance to surgical-site infection
Free from infection transmission hazard
Affordability
Availability

Features of the optimal vascular graft

If one considers the features of an ideal vascular conduit an allograft should demonstrate the properties of biocompatibility as shown in Table 5.1. Indeed much of the reluctance amongst clinicians to embrace the use of allografts stems from limitations of some of these attributes compared with prosthetic or autologous alternatives.

History of allograft use

The earliest reported use of vascular allografts dates from the beginning of the twentieth century. Pioneers in this field were keen to repair arteries using preserved conduits. Initial allograft experiments were conducted by Hopfner in 1903 using a canine model [2]. In his experiments the femoral artery of one animal was transplanted into the carotid position in another. These were fresh allografts, no attempt at preservation was made in these experiments. Around the same time, Alexis Carrel and Claude Guthrie, arguably the founders of modern vascular surgery, reported their experiments in a variety of animal models. In their experiments the vessels were stored in Locke's solution at 0–1°C for periods up to 24 days [3, 4]. Graft patency was demonstrated many months later by these investigators. Carrel went on to attempt freezing, drying and other preservation methods [5]; however, these experiments were unsuccessful as the implanted vessels rapidly thrombosed [6].

Surprisingly, interest in vascular allografts waned over the next four decades. It was not until 1951 that a landmark in vascular surgery was reached when Charles Dubost performed the first repair of an abdominal aortic aneurysm in Paris, using a preserved deceased donor allograft with a successful outcome at five months postoperatively [7].

Such was the pace of development in the early post-war period that within three years of this landmark, Blakemore and Voorhees had successfully repaired an aortic aneurysm using a novel prosthetic graft made from Vinyon-N cloth [8].

Early preservation methods

By the mid-1950s, retrieval and processing protocols were adopted that allowed surgeons ready access to allografts. Numerous positive reports followed; perhaps the most prolific of these were the publications from Michael DeBakey and colleagues in Houston [9, 10]. During this time surgeons made a choice between fresh or preserved vessels. Fresh allografts were typically held in cool storage at 4°C for up to 6 weeks in physiological solutions such as Ringer's lactate with 10% homologous serum and antimicrobial agents [11]. It was recognized that fresh allografts could not be kept indefinitely and long-term storage methods were advocated which included freeze-drying and lyophilization, and early attempts at cryopreservation [12, 13]. Sterilization of the grafts was attempted by a variety of methods which included formalin fixation, immersion in antiseptics and both ethylene oxide permeation and irradiation [14, 15]. With regard to "cryopreservation" techniques, these were crude with little understanding of cryobiology. The rate at which both cooling and especially re-warming were performed was generally uncontrolled. It was not until recognition of the importance of cryoprotectants and the vitreous, glass-transition phase that controlled-rate freezing and re-warming were introduced.

Cryoprotectant solutions such as dimethylsulfoxide (DMSO) were introduced in the 1970s in an attempt to preserve cellular integrity and function [16]. This remains the standard today, although it is not clear that cell function is a prerequisite for the allograft to work as a successful conduit (see Plate 5.2). Indeed, in the earliest xenograft experiments by Carrel, he noted that although the allograft became hyalinized it continued to function for many months [6].

Decline in the 1960s and 1970s owing to late aneurysmal formation and degradation

In common with many innovations in medicine, a period of enthusiasm and high uptake was followed by a period of conservatism and retrenchment as the late complications of these early cryopreserved and fresh allografts became apparent. By 1960 arterial allograft use in vascular surgery had been almost completely replaced by prosthetic grafts. In 1970 Knox and Miller wrote, "The era of the use of arterial homografts is now long passed" (Knox 1970) [17], although they noted in their long-term follow up that only a few of their patients developed complications related to the allograft.

Resurgence in the 1990s

At the beginning of the 1990s there was a resurgence of interest in vascular allografts in the face of increasingly troublesome poly-resistant bacterial strains such as methicillin-resistant *Staphylococcus aureus* [18]. Initially, fresh arterial allografts were favored but as a new understanding of cryobiology-developed cyropreserved allografts regained a place in vascular surgeons' armamentarium.

Despite the improved understanding of the cryopreservation process, there remained reluctance among some surgical communities to adopt allo-grafts as a treatment option for arterial infection. Perhaps the reassuring reports for in situ prosthetic graft reconstruction have dissuaded some surgeons from trialing allografts in their patients.

Cryopreserved allograft vessels today

Techniques used today in the provision of suitable cryopreserved allograft vessels are detailed. Donor selection, procurement, processing, preservation, storage, and distribution protocols have been developed to optimize tissue quality; however, many donated allogeneic vessels, primarily iliac arteries or veins, are not cryopreserved but instead are retained and stored at 4°C by organ-retrieval teams to be used in organ transplant procedures. Alter-natively, cryopreserved allograft vessels can be inventoried and be readily available for use. After thawing, they handle extremely well in the operating room; their characteristics are indistinguishable from healthy native arteries (Plate 5.1). Caution is nevertheless required to avoid placing tension on the anastomosis and rigorous efforts to debride the surgical field are required to prevent re-infection of the host vessels, which tend to be more susceptible to enzymatic digestion caused by bacterial infection. Accompanying the use of allograft vessels, long-term antimicrobial therapy including anti-fungal agents is considered by most surgeons to be mandatory.

Indications for use/clinical situations

Vascular allografts are currently used in a variety of clinical situations. In principle, allografts are used when autologous tissues are unavailable or unsuitable and prosthetic materials are either not available or considered to present too great a risk of failure due to thrombosis or infection.

Vascular infection

Primary arterial infection can arise in the major arteries from a wide variety of sources. Certain bacteria, such as *Salmonella* species, appear to have a predilection for the aorta. Acute bacterial infection often presents with malaise and pain originating from the infected vessel. Septic emboli or distal ischemia can occur, but arterial disruption and hemorrhage is the most feared complication. Early intervention to prevent this complication is mandated and often life-saving.

Arterial Infection

The variety of organisms reported to cause arterial of vascular graft infection is immensely wide-ranging; however, a few species predominate. In primary arterial infection, *Salmonella* species and *Staphylococcus* species are commonest. In graft infection, *Staphylococcus* species, coliforms, and others are found. In many cases no infective agent can be positively identified, although recently polymerase chain reaction techniques have been used to identify a culprit organism, when culture methods have been negative [19].

Imaging modalities

Contrast-enhanced computed tomography (CT) imaging is the most useful investigation in establishing the extent of acute arterial infections and assists with planning intervention. Low-grade chronic sepsis is sometimes difficult to confirm and 18-fluoro-2-deoxy-glucose positron emission tomography (18 FDG PET) combined with CT has been found to be very useful in detecting persistent arterial infections [20].

With graft infections, often indolent use of indium-111-labeled leukocyte imaging has been used in certain vascular units. This diagnostic modality, because of its high false-negative rate, should be used in combination with conventional CT imaging.

Prosthetic graft infection

Prosthetic graft infection occurs in approximately 1% of patients undergoing aortic aneurysm surgery. Risk factors for infection include emergency surgery for ruptured aneurysm, pre-existing sepsis, and diabetes. In 2003, Chang et al. determined that operative duration was the most important factor in the development of postoperative infection in their series of lower extremity bypass procedures [21]. They did not find an association with other presumed risk factors such as increasing age, presence of diabetes, obesity, extremity ulceration, or gangrene.

The infection may become apparent in the immediate postoperative period but can be delayed presenting years or even decades later. The mechanism of infection is likely to be due to a breach in the aseptic protocol in the early phase, owing to hematogenous seeding of the prosthetic graft later or contact with viscera and subsequent erosion of visceral continuity. Treatment options will depend on the clinical status and pre-morbid condition of the patient, and the severity of the arterial infection at presentation. Infected peripheral grafts are usually resected and the resultant distal tissue ischemia managed with re-grafting with autologous tissue if available, cryopreserved allografts, endovascular intervention, or amputation. The treatment of aortic graft infection is a formidable surgical challenge and requires careful planning and considerable intensive-care support. Most surgeons would currently opt for autologous tissue reconstruction, harvesting the superficial femoral vein and constructing a vessel conduit to bridge the vascular defect. When autologous tissue is not available, opinion diverges on the next best option. Some surgeons achieve good results with rifampicin-bonded prosthetic grafts whereas others prefer cryopreserved allografts. Yet others elect for extra-anatomic routing of prosthetic grafts and resection of infected graft and ligation of in-line arterial flow. A lack of ready availability has prevented surgeons in many regions of the world from developing familiarity with allografts, which might explain why some territories, for example Benelux, use large numbers of these grafts whereas in the UK allograft use remains in single figures each year.

In a recent review of prosthetic aortic graft infection, O'Connor and colleagues concluded that autologous vein, cryopreserved allograft or rifampicin-bonded prosthetic grafts fared comparably, whereas extra-anatomic, axillo-femoral, and prosthetic grafting had inferior outcomes [22]. Their review noted that autologous vein and cryopreserved allografts were similarly resistant to re-infection, whereas rifampicin-bonded prosthetic grafts were associated with fewer lower limb amputations and graft failures. Late mortality was equivalent for autologous vein and cryopreserved allografts. When each option is available, the choice of conduit can be difficult.

Previous experience with each conduit is often a determinant. However, more virulent infections such as with methicillin-resistant *Staphylococcus aureus* or *Escherichia coli* might lead one to select a biological graft. In a stable patient, with good quality superficial femoral vein, this is likely to be the best option. In patients who are unstable, or in whom the veins are compromised, cryopreserved allografts appear to be the viable solution. Finally, there is still use in these often very ill patients for a staged approach using extra-anatomic bypass and aortic or aortic graft resection.

It is reassuring that, in this meta-analysis, cryopreserved allografts were found to be associated with low complication and late mortality rates [22].

Solid-organ transplantation

The use of vascular allografts is inherent in solid-organ transplantation, as all solid organs require anastomosis to the recipient's arterial and venous circulation. In deceased donor organ transplantation, the donor organ will normally be procured with adequate donor vessel length to allow primary anastomosis with the recipient's vessels. However, in live-donor organ transplantation, the length of vessels that can be harvested without compromising the donor is more limited and an interposition vascular allo-graft is commonly used to connect the donor organ to the recipient's circulation.

The limited supply of deceased donor organs has led to considerable development of live-donor procedures to provide lung, kidney, and partial-liver organ grafts. In these cases the graft cannot be retrieved with a vascular pedicle comparable to the deceased donor organ and an interposition conduit is required. Concerns about immunogenicity are largely irrelevant as recipient immunosuppression is required when using solid organ grafts. Fresh, hypothermic vascular allografts are most commonly used by transplant surgeons to facilitate organ implantation. Although cryopreserved allografts have gained a foothold in this situation, the ease of availability of fresh deceased donor tissue limits the applicability of cryopreserved tissues. In liver transplantation, cryopreserved saphenous and iliac vein have been reported to have an unacceptably high late-failure rate due to thrombosis when used for portal vein reconstruction [23].

Tumour resection/reconstruction

Vascular involvement and perivascular invasion is a common feature of many advanced malignant and benign tumors. Arterial, and less commonly venous, reconstruction is therefore indicated to facilitate full resection of these lesions. In patients in whom there is no established focus of infection or sepsis, prosthetic graft materials can be safely used. However, in the rare instance of fungating tumors, involving the femoral vessels for example, an allograft can be used as the risk of prosthetic graft infection would be prohibitive.

Tracheal reconstruction

Recently, interest in the use of arterial allografts for use in tracheal and carinal trachea reconstruction has led to animal experimentation and small clinical series. In 1999 Carbognani et al. reported the outcome of tracheal replacement with cryopreserved aortic allografts in a canine model [24]. Chahine et al. first reported the use of an aortic allograft to reconstruct the trachea in three pediatric patients [25]. Recently this concept has been extended experimentally to bronchial reconstruction to facilitate sleeve lobectomy and avoid the need for pneumonectomy with promising results [26].

Pediatric congenital cardiac disease

In infants with hypoplastic left heart syndrome, cryopreserved femoral and saphenous vein allografts have been explored for neoaortic reconstruction in the Norwood stage I operation. In this condition the left heart is hypoplastic, the pulmonary artery has to be reconstructed, and cryopreserved vein containing a venous valve, or a monocusp with pulmonary artery fashioned from an allograft pulmonary valve/outflow tract, can be a promising conduit when constructs from autologous tissues are inadequate [27]. Reports of the outcome of this procedure are sparse in the literature. There is a concern that using allograft tissue could cause immune sensitization, which might make subsequent cardiac transplantation less favorable.

Use in dialysis access

The demographics of patients on dialysis in the USA have shifted to older and sicker patients. The use of primary arterial–venous fistula with the obligatory maturation period is preferred; however, when it becomes necessary to use prosthetic grafts for access there is a significant risk of infection. Use of cryopreserved arterial conduits has been used with varying success when alternative sites are unavailable [28, 29].

Evidence for use

Although cryopreserved allografts have been widely used over the past two decades, there is a paucity of literature about the outcome of these procedures. This probably reflects the fact that most cases are sporadic and individual surgeons have relatively small case series that go unreported.

Systematic follow-up of patients has been haphazard and incomplete in all but a few centers. In Europe the largest reported series show promising outcomes [30]. Perhaps the sporadic use of these grafts can be best explained by the relative ease of acquiring these grafts rather than harvesting autologous tissue or arduous extra-anatomic reconstructions. Additionally the supple handling of these grafts can be attractive compared with splicing together autologous tissues from the same patient when faced with excising the infected graft.

Clinical trials

As has been described already in this chapter, the development of cryopreserved vascular allografts was largely in the era when controlled clinical trials were rare. The sporadic nature of vascular infections means that few groups of surgeons accumulate large series of cases. There are a few notable exceptions; these are reviewed below.

Aortic replacement

The largest reported series of arterial allografts reported in the modern literature comes from Edouard Kieffer's group in Paris, France [30]. Between 1988 and 2002, 179 patients with prosthetic aortic graft infection received arterial allografts in their institution. Before 1996, fresh allografts were used to treat 111 patients, thereafter cryopreserved allografts were used in the remaining 68 patients. The early postoperative mortality was 20% overall. There was a striking reduction in the rate of graft-related complications once cryopreserved allografts were used. In the fresh allograft series there were four (2.2%) deaths due to rupture, which included three recurrent aorto-enteric fistulas. Most deaths were due to overwhelming sepsis or myocardial infarction.

In 2002, Paul Vogt and colleagues reported their experience with the use of arterial allografts and detailed the considerations at operation that they believed were causal in graft failure and tips to avoid them [31]. Modes of graft failure are summarized in Table 5.2.

In their series of 49 patients, 21 presented with a mycotic aneurysm and 28 with a prosthetic graft infection in the thoracic or abdominal aorta. Cryopreserved allografts were used in each case. In eight patients there were technical problems with the allograft. These were mostly in their early experience; seven occurred in their first 10 patients. They encountered only one technical problem in their remaining 39 cases. They reviewed each procedure and identified the modifications they made to the procedure which they felt accounted for their improved outcomes. In essence these were to

Table 5.2 Modes of arterial allograft failure

Immediate
Graft disruption
Suture pull-out
Side-branch blow-out

Early
Infective
Mycotic aneurysm formation
Persistent infective arteritis
Thrombosis

Delayed
Graft thrombosis
Aneurysmal degeneration

avoid any tension on the anastomotic suture line, securely transfixing any side branches, thorough debridement of the tissue bed in to which the allograft was placed, and adequate postoperative drainage to minimize the re-emergence of surgical-site sepsis. The suture lines were further reinforced with allograft strips as buttress material and gentamicin-containing fibrin glue. Overall they achieved a 30-day mortality rate of 6%, falling to 2.6% in the last 39 patients.

The most recent publication on the use of these grafts is from Teebken's group in Hannover, Germany [32]. They reviewed the outcomes of an eight-year experience using cryopreserved arterial allografts for in situ reconstruction of the aorta in 57 patients. Most (39/57; 55%) of their patients presented with prosthetic graft infection. They achieved a 30-day mortality rate of 9% and three-year survival rate of 81%. Five patients (9%) required re-operation, four of which were for graft related complications, three bleeding, and one aneurysmal degeneration. In each case the patient was found to be free from infection at re-operation.

Peripheral graft infection

Guy Leseche and colleagues in Clichy, France, reported their experience in 2005 in treating seventeen patients with major peripheral arterial graft infection in whom graft excision was required and who would probably have suffered limb loss if not offered reconstruction [33]. In their series they used deceased donor allografts stored at −80°C. There were no peri-operative deaths; however, two allografts disrupted at the proximal anastomosis necessitating re-operation. In one case the allograft was salvaged, in the other a prosthetic implant was used. In late follow-up, four allografts thrombosed and one graft became aneurysmal. There was no persistent infection in their patients. At 18 months primary and secondary allograft patency was 68% and 86%. Overall limb salvage was 82% at five years.

Cryopreserved aortic allograft registry

In the USA, the results of the Cryopreserved Aortic Allograft Registry were reported in 2002 [34]. This multi-centre registry received data from 31 centres on fifty-six patients receiving in situ aortic replacement. Thirty-day mortality was 13% of which one patient died of immediate graft rupture, whereas a further two suffered graft-related mortality due to persistent inf-arction and hemorrhage. Graft related morbidity was encountered in 14/55 patients (25%) in the follow-up period. The opinion of the authors of this report was that the rate of complications did not justify the use of cryopre-served allografts in preference to other established techniques. Data pub-lished from the Italian Homograft registry reveal similar results to the single centre series from elsewhere in Europe, with promising results reported in 44 patients having prosthetic graft infections [35].

It is lamentable that no further reports from these registries have been published since to indicate the expansion of these programs and the longer-term outcome from these complex procedures.

Contemporary perspective

Current opinion, especially in the USA, is largely in favor of in situ recon-struction with autologous femoral veins, followed by rifampicin-soaked prosthetic grafts, with cryopreserved allografts used less frequently [36–41]. However, the neo-aorto iliac system (NAIS) is most often performed in larger centers that tend to be the referral base for these complicated cases. Private practice vascular surgeons are less likely to take on this technical tour de force and often seek transfer of such patients to larger centers. Endovascular intervention has also gained ground, with surgeons initially adopting this as a temporizing measure finding that it can be used as a definitive therapy in low-grade infections [42, 43].

These findings are echoed by Nevelsteen et al. who reported their experi-ence with cryopreserved allografts in 30 patients between 1990 and 1997 [44]. Early allograft rupture occurred in two patients. Six patients (27%) developed late allograft related complications.

Recently there has been interest in silver-ion coated prosthetic grafts that will resist development of a bacterial biofilm [45]. Early experience with these grafts seems comparable with rifampicin-bonded prosthetic grafts although no randomized-controlled trial data have been published so far [46].

The consensus amongst the authors reporting their experience is that adequate surgical debridement of the infected artery and adjacent tissue bed, followed by healthy tissue cover with omentum or muscle flap and tube drainage is mandatory. Prolonged antibiotic treatment for infective agents, including anti-fungal therapy, is also recommended.

Evidence for saphenous vein grafts

Cryopreserved greater saphenous vein has been used for peripheral arterial reconstruction for about two decades. Carpenter and Tomaszewski reported a prospective trial in which 40 patients underwent cryopreserved venous allograft bypass [47, 48]. Biopsies were taken from allografts requiring explantation for graft failure. During the follow-up period 22 allografts were removed, of which 19 were suitable for immunohistochemical study. One-third of the allografts had moderate or severe transmural infiltrates, predominantly comprising activated T-lymphocytes, whereas macrophages, B cells, and natural killer cells were infrequently identified. They concluded that allografts are susceptible to cell-mediated inflammation, indicating chronic rejection. However, they also noted that most grafts failed for technical reasons without evidence of rejection. Furthermore they also reported that low-dose azathioprine had no effect on the immune response to the allografts or failure rate overall. Additionally, Posner et al. demonstrated that with more aggressive immunosuppression and the combination with warfarin that patency rates could be improved. However, the grafts themselves failed (rupture, blowout) in greater frequency the longer the grafts survived [49].

The most recent report in the literature, from Zehr et al., reports a series of 54 cases over a six-year period [50]. Overall limb salvage and graft patency rates were similar to other bypass conduits, 67% and 63% respectively at 12 months. Of particular interest is their finding that ABO blood-group-compatible allografts displayed significantly superior limb salvage rates than mismatched grafts, 30/34 versus 6/20. It should be pointed out that perhaps allograft can be used if autologous tissue is limited and the goal of therapy is short-term limb salvage. An ideal example would be under the clinical scenario where the surgeon is attempting to heal a wound and an open conduit for 12–18 months is an acceptable outcome.

Immunology

Although the immunological response to solid organ allografts has been well characterized since the introduction of renal transplantation in the 1950s, the immunological response to vascular allografts has been less intensively studied. For non-autologous grafts to be accepted by the host, either immunosuppression or immunotolerance of the host, or non-antigenicity of the graft must be achieved. At present ABO group matching is not considered routine and HLA-typing is not undertaken [51].

Xenografts

The host response to xenotransplantation leads to hyperacute rejection in solid organ transplantation and is largely mediated by the anti-Gal antibody, which is almost ubiquitous in non-primate mammals and even in New World monkeys [52]. It is widely expressed as a calcium-bound membrane protein and therefore strategies to mask its presence have been unsuccessful. Anti-Gal knockout transgenic animals have been bred but the presentation of other xenotypic antigens still leads to rejection. Therefore, vascular xenografts are limited to glutaraldehyde cross-linked heart valves in the cardiovascular setting.

Fate of cryopreserved allografts

Although cryopreservation was originally developed to maximize cellular viability in the allograft, there is a marked attenuation in cell function after the cryopreservation process. Indeed it now appears that graft cell viability is not required for the role of arterial conduit replacement and it seems likely that it is the allogeneic cell antigens that drive the host immune response to reject the graft over time.

Cryopreservation appears to mediate the host response to implanted vascular allografts, but does not abolish it completely. This host-reaction appears to be more intense in infants and children indicating that immunotolerance might be acquired over a person's lifetime. In the arterial system, chronic cell-mediated rejection leads to calcification and aneurysmal degradation of some allografts [53]. Ectopic calcification is a phenomenon not confined to the arterial tree but is found in many tissues.

The process by which arteries become aneurysmal is not fully elucidated but imbalance in the expression of matrix metalloproteinases is considered by many to be the mechanism underlying vessel aneurysm. Cell-matrix proteins are degraded and collagen turnover increased leading to relative weakening of the vessel wall and subsequent dilatation. This process is probably replicated in the allograft vessel wall with a cell-mediated immune response driving a chronic inflammatory process.

One of the major concerns shared by many vascular surgeons is the possibility of late aneurysmal degeneration necessitating life-long follow-up and potential major revision surgery. Overcoming this problem would go a long way to increasing the acceptability of these grafts in the future.

The global picture

Outside of North America and continental Europe the uptake of vascular allografts is extremely sporadic. There is no significant allograft use in the UK, Australasia, or the developing regions of southern Asia and Africa. A few reports from Russia and South America can be found in the literature but these are limited to single case-reports and small series. There has been very little published activity in Japan, China, Singapore, or Taiwan.

Future of allograft use

Decellularization

One of the main reasons surgeons are reluctant to use cryopreserved allografts stems from the experience of the mid-twentieth century when aneurysmal degradation of cryopreserved allografts was widely reported [54, 55]. This was increasingly recognized in the 1960s and 1970s in patient who had received grafts up to a decade earlier.

The consequence of late aneurysmal degradation is potentially fatal as the first presentation is often with catastrophic internal hemorrhage.

Although these experiences date back to an era in which cryopreservation methods differed significantly from current practice, the wariness among the vascular surgical community has persisted. Late aneurysmal degradation cannot be entirely explained by cryopreservation technique but is more likely to represent a chronic cell-mediated inflammatory immune reaction to the allograft. So far, very little work has been done with vascular allografts but there have been several important publications relating to the late degradation of allograft heart valves. Processing techniques in which the structural integrity of the valves is maintained but the cellular component is removed have demonstrated remarkable amelioration of the development of calcific degeneration in valve cusps [56].

Tissue engineering

Although satisfactory conduits have been developed to replace the larger arteries, the ideal small-caliber arterial graft has yet to be found. At the moment autologous superficial veins remain the best option for peripheral arterial bypass, but these are not always available, and even then do not offer especially rewarding long-term results. The current prosthetic alternatives fare less well, so the search for a better solution continues. Conduits of 2–4 mm diameter, equivalent to the native coronary and leg arteries, would expand the possibilities of vascular reconstruction immeasurably.

At the core of this problem is the failure of prosthetic grafts to heal. Unlike animal models, cellular pannus ingrowth is restricted to the first few millimeters in prosthetic grafts implanted in humans. For a small-caliber graft to function well, it requires a normally functioning endothelial lining. Most small-caliber grafts have been plagued by unacceptably high-rates of early thrombosis and it is this lack of endothelial function that is seen by many as the cause. Researchers in tissue engineering have spent the past two decades attempting to establish a healthy endothelium on a variety of artificial scaffolds. Interestingly, decellularized vascular allografts could offer the optimal substrate on which to build. Normal vascular endothelial function is key to the regulation of the circulation. Establishment of a healthy neointima in the allograft ought to minimize the risks of thrombosis, inflammatory response, and help to induce immunotolerance of the allograft tissues.

Limitations

The availability of allografts is limited by the size of the donor pool, adequate vessel lumen size (mostly available from male donors), and, in some countries, from competition for these valuable conduits with the solid-organ transplant teams.

Donor-pool insufficiency

The number of potential deceased donors may diminish in the developed world owing to progressive improvements in road safety, and more successful interventions in trauma and neurosurgery. Many potential donors are found to have pre-existing atherosclerosis, which limits the suitability of their vessels for banking. Significant atheroma is found in most male cadavers over the age of 45 in the UK. Because most vascular tissue donors are non-heart beating, the logistics required to recover good quality vessels with an acceptably short ischemic time before processing means that a national or supra-regional programme is required [57]. Establishment of such a program is dependent not only on the banking services but also on the willingness of vascular surgeons to overcome their reticence to adopt these grafts for their patients.

Cost containment

One of the greatest difficulties facing health care systems is the ever-increasing expectations and demands on services from an ageing population being met by a finite funding resource. In this context, cryopreserved allografts appear expensive compared with autologous tissue or prosthetic grafts. As discussed earlier, vascular allografts are generally regarded as a last-resort option, the alternatives ultimately being palliation to terminal care or major amputation. Several series have demonstrated that surgical reconstruction is more cost-effective than amputation and although no data exist for the cost effectiveness of vascular allografts, a similar benefit is likely. Restriction of the use of allografts on financial grounds would be unpalatable to many, as they have become an established therapy for some of the most challenging cases vascular and transplant surgeons face. The patient's quality of life is also a factor to consider.

Competing technologies

Reduction in volume of open arterial procedures might lead to a reduction in post-procedural complications. Endovascular therapies are associated with a remarkably low infective complication rate. In addition, improvement in the applicability of endovascular therapies in complex cases can be expected to widen the application of these minimally invasive options to treat patients effectively with established arterial and graft infections. While many believe that, in the face of fulminant sepsis, endovascular stent-grafting can be used as a bridge to definitive surgical repair, and there is an increasing trend to consider this as an effective treatment in its own right in cases of less virulent infections.

At this time it is unclear whether vascular allograft banking will be re-established or once again consigned to history.

KEY LEARNING POINTS

- The use of allografts in vascular surgery spans the past 100 years and enthusiasm for allografts has waxed and waned as developments in allograft processing have competed with the availability of improved prosthetic vascular grafts and stents.

- In principle, allografts are used today when autologous tissues are unavailable or unsuitable and prosthetic materials are either not available or considered to present too great a risk of failure due to thrombosis or infection.

- The goal is to use a replacement or repair conduit that allows the passage of blood without restriction to flow or activation of the coagulation, inflammation, or immune pathways (i.e., it must be biocompatible).

- Cryoprotectant solutions, such as addition of dimethylsulfoxide (DMSO), have been used to attempt to preserve allograft vessel cell integrity and function, although it is not clear that cell function is a prerequisite for the allograft to work as a successful conduit.

- Regarding use of allografts, a major concern shared by many vascular surgeons is the possibility of late aneurysmal degeneration necessitating lifelong follow-up and potential major revision surgery.

- Competing technologies, using minimally invasive options, may reduce incidence of open arterial procedures, leading to reduction in post-procedural complications.

- Thus it is unclear whether vascular allograft banking will find a role and be re-established or once again consigned to history.

References

1. Cooper A. Lectures on Surgery. Boston, Wells and Lilly 1825; 2, 56.
2. Watts S. The suture of blood vessels. Implantation and transplantation of vessels and organs. An historical and experimental study. Ann Surg 1907;46:373–404.
3. Carrel A. Results of the transplantation of blood vessels, organs and limbs. JAMA 1908;51:1662.
4. Klotz O, Permar HH, Guthrie CC. End results of arterial transplants. Ann Surg 1923;78:305–20.
5. Carrel A. Latent life of arteries. J Exp Med 1910;12:460–86.
6. Carrel A. Ultimate results of aortic transplantations. J Exp Med 1912;15:389–92.
7. Dubost C, Allary M, Oeconomos N. Resection of an aneurysm of the abdominal aorta: reestablishment of continuity by a preserved human arterial graft, with result after five months. Arch Surg 1952;64:405–8.
8. Blakemore AH,Voorhees AB Jr. The use of tubes constructed from vinyon "N" cloth in bridging arterial defects–experimental and clinical. Ann Surg 1954;140:324–33.
9. DeBakey ME, Creech O, Cooley DA. Occlusive disease of the aorta and its treatment by resection and homograft replacement. Ann Surg 1954;140:290–307.
10. DeBakey ME, Creech O, Morris GC. Aneurysm of thoracoabdominal aorta involving the celiac, superior mesenteric, and renal arteries. Report of four cases treated by resection and homograft replacement. Ann Surg 1956;144:549–72.
11. Gross RE. Treatment of certain aortic coarctations by homologous grafts. Ann Surg 1951;134:753–68.
12. Hufnagel CA, Rabil PJ, Reed L. A Method for the Preservation of Arterial Homo- and Heterografts. Surgical Forum, IV: 162. Philadelphia, WB Saunders Co., 1953, pp. 162–8.
13. Rob CG. The preservation of arterial grafts by freeze-drying. Proc R Soc Med 1954;47:368–70.
14. Cockett FB, Kinmonth JB. Preservation of Arterial Homografts. Br Med J 1962;21:194.

15. Foster JH, Lance EM, Scott HW. Experience with ethylene oxide treated freeze-dry arterial homografts in 110 consecutive patients. Ann Surg 1958;148:230–8.

16. Weber TR, Lindenauer SM, Dent TL, Allen E, Salles CA, Weatherbee L. Long-term patency of vein grafts preserved in liquid nitrogen in dimethyl sulfoxide. Ann Surg 1976;184:709–12.

17. Knox WG, Miller RE. Long-term appraisal of aortic and arterial homografts implanted in years 1954–1957. Ann Surg 1970;172:1076–8.

18. Murphy GJ, Pararajasingam R, Nasim A, Dennis MJ, Sayers RD. Methicillin-resistant *Staphylococcus aureus* infection in vascular surgical patients. Ann R Coll Surg Engl 2001;83:158–63.

19. Whitfield CG, Lonsdale RJ, Rahbour G, Parsons H, Dodd PD. Infective abdominal aortic aneurysm due to haemophilus influenza identified via the polymerase chain reaction. Eur J Vasc Endovasc Surg 2008;36:28–30.

20. Bruggink JL, Glaudemans AW, Saleem BR, et al. Accuracy of FDG-PET-CT in the diagnostic work-up of vascular prosthetic graft infection. Eur J Vasc Endovasc Surg 2010;40:348–54.

21. Chang JK, Calligaro KD, Ryan S, Runyan D, Dougherty MJ, Stern JJ. Risk factors associated with infection of lower extremity revascularization: analysis of 365 procedures performed at a teaching hospital. Ann Vasc Surg 2003;17:91–6.

22. O'Connor S, Andrew P, Batt M, Becquemin JP. A systematic review and meta-analysis of treatments for aortic graft infection. J Vasc Surg 2006;44:38–45.

23. Kuang AA, Renz JF, Ferrell LD, Ring EJ, Rosenthal P, Lim RC, Roberts JP, Ascher NL, Emond JC. Failure patterns of cryopreserved vein grafts in liver transplantation. Transplantation 1996;62:742–7.

24. Carbognani P, Spaggiari L, Solli P, et al. Experimental tracheal transplantation using a cryopreserved aortic allograft. Eur Surg Res 1999;31:210–5.

25. Chahine AA, Tam V, Ricketts RR. Use of the aortic homograft in the reconstruction of complex tracheobronchial tree injuries. Pediatr Surg 1999;34:891–4.

26. Radu DM, Seguin A, Bruneval P, Fialaire Legendre A, Carpentier A, Martinod E. Bronchial replacement with arterial allografts. Ann Thorac Surg 2010;90:252–8.

27. Sinha P, Moulick A, Jonas RA. Femoral vein homograft for neoaortic reconstruction in Norwood stage 1 operation. Ann Thorac Surg 2009;87:1309–10.

28. Bolton WD, Cull DL, Taylor SM, Carsten CG, Snyder BA, Sullivan TM, Youkey JR, Langan EM, Gray BH. The use of cryopreserved femoral veins grafts for hemodialysis access in patients at high risk for infection: A word of caution. J Vasc Surg 2002;36:464–8.

29. Matsuura J, Johansen KH, Rosenthal D, Clarke MD, Clarke KA, Kirby LB. Cryopreserved femoral vein grafts for difficult hemodialysis access. Ann Vasc Surg 2000;14:50–5.

30. Kieffer E, Gomes D, Chiche L, Fleron M-H, Koskas F, Bahnini A. Allograft replacement for infrarenal aortic graft infection: Early and late results in 179 patients. J Vasc Surg 2004;39:1009–17.

31. Vogt PR, Brunner-LaRocca HP, Lachat M, Ruef C, Turina MI. Technical details with the use of cryopreserved arterial allografts for aortic infection: influence on early and midterm mortality. J Vasc Surg 2002;35:80–6.

32. Bisdas T, Bredt M, Pichlmaier M, et al. Eight-year experience with cryopreserved arterial homografts for the in situ reconstruction of abdominal aortic infections. J Vasc Surg 2010;52:323–30.

33. Castier Y, Francis F, Cerceau P, Besnard M, Albertin J, Fouilhe L, Cerceau O, Albaladejo P, Lesèche G. Cryopreserved arterial allograft reconstruction for peripheral graft infection. J Vasc Surg 2005;41:30–7.

34. Noel AA, Gloviczki P, Cherry KJ, et al. and members of the United States cryopreserved aortic allograft registry. Abdominal aortic reconstruction in infected fields: early results of the United States cryopreserved aortic allograft registry. J Vasc Surg 2002;35:847–52.

35. Chiesa R, Astore D, Piccolo G, et al. Fresh and cryopreserved arterial homografts in the treatment of prosthetic graft infections: experience of the Italian Collaborative Homograft Group. Ann Vasc Surg 1998;12:457–62.

36. Reilly LM, Stoney RJ, Goldstone J, Ehrenfield WK. Improved management of aortic graft infection: the influence of operation sequence and staging. J Vasc Surg 1987;5:421–31.

37. Daenens K, Fourneau I, Nevelsteen A. Ten-year experience in autogenous reconstruction with the femoral vein in the treatment of aortofemoral prosthetic infection. Eur J Vasc Endovasc Surg 2003;25:240–5.

38. Gibbons CP, Ferguson CJ, Fligelstone LJ, Edwards K. Experience with femoropopliteal vein as a conduit for vascular reconstruction in infected fields. Eur J Vasc Endovasc Surg 2003;25:424–31.

39. Hayes PD, Nasim A, London NJM, et al. In situ replacement of infected aortic grafts with rifampicin-bonded prostheses: the Leicester experience (1992 to 1998). J Vasc Surg 1999;30:92–8.

40. Teebken OE, Pichlmaier MA, Brand S, Haverich A. Cryopreserved arterial allografts for in situ reconstruction of infected arterial vessels. Eur J Vasc Endovasc Surg 2004;27:597–602.

41. Walker WE, Cooley DA, Duncan JM, Hallan GR, Ott DA, Reul GJ. The management of aortoduodenal fistula by in situ replacement of the infected abdominal aortic graft. Ann Surg 1987;205:727–31.

42. Lonn L, Dias N, Veith Schroeder T, Resch T. Is EVAR the treatment of choice for aortoenteric fistula? J Cardiovasc Surg 2010;51:319–27.

43. Kan CD, Lee HL, Luo CY, Yang YJ. The efficacy of aortic stent grafts in the management of mycotic abdominal aortic aneurysm–institute case management with systemic literature comparison. Ann Vasc Surg 2010;24:433–40.

44. Nevelsteen A, Lacroix H, Suy R. Autogenous reconstruction with the lower extremity deep veins: an alternative treatment of prosthetic infection after reconstructive surgery for aortoiliac disease. J Vasc Surg 1995;22:129–34.

45. Klueh U, Wagner V, Kelly S, Johnson A, Bryers JD. Efficacy of silver-coated fabric to prevent bacterial colonization and subsequent device-based biofilm formation. J Biomed Mater Res 2000;53:621–31.

46. Batt M, Magne JL, Alric P, Muzj A, Ruotolo C, Ljungstrom KG, Garcia-Casas R, Simms M. In situ revascularization with silver-coated polyester grafts to treat infection: early and midterm results. J Vasc Surg 2003;38:983–9.

47. Carpenter JP, Tomaszewski JE. Immunosuppression for human saphenous vein allograft bypass surgery: a prospective randomized trial. J Vasc Surg 1997;26:32–42.

48. Carpenter JP, Tomaszewski JE. Human saphenous vein allograft bypass grafts: immune response. J Vasc Surg 1998;27:492–9.

49. Posner MP, Makhoul RG, Altman M, Kimball P, Cohen N, Sobel M, Dattilo J, Lee HM. Early results of infrageniculate arterial reconstruction using cryopreserved homograft saphenous conduit (CADVEIN) and combination low-dose systemic immunosuppression. J Am Coll surg 1996;183:208–16.

50. Zehr BP, Niblick CJ, Downey H, Ladowski JS. Limb salvage with cryovein cadaver saphenous vein allografts used for peripheral arterial bypass: role of blood compatibility. Ann Vasc Surg 2011;25:177–81.

51. Jashari R, Daenen W, Meyns B, Vanderkelen A. Is ABO group incompatibility really the reason of accelerated failure of cryopreserved alllografts in very young patients? Echocardiography assessment of the European Homograft Bank (EHB) cryopreserved allografts used for reconstruction of the right ventricular outflow tract. Cell Tissue Bank 2004;5:253–9.

52. Machera BA, Galilic U. The Galα1,3Galβ1,4GlcNAc-R (α-Gal) epitope: a carbohydrate of unique evolution and clinical relevance. Biochim Biophys Acta 2008;1780: 75–88.

53. Smith JM, Dernbach TA, Cooley DA. Treatment of aortic insufficiency with a descending aortic valvular homograft: 19-year follow-up and historical perspective. Cardiovasc Dis 1980;7:206–13.

54. Harrington RW, Pallette EC, Pallette EM. Arterial homografts – long term observation of results. Calif Med 1962;96:384–7.

55. Provan JL. Late aneurysm formation in arterial homografts: report of four cases of femoral aneurysm. J Thorac Cardiovasc Surg 1964;48:282–8.

56. Miller DV, Edwards WD, Zehr KJ. Endothelial and smooth muscle cell populations in a decellularized cryopreserved aortic homograft (SynerGraft) 2 years after implantation. J Thorac Cardiovasc Surg 2006;132:175–6.

57. Wusterman MC, Pegg DE, Warwick RM. The banking of arterial allografts in the United Kingdom. A technical and clinical review. Cell Tissue Bank 2000;1: 295–301.

6 The Use of Allograft Heart Valves and Conduits

Richard A. Hopkins[1], Gabriel L. Converse[1], and Ulrich Stock[2]

[1]Children's Mercy Hospital and Clinics, Kansas City, MO, USA
[2]University Hospital Frankfurt, Frankfurt, Germany

The past

Short history of allograft heart valve and conduit use

Lam reported in 1952 the technical feasibility of transplanting canine aortic valve homografts into the descending aorta of recipient dogs [1]. They also noted that, given the continuous diastolic flow present in the descending aorta, the cusps were not "used," and were constantly in the open position, subsequently deteriorating. However, if they induced aortic insufficiency in the recipient dog, this forced the transplanted valve to function and valve integrity was greatly enhanced. This fascinating study still has relevance today and was the basis on which Murray and others developed the technique for clinical implantation of human homografts [2]. Murray's publication in 1956 reported the successful use of fresh aortic valve homografts transplanted into the descending thoracic aorta for management of native aortic valve insufficiency. His initial operations preceded by five years the availability of the Starr-Edwards mechanical aortic valve prostheses. The Murray operation was only partly hemodynamically successful, but he reported remarkable durability of performance for the implanted homograft valves. Many of these valves remained functional for 13–20 years without calcification. Professor Gunning cited an unsuccessful operation in 1961 by Dr Bigelow and Dr Heimbecker as the first clinical insertion of an aortic valve homograft in the orthotopic position [3], but the first two survivors of such a procedure were reported independently by Ross of England and Barratt-Boyes in 1962 [4]. Initial excellent results with fresh deceased donor

Tissue and Cell Clinical Use: An Essential Guide, First Edition. Edited by Ruth M. Warwick and Scott A. Brubaker.
© 2012 Blackwell Publishing Ltd. Published 2012 by Blackwell Publishing Ltd.

homografts prompted an enormous focus on the use of such tissue despite the parallel progress in manufactured prosthetic valves. Limitation of donor availability led to multiple preservation methods to increase storage time and to establish homograft valve "banks." Many storage and preservation techniques were tried including freeze-drying, antibiotic sterilization with prolonged refrigeration, radiation, and various preservative treatments such as glutaraldehyde and formaldehyde. Unfortunately, although such harsh methods tended to increase the availability, they resulted in shortened functional survival of the homograft valves and caused significant disenchantment with the technique during the 1960s and 1970s [5]. Given the historical vocabulary, in reference to valves and valved conduits, the terms "homograft and allograft are used interchangeably.

Thus, to interpret the literature properly, it is important to remember that beginning in 1962, there have been four eras related to the methods of procurement, treatment, and storage of aortic and pulmonary valve homografts. The first era was defined by fresh aseptic deceased donor harvests with immediate transplantation (within hours of retrieval, or at most after a few days of refrigeration at 4°C typically in tissue culture media). The second era consisted of clean procurement with harsh sterilization and storage techniques clearly resulting in poor durability. The third era was defined by aseptic procurement with gentle antibiotic sterilization and wet 4°C storage for up to six weeks ("fresh-wet-stored valves"). These valves, as prepared, were likely minimally viable and for which there was extensive use and experience during the 1970s and early 1980s. The fourth method, introduced in the mid 1980s, involved cryopreservation after aseptic recovery with short, warm ischemic times – typically at multi-organ and tissue procurement during the organ transplant era and in the USA, according to the standards of the American Association of Tissue Banks (AATB) and similar organizations elsewhere in the world. These valves were characterized by relatively short, warm ischemic times, controlled cold ischemic times during transport and dissection, gentle antibiotic treatment, and scientifically valid cryopreservation techniques modified for the complex tissue structures of semilunar heart valves [6]. Storage was, generally, in the vapor phase of liquid nitrogen using a cryoprotectant. This methodology finally brought to fruition long-term cryostorage, banking, distribution, and transport methods that allowed these valves to be used virtually anywhere in the world, and led to an explosion of surgical techniques designed to exploit the positive features of allografts. Specifically, these valves provide optimal hydraulic function with central nonobstructive flow resulting in excellent hemodynamics performance, even in small sizes. Larger effective valves for small recipient annuli could be implanted, truly revolutionizing conduit surgery and allowing valve insertions in younger and smaller patients than had ever been possible before. Thromboembolism and hemolysis rates were reduced over prosthetic valves. The technical feasibility of these implants became apparent to congenital heart surgeons everywhere. Calcification appeared commonly to affect the conduit wall, but other than in the youngest patients, it seemed that calcification more slowly involved the leaflets, at least during the initial two to seven years of implantation (depending on age of recipient). Finally, resistance to endocarditis, an infection of the inner lining of the heart, appeared to be enhanced over glutaraldehyde-fixed bioprosthetic valves and mechanical valves. From a materials property standpoint, such allograft valve implants became preferred by surgeons as a flexible prosthesis useful for complex ventricular outflow tract reconstructions.

Limitations of use

The first limitation is the availability of tissue in appropriate sizes. Because these are transplantable gifted tissues, the resource is limited and depends on adequate donation rates. The most critical and effective use of homografts has been in the right ventricular outflow tract (RVOT) conduit position for which there are relatively poor alternatives. As a consequence, the highest priority sizes (from 10 to 24 mm diameter pulmonary valves) are highly prized and often scarce. The second main limitation is the finite durability of the graft. This appears to be a serious problem for recipients of ages less than three years. Decreased durability with subsequent conduit replacements in the same patient suggests that perhaps immune factors might intensify following subsequent reoperations with multiple allograft implants. Additionally, aortic homografts appear to calcify more rapidly than pulmonary homografts whether placed in the hemodynamic pulmonary circulation or systemic circulation. Thus, the usage rates for optimally sized pulmonary allograft tissue are extremely high, whereas many homograft banks eventually discard aortic valve tissue due to "shelf life" expiration. The homograft as currently processed and used is not a permanent replacement and should be viewed as a staging procedure that, by containing a functioning valve mechanism, helps to protect medium- and long-term ventricular function, even at the cost of a second operation.

Alternatives to allografts

Allograft tissues are currently the optimal choice for all right ventricular outflow reconstructions in children, and probably for many complex left ventricular outflow tract repairs as well. The primary reasons for using other options are the lack of allograft availability or in instances in which a rigid conduit offers an advantage against compression or distortion. Other alternatives are available. For the systemic circulation, xenogeneic glutaraldehyde crosslinked bioprostheses are available in stented models as well as stentless versions, and are especially useful for left ventricular outflow tract reconstructions. In particular, the stentless porcine valves have been especially useful in the adult population in the age group between 40 and 65. For right-sided reconstructions, the stentless valves have been used, but in most reports exhibit a more rapid calcific failure profile than homografts. Bovine superior vena cavae (including the caval valve) have been used as right-sided conduits, and seem to offer some promise for staging operations in very young patients, or in patients who have received multiple homografts and have presumably become sensitized to ABO or human leukocyte antigen (HLA). Such patients with preformed antibodies (alloantibodies) appear to have markedly reduced homograft durability. Dacron conduits containing a selection of valves have been used with varying levels of success as pulmonary valve conduits. Mechanical valves require anticoagulation and porcine valves appear to have accelerated calcification in younger patients.

The present

Clinical issues about the need for matching

Immune mechanism of inflammation is recognized as critical to the durability of bioprosthetic, cryopreserved allografts and even native aortic valves [7]. Allograft valves (and xenogeneic bioprosthetic valves) typically fail owing to inflammation, fibrosis, and ultimate calcification. Subsequent reoperations with allografts seem to have shorter durability than the initial conduits, suggesting adaptive immune mechanisms [6]. Numerous studies now indicate, in addition to younger recipient age, HLA and ABO discordance stimulates adaptive immune rejection and is more provocative of the innate immune system than biologic materials that do not contain such antigens [8, 9]. Several centers are now ABO matching homografts, which may improve durability for younger patients [10, 11]. The major constraint for adhering to ABO matching is the lack of adequate resource material. Theoretically, at least three options exist to address the immune response: (1) introduction of processing methods to reduce antigen-rich materials from the valves before cryopreservation – HLA antigens reside primarily on and in the cells, and thus, a thorough decellularization procedure would accomplish that goal; (2) immunosuppression of the recipient; and (3) ABO and HLA tissue matching of all homografts to the recipient (analogous to whole organ transplants). Although a few pilot trials have been attempted with immunosuppression, given the young age and health concerns of the recipients, this is a particularly unattractive option for long-term suppression of immune mediated inflammatory damage. Tissue matching is not feasible and thus, the most attractive option is to bioengineer the allograft tissues to create scaffolds that are antigen-free or at least antigen-reduced. An extension of this approach would be actually to reintroduce cells of recipient origin, thus creating a truly tissue engineered heart valve [11–13].

Biomechanics of transplantable semilunar heart valves

The quasi-static and time-dependent biomechanical properties of valvular tissues are widely reported in the literature. Testing is often conducted under uniaxial, biaxial, and, to a lesser extent, flexural loading conditions. Seebacher's group reported failure tensions of approximately 800 and 400 N/mm for human pulmonary valve conduit tissue loaded under uniaxial tension in the circumferential and longitudinal specimen directions, respectively [14]. Porcine aortic valve leaflet tissue has been reported to exhibit decreased radial stretch, but increased stiffness, compared to pulmonary valve leaflet tissue under biaxial loading [15]. Another laboratory reported the biaxial stress-relaxation and creep behavior of porcine aortic valve leaflet tissue, finding 28 and 33% relaxation over a three-hour period in the longitudinal and radial specimen directions, respectively; negligible creep was observed over the same period [16]. Thus, the observed mechanical behavior of the aortic valve leaflet does not strictly follow the traditional criteria for a viscoelastic material and is functionally well adapted to the requisite hemodynamic loading.

The effects of decellularization on the biomechanical properties of valvular tissues are not widely reported in the literature but do tend to vary between tissue types and decellularization protocols. In one study, detergent-based decellularization resulted in little change to the uniaxial tensile properties of porcine pulmonary valve conduit tissue [14]. Liao and colleagues studied the effects of multiple decellularization protocols on the biomechanics of porcine aortic valve leaflet tissue using biaxial tension conditions and reported increased extensibility for decellularized tissue, compared to native tissue, which was attributed to increased mobility of collagen fibers following decellularization [17]. The degree of increased extensibility was affected by the specific detergent or enzymatic agent used for decellularization. These findings illustrate the necessity of performing biomechanical characterization of manipulated valvular tissues as compared to native, using multiple testing procedures performed with both quasi-static and time dependent protocols, as well as using uniaxial and biaxial loading conditions. The material properties of the functional components of semilunar heart valves (e.g., leaflets, sinus wall, conduit) can be specifically tested separately and then as intact valves (hydraulic and hydrodynamic testing) to assess risk of specific failure modes.

Antibiotics, anticoagulants, and immunomodulation

Since the first clinical introduction in 1962 [18], transplantation of allograft heart valves has demonstrated exceptionally good initial hemodynamic characteristics, hardly any thromboembolic events without anticoagulation, and better resistance to endocarditis compared to bioprosthetic or mechanical valve substitutes [19, 20].

Initially, valves were collected and immediately transplanted as so-called homovitals [21]. Owing to logistic issues, grafts were subsequently stored at 4°C in tissue culture medium with antibiotics for up to six weeks before implantation [22]. Eventually, to enable long-term storage and improve safety by means of microbiology and virology testing, cryopreservation with controlled rate freezing and storage in vapor phase nitrogen was introduced [23]. The process of storage and shipping remains essentially unchanged since the mid-1980s. The three main concerns regarding clinical application of allograft valves are cell and tissue viability, immunomodulation, and extracellular matrix disruption as a consequence of the cryopreservation process.

According to international guidelines, such as those found in the AATB's Standards for Tissue Banking, valves undergo an antibiotic decontamination step after their dissection, morphological evaluation, measurements, competence testing and sampling for microbiology testing [24]. A considerable number of allografts arriving at tissue banks are contaminated. Main contaminants originate from skin, gastrointestinal or respiratory tracts with staphylococci and streptoccci as the most frequent microorganisms. Antibiotic cocktails may contain bacteriostatic, bactericidal, and antifungal agents to eliminate or reduce this microbial load. The decontamination step reduces the rate of contamination from initially 23% to 0–10% [25]. Side effects of the antibiotics include cell toxicity.

A broad misconception is the idea that surviving endothelial or interstitial valve cells will positively influence long-term function. In fact, it has been shown that surviving donor cells are not capable of maintaining normal leaflet architecture, and might contribute to failure by increasing the loss of leaflet flexibility [26, 27]. At time of implantation, cryopreserved allografts normally demonstrate endothelium with focal dropout in a variable pattern. Only a week after implantation the endothelium is almost completely lost and, after 2–11 months, virtually no interstitial tissue cells are observed [28]. Yacoub et al. have published results indicating that surviving endothelial cells on heart valve allografts mediate immunogenicity [29]. Human valvular endothelial cells, but not fibroblasts, are capable of directly stimulating CD4-positive T cells. After incubation in antibiotics they were able to significantly attenuate this CD4$^+$ T cell stimulation.

If remaining cells might be a contributing factor for graft failure, the careful removal of all potentially immunogenic cells before transplantation appears logical. Preliminary data on patients treated with decellularized and cryopreserved allografts with a mean follow-up of 52 months have recently demonstrated that decellularization did not significantly improve outcome in terms of pressure gradients and structural deterioration compared to non-decellularized allografts [30]. Disastrous clinical results with acellular xenograft heart valves suggest xenogeneic proteins or carbohydrate (e.g., α-galactose) mediated immunoreactivity may contribute beyond the donor-cell-mediated inflammation [31].

Indications for valve allografts

The development of the extra cardiac conduit for reconstruction of continuity between the "blue" ventricle and the pulmonary artery has revolutionized the surgery of complex congenital heart disease. In infants with anomalies such as tetralogy of Fallot, non-valved reconstruction of the RVOT has been well tolerated with relatively low, early reoperation rates. Usually with progressive right ventricular dilatation, most patients require later replacement of a pulmonary outflow valve. Other anatomic situations including pulmonary atresia, with or without other defects, have been repaired during childhood and infancy, and have done best with right ventricular outflow reconstructions with allograft valves. Neonatal and infant reconstructions that are optimally accomplished with allograft valved conduits include truncus arteriosus, absent pulmonary valve syndrome, and Ross operations. A functioning right ventricular outflow valve is recommended for either primary or secondary reconstructions when there is the following: (1) symptomatic right ventricular dysfunction; (2) fixed pulmonary hypertension; (3) hypoplastic pulmonary arteries; (4) pulmonary insufficiency with right ventricular dilatation; (5) tricuspid regurgitation; (6) echocardiographic evidence of small right ventricular volume or poor performance; (7) absent pulmonary valve syndrome; (8) peripheral pulmonary arterial stenosis; and (9) highly reactive pulmonary circulations. Systemic ventricle outflow valve implantations (e.g., aortic valve replacement, left ventricular outflow tract reconstructions) have more options than to right-sided reconstructions. However, there are numerous anatomic situations that favor the insertion of allograft valves. When possible, the autotransplant (Ross operation) in which the native pulmonary valve is transplanted as a neo-aortic valve has typically had better durability than any prosthetic options. It is a reportable event for a pulmonary valve functioning as a neo-aortic valve to fail owing to stenosis and calcification. However, the limitations of the Ross operation include annular and sinotubular junction dilatation with distortion of valve leaflet coaptation and subsequent systemic valve insufficiency. Surgical methods have been developed, which can minimize the development of valve insufficiency. In general, allograft valve implants are at least considered for the following indications: (1) all aortic valve replacements and left ventricular outflow tract reconstructions in patients with more than a 15-year life expectancy in whom anticoagulation is undesirable (e.g., children, young women of childbearing age and young active adults); (2) aortic root replacement; (3) aorta ventriculoplasty; (4) small aortic annulus; (5) bacterial endocarditis; and (6) reoperation for failure of an aortic valve prosthesis, particularly in patients with accelerated degeneration of porcine bioprostheses. Older patients may be well suited for stentless or stented xenografts, whereas younger active patients should be considered for Ross autotransplants. Relative contraindications for the insertion of an allograft valve in the left ventricular outflow tract include the following: (1) severe asymmetric annular calcification precluding uniform seating of the valve; (2) lack of availability; (3) active immune complex rheumatoid-like diseases (e.g., lupus, rheumatoid arthritis, collagen vascular disease, etc.); (4) aortic root ectasia exceeding a diameter of 30 mm; (5) aortic valve replacement being a small component of the total amount of cardiac surgery necessary in which cross-clamp times would be expected to exceed 120 minutes; (6) severe left ventricular dysfunction; and (7) connective tissue disorder such as Marfan's syndrome or cystic medial necrosis.

Clinical utility and potential pitfalls in use of allograft heart valves

The durability of contemporary cryopreserved allograft valves varies from 50 to 90% at 10–15 years [32]. In particular, in pediatric patients, allograft function is limited by earlier and faster structural deterioration necessitating more frequent reintervention procedures [33, 34]. The actual reasons for the variable failure rate remain unclear but one concern was attributed to the adequacy of thawing and dilution (of cryoprotectant) protocols. Several different methods for thawing homograft materials have been validated. The specific recommended protocol is included with the homograft product by the responsible tissue processing facility. The normal thawing process starts from the outside and proceeds to the inside. At the point when the ice surrounding the graft has melted, an ice core inside the allograft valve remains but is not visible. It is absolutely essential to not squeeze the valve at this time to attempt to speed the thawing process, as the ice core will cause damage to the delicate leaflets. Next, a thorough but extremely gentle washing process is required to remove residual cell toxic cryoprotectants (dimethyl sulfoxide, DMSO). Until use, the valve is then placed in heparinized oxygenated blood or tissue culture medium on the operating room table.

Pulmonary valve allografts are either used as pulmonary substitutes during the Ross procedure or as stand-alone implants for reconstruction of diseased RVOTs. Surgical implantation techniques such as inversion of the allograft for facilitated implantation imply significant tissue stress, and might contribute to early graft failure and should be omitted [35]. The removal of adjacent and excessive muscle from the RVOT in pulmonary allografts to reduce shrinking after implantation has been investigated, with evidence that transvalvular pressure gradients can be significantly reduced within the first two years after operation by homograft muscle reduction [36].

For aortic allograft valves there are currently two surgical implantation techniques favored. The full root technique requires removal of the aortic root with reimplantation of the coronary arteries [37]. The subcoronary implantation option inserts the trimmed valve within the native aortic root [38, 39].

Valve allografts are typically recovered from non-heart-beating or deceased donors. With respect to organ scarcity and legislative restrictions, some European or South American countries also retrieve allograft valves from explanted hearts of transplant recipients with a cardiomyopathy [40, 41]. This should be discouraged as a recent study on human and porcine heart valves revealed that the structural deterioration observed in cardiomyopathic heart is not restricted to the myocardium, but also affects the valvular histoarchitecture with disrupted collagen and elastic fiber network [42].

A variety of studies have compared the two major implant methods for survival, freedom from structural valve disease, and reoperation [37, 43–48]. Root replacement may be associated with an increased risk of perioperative death after adjustment for covariates using propensity analysis [49]. Long-term function and structural deterioration in contrast is not influenced by either technique [50].

Lessons learned from stentless aortic valve surgery include the need for accurate valve sizing (to avoid patient-prosthesis mismatch), better outcomes related to surgeon experience, and consequences of patient-related factors such as: diabetes mellitus; atrial fibrillation; peripheral vascular disease; renal dysfunction; female gender; age greater than 80 years; and, patients less than 165 cm height with body mass index greater than 24 [51].

Processing methods affect immunological reactions

Standard freezing technologies have been shown to variously impact extracellular matrix integrity [50]. This damage is attributed to interstitial crystallization. Because the destruction of the amorphous and fibrillar matrix structures may predispose cryopreserved valve grafts to structural failure, alternative preservation techniques have been explored. Vitrification, so called ice-free cryopreservation, only requires storage at −80°C rather than below −135°C to maintain these valves above the glass transition temperature (approximately −124°C) of the cryoprotectant formulation [51]. This may enable the promotion of amorphous solidification rather than crystallization, and might avoid the risk of tissue cracking that may occur in cryopreserved tissues during storage. Unpublished results from the Stock laboratory revealed that after implantation in the orthotopic pulmonary position in sheep, vitrified valves resulted in cell-free matrices, while maintaining crucial extracellular matrix components such as elastin and collagen, translating into superior hemodynamics, in contrast, to standard cryopreserved valves that exhibited extracellular matrix damage, and in vivo T-cell inflammation of the stroma with significant leaflet thickening.

The future

What does the future hold in the field of allograft heart valve usage?

The quest for the ideal cardiac valve replacement has been ongoing for approximately five decades. An approved, viable, biological heart valve containing functional leaflet cells, which are retained for the life of the patient, is currently not available. None of the clinical options is perfect, and all exhibit aspects of prosthetic valve disease, and sometimes with both accelerated and catastrophic fibrocalcific failure. Currently, heart valves and cardiovascular patch materials that have been decellularized are available, which appear to have antigen reduction as a primary rationale for improved durability. The putative mechanism would be a reduction in immune-driven inflammatory degradation of the materials. Early results are promising, but the duration of clinical usage has been too short for any definitive conclusions [30, 52, 53]. Earlier versions of decellularized heart valves that appear to have had retained necrotic cell debris or that are derived from xenogeneic sources were actually more inflammatory with less durability than traditional cryopreserved ("viable") allograft valves [10, 31]. The myth of retained cell viability in traditional cryopreserved homografts has been clearly debunked, and in fact, it now seems likely that a reduction in cell viability and processing related removal of endothelium and other high HLA antigen-containing cell types is in fact preferable to enhanced donor cell "viability" retention. Thus, improvement in "de-antigenization" using either decellularization methods or antigen masking techniques may provide scaffolds of semilunar heart valves that will enhance or prolong functional durability. However, current evidence suggests that the leaflets do not recellularize automatically in vivo, and thus even passive wear and tear could ultimately cause material fatigue and valve failure. Thus, the ultimate solution may be to tissue engineer a heart valve as a viable personal heart valve based upon decellularized allografts and cells obtained from the putative recipient. This has now been accomplished on a very limited basis clinically, and increasingly in experimental surgery animal studies [53–55].

High-technology applications are often considered incongruent with Third World medical care. But where cardiac surgery can be performed, the use of allografts rather than manufactured prostheses is an appealing approach given the better hemodynamics in young, active individuals, the lack of need for anticoagulation and the reduced incidence of bacterial endocarditis. This will be even more compelling if durability can be enhanced by bioengineering or advanced processing methods.

It is likely that development of such tissue engineered heart valves will markedly increase the demand for gifted heart valve tissues. Counterbalancing this resource requirement could be the relaxation of procurement criteria in regards to time from death. The original professional guidelines were established based upon cell viability of valve interstitial cells in appropriately cooled deceased donors (i.e., 24 hours) [56–60]. Because the scaffold requirements for a tissue engineered heart valve would not include native cell viability but rather on the kinetics of matrix degradation, it is quite likely that more valves could be available.

Application in a cost-constrained environment

Any additional processing methodologies that are used to reduce the antigenicity of transplantable tissues or to otherwise increase safety, will add to the cost of producing such materials. Regulatory requirements, liability insurance, research and development costs will also constrain the expansion and diversification of processing methodologies. However, with the current average cryopreserved allograft replacement interval being approximately five to seven years, one can calculate the need for up to five reoperations per patient treated in early childhood. If advanced processing methods or tissue engineering technologies reduce the need for reoperations, even a doubling or tripling of the cost of such "smart" valves would be justified on an overall health care cost reduction basis, but more importantly by the reduction in patient mortality and morbidity.

CASE STUDY 6.1

Outgrowing a pediatric pulmonary valved conduit replacement for tetralogy of Fallot

A full-term male child presented four days after birth with progressive cyanosis. Echocardiography confirmed the diagnosis of tetralogy of Fallot with virtual pulmonary atresia. The child was stabilized with prostaglandin infusion for maintenance of ductus arteriosus patency and underwent modified Blalock-Taussig shunting by right thoracotomy the next day. At six months of age the child underwent a classic tetralogy of Fallot repair with a transannular patch, closure of the ventricular septal defect and ligation of the shunt. At age four the child was noted on cardiology follow up to have severe pulmonary regurgitation and increasing right ventricular dimensions. Surgical repair was undertaken and a size 13 cryopreserved allograft pulmonary valved conduit was inserted between the right ventricle and the pulmonary artery confluence. The child's congestive heart failure resolved and he resumed normal growth and development. At age seven the patient again developed signs of right ventricular heart failure. Reevaluation demonstrated that this time the right ventricular dysfunction was due to pressure overload (peak right ventricle pressure = systemic) as a consequence of outgrowing his conduit. There was residual valve leaflet function and thus only mild regurgitation. The child was returned to the operating room and underwent resection of the first homograft, which was then

(Continued)

replaced with a second homograft size 18mm internal annulus diameter. All signs of heart failure resolved and he resumed normal growth and development. At age 17 he again returned with signs of both pulmonary stenosis and pulmonary insufficiency with progressive right-sided congestive heart failure. Evaluation demonstrated conduit stenosis at the level of the leaflets which were immobile and calcified. There was also 4+ pulmonary regurgitation and mild to moderate tricuspid regurgitation. The patient was returned to the operating room for his third median sternotomy and had re-replacement of the conduit with a size 25mm pulmonary cryopreserved valved conduit and a tricuspid annuloplasty repair. The patient is currently active, working full time, has fathered a child, and has no evidence of heart failure and reports normal exercise tolerance. Echocardiography demonstrates excellent function of all cardiac valves. Dimensions of the right ventricle are at the high end of normal.

CASE STUDY 6.2

Adult bicuspid aortic stenosis

A 21-year-old female senior attending college on an athletic scholarship (as a middle-distance runner) presented in acute heart failure with no prior history other than various reports of an audible heart murmur heard by various medical practitioners. Upon presentation, she was found to have bicuspid aortic valve with stenosis hemodynamics demonstrating a calculated valve area of $0.9\,cm^2$. The patient had been relatively inactive for the preceding four months owing to an episode of mononucleosis but had previously been able to compete with no symptoms. The patient was scheduled to be married after graduation and contemplated multiple pregnancies. Therefore for surgical replacement of her aortic valve she was offered various prosthetic options as she did not want the anticoagulation (teratogenic) required for a mechanical valve nor the limited durability of porcine bioprosthetic valves and thus chose an allograft valve transplant. At surgery, her valve could not be repaired and appeared to have sustained an occult episode of bacterial endocarditis which had spontaneously healed but which resulted in fibrous scarring of the leaflets increasing the severity of the bicuspid stenosis deformation. Her aortic root was excised which allowed placement of a large, non-restrictive (to allow for exercise induced major increases in cardiac output) 22mm aortic valve allograft with coronary button reimplantation. Given her size, 62kg and height of 5'6", this established supra-normal left ventricular outflow geometry with minimal gradient and normal effective orifice area. The patient made a full recovery and was able to return to spring track competition, ultimately being ranked 105th in the country in the 5000 meter event. Two years after graduation from college she gave birth to the couple's first child. Her husband is an extremely active individual as well and they pursue a lifestyle that involves mountain climbing, white water rafting, half marathons, and liberal use of golf courses, tennis and basketball courts. Currently her only medication is a daily baby aspirin.

CASE STUDY 6.3

Prosthetic valve re-replacement

A 17-year-old male presented with acute congestive heart failure with a history of a bi-leaflet prosthetic mechanical valve replacement at age 14 for bacterial endocarditis complicating a congenital bicuspid aortic valve. He was maintained on coumadin but was irregularly compliant. Emergency echocardiography suggested thrombosis with one leaflet frozen in the closed position creating severe acute aortic stenosis. Patient developed mild pulmonary edema and required tracheal intubation. Laboratory studies demonstrated normal clotting times. He was begun on heparin and intravenous clot lysis therapy (tissue plasminogen activator) with no resolution. After 16 hours of therapy, he began to develop decreasing urine output and was therefore taken to the operating room for surgical intervention on cardiopulmonary bypass. At the time of surgery one leaflet was found to be involved in a combination of pannus type fibrous scar tissue as well as acute and chronic thrombus. The size 19 valve was excised. Because he was a relatively large individual with a body surface area greater than $2.0\,m^2$, aortic annulus enlargement was accomplished with an annuloplasty enlargement (Nick's type) and a size 24 aortic valve cryopreserved allograft inserted as a root, reimplanting his coronary artery buttons and replacing the native aortic root which was moderately deformed and somewhat hypoplastic for his size. This restored normal left ventricular outflow tract hemodynamics with a peak gradient of 8 mmHg. His acute heart failure rapidly resolved. No further anticoagulation was required other than a daily baby aspirin and he returned to an active and typical teenage lifestyle.

CASE STUDY 6.4

Re-replacement of mechanical valve with a human valve

A 56-year-old musician presented with fever, chills, and hypotension six months after receiving a mechanical aortic valve replacement. Anticoagulation had been well maintained with minimal adjustments required to his Coumadin dosage. Three weeks earlier he had developed acute rectal hemorrhoid symptoms with anal fissure. Echocardiograph suggested endocarditis involving the prosthetic valve with partial loss of annulus prosthetic valve ring integrity due to annular abscess (valve dehiscence). The patient was begun on antibiotics and anti-congestive heart failure therapy and in 48 hours returned to the operating room. The previously placed prosthesis had disruption of over 50% of the sutures due to an annular abscess. The prosthesis was removed and the annulus extensively debrided. There was essentially total loss of continuity between the base of the fibrous skeleton of the heart

(Continued)

and the base of the aorta. Therefore the aortic root was excised leaving the coronaries on very large buttons. A 25 mm aortic allograft was then sutured into the aortic outflow tract using a portion of the attached anterior leaflet of the mitral valve to buttress the defect left by the abscess that burrowed into the septum beneath the aortic annulus. Coronary buttons were reimplanted. The patient recovered from surgery without difficulty and was treated with a six-week course of intravenous antibiotics with no subsequent evidence of recurrent bacterial endocarditis. He no longer requires anticoagulation. He is very strict about the use of subacute bacterial endocarditis prophylaxis. As a musician, he has also noted the additional benefit of the disappearance of the regular clicking metronome in his chest that, in retrospect, had actually been both annoying and quite disruptive to his professional activities.

KEY LEARNING POINTS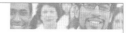

- Cryopreserved allograft valves have finite durability.
- Allografts have optimal hydraulic and hemodynamic performance.
- Allograft antigenticity is primarily attributable to residual cells and cell debris.
- ABO matching for current generation cryopreserved allograft valve transplants is optimal.
- Tissue engineering solutions to current limitations of cryopreserved heart valves are in the near future.

References

1. Lam CR, Aram HH, Munnell ER. An experimental study of aortic valve homografts. Surg Gynecol Obstet 1952;94:129–35.
2. Murray G. Homologous aortic-valve-segment transplants as surgical treatment for aortic and mitral insufficiency. Angiology 1956;7:466–71.
3. Gunning AJ. Ross' first homograft replacement of the aortic valve. Ann Thorac Surg 1992;54:809–10.
4. Hopkins RA, St Louis J, Corcoran PC. Ross' first homograft replacement of the aortic valve. Ann Thorac Surg 1991;52:1190–3.
5. Merin G, McGoon DC. Reoperation after insertion of aortic homograft as a right ventricular outflow tract. Ann Thorac Surg 1973 16:122–6.
6. Hopkins RA, Hopkins RA. Cardiac reconstructions with allograft tissues. New York: Springer-Verlag; 2005.
7. Shaddy RE, Hawkins JA. Immunology and failure of valved allografts in children. Ann Thorac Surg 2002;74:1271–5.
8. Sherif HM. Calcification of left-sided valvular structures: evidence of a pro-inflammatory milieu. J Heart Valve Dis 2009;18:52–60.

9. Caldarone CA, McCrindle BW, Van Arsdell GS, et al. Independent factors associated with longevity of prosthetic pulmonary valves and valved conduits. J Thorac Cardiovasc Surg 2000;120:1022–31.

10. Simon P, Kasimir M-T, Rieder E, Weigel G. Tissue Engineering of heart valves – immunologic and inflammatory challenges of the allograft scaffold. Progr Pediatr Cardiol 2006;21:161–5.

11. Taylor PM, Cass AEG, Yacoub MH. Extracellular matrix scaffolds for tissue engineering heart valves. Progr Pediatr Cardiol 2006;21:219–25.

12. Hopkins R. From cadaver harvested homograft valves to tissue-engineered valve conduits. Progress in Pediatric Cardiol 2006;21:137–52.

13. Christenson JT, Kalangos A. Blood group antigenicity and clinical durability of cryopreserved homografts. Progr Pediatr Cardiol 2006;21:227–31.

14. Seebacher G, Grasl C, Stoiber M, et al. Biomechanical properties of decellularized porcine pulmonary valve conduits. Artif Organs 2008;32:28–35.

15. Christie GW, Barratt-Boyes BG. Mechanical properties of porcine pulmonary valve leaflets: how do they differ from aortic leaflets? Ann Thorac Surg 1995;60 (2 Suppl):S195–9.

16. Stella JA, Sacks MS. On the biaxial mechanical properties of the layers of the aortic valve leaflet. J Biomech Eng 2007;129:757–66.

17. Liao J, Joyce EM, Sacks MS. Effects of decellularization on the mechanical and structural properties of the porcine aortic valve leaflet. Biomaterials 2008;29: 1065–74.

18. Ross DN. Homograft replacement of the aortic valve. Lancet 1962;ii:487.

19. O'Brien MF, Stafford EG, Gardner MA, Pohlner PG, McGiffin DC. A comparison of aortic valve replacement with viable cryopreserved and fresh allograft valves, with a note on chromosomal studies. J Thorac Cardiovasc Surg 1987;94: 812–23.

20. Tuna IC, Orszulak TA, Schaff HV, Danielson GK. Results of homograft aortic valve replacement for active endocarditis. Ann Thorac Surg 1990;49:619–24.

21. Gonzalez-Lavin L, McGrath LB, Amini S, Graf D. Homograft valve preparation and predicting viability at implantation. J Card Surg 1988;3(3 Suppl):309–12.

22. Jonas RA, Ziemer G, Britton L, Armiger LC. Cryopreserved and fresh antibiotic-sterilized valved aortic homograft conduits in a long-term sheep model. Hemodynamic, angiographic, and histologic comparisons. J Thorac Cardiovasc Surg 1988;96:746–55.

23. Watts LK, Duffy P, Field RB, Stafford EG, O'Brien MF. Establishment of a viable homograft cardiac valve bank: a rapid method of determining homograft viability. Ann Thorac Surg 1976;21:230–6.

24. Pearson K, Dock N, Brubaker S. Standards for Tissue Banking, 12 edition. McLean, VA: American Association of Tissue Banks; 2008.

25. Jashari R, Tabaku M, Van Hoeck B, Cochez C, Callant M, Vanderkelen A. Contamination of heart valve and arterial allografts in the European Homograft Bank (EHB): comparison of two different antibiotic cocktails in low temperature conditions. Cell Tissue Bank 2007;8:247–55.

26. Armiger LC. Postimplantation leaflet cellularity of valve allografts: are donor cells beneficial or detrimental? Ann Thorac Surg 1998;66(6 Suppl):S233–5.

27. Armiger LC. Viability studies of human valves prepared for use as allografts. Ann Thorac Surg 1995;60(2 Suppl):S118–20; discussion S20–1.

28. Mitchell RN, Jonas RA, Schoen FJ. Pathology of explanted cryopreserved allograft heart valves: comparison with aortic valves from orthotopic heart transplants. J Thorac Cardiovasc Surg 1998;115:118–27.

29. Johnson DL, Sloan C, O'Halloran A, Yacoub MH. Effect of antibiotic pretreatment on immunogenicity of human heart valves and component cells. Ann Thorac Surg 1998;66(6 Suppl):S221–4.

30. Bechtel JF, Stierle U, Sievers HH. Fifty-two months' mean follow up of decellularized SynerGraft-treated pulmonary valve allografts. J Heart Valve Dis 2008;17: 98–104.

31. Simon P, Kasimir MT, Seebacher G, et al. Early failure of the tissue engineered porcine heart valve SYNERGRAFT(TM) in pediatric patients. Eur J Cardiothorac Surg 2003;23:1002–6.

32. Mitchell RN, Jonas RA, Schoen FJ. Structure–function correlations in cryopreserved allograft cardiac valves. Ann Thorac Surg 1995;60(2 Suppl):S108–12; discussion S13.

33. Bonhoeffer P, Boudjemline Y, Saliba Z, et al. Percutaneous replacement of pulmonary valve in a right-ventricle to pulmonary-artery prosthetic conduit with valve dysfunction. Lancet 2000;356:1403–5.

34. Joudinaud TM, Baron F, Raffoul R, et al. Redo aortic root surgery for failure of an aortic homograft is a major technical challenge. Eur J Cardiothorac Surg 2008;33:989–94.

35. O'Brien MF, McGiffin DC, Stafford EG. Allograft aortic valve implantation: techniques for all types of aortic valve and root pathology. Ann Thorac Surg 1989;48:600–9.

36. Schmidtke C, Dahmen G, Graf B, Sievers HH. Pulmonary homograft muscle reduction to reduce the risk of homograft stenosis in the Ross procedure. J Thorac Cardiovasc Surg 2007;133:190–5.

37. Takkenberg JJ, Klieverik LM, Bekkers JA, et al. Allografts for aortic valve or root replacement: insights from an 18-year single-center prospective follow-up study. Eur J Cardiothorac Surg 2007;851–9.

38. Hickey E, Langley SM, Allemby-Smith O, Livesey SA, Monro JL. Subcoronary allograft aortic valve replacement: parametric risk-hazard outcome analysis to a minimum of 20 years. Ann Thorac Surg 2007;84:1564–70.

39. Nowicki ER, Pettersson GB, Smedira NG, Roselli EE, Blackstone EH, Lytle BW. Aortic allograft valve reoperation: surgical challenges and patient risks. Ann Thorac Surg 2008;86:761–8.

40. Da Costa ML, Ghofaili FA, Oakley RM. Allograft tissue for use in valve replacement. Cell Tissue Bank 2006;7:337–48.

41. Hunt CJ, Caffrey EA, Large SR. Factors affecting the yield of cardiac valve allografts from living unrelated donors. Eur J Cardiothorac Surg 1998;13:71–7.

42. Schenke-Layland K, Stock UA, Nsair A, et al. Cardiomyopathy is associated with structural remodelling of heart valve extracellular matrix. Eur Heart J 2009;30: 2254–65.

43. Lund O, Chandrasekaran V, Grocott-Mason R, et al. Primary aortic valve replacement with allografts over twenty-five years: valve-related and procedure-related determinants of outcome. J Thorac Cardiovasc Surg 1999;117:77–90.

44. O'Brien MF, Harrocks S, Stafford EG, Gardner MA, Pohlner PG, Tesar PJ, et al. The homograft aortic valve: a 29-year, 99.3% follow up of 1,022 valve replacements. J Heart Valve Dis 2001;10:334–44; discussion 5.

45. Kirklin JK, Smith D, Novick W, et al. Long-term function of cryopreserved aortic homografts. A ten-year study. J Thorac Cardiovasc Surg 1993;106:154–65; discussion 65–6.

46. Shapira OM, Shemin RJ. Aortic valve replacement with cryopreserved allografts: mid-term results. J Card Surg 1994;9:292–7.

47. Jones EL, Shah VB, Shanewise JS, et al. Should the freehand allograft be abandoned as a reliable alternative for aortic valve replacement? Ann Thorac Surg 1995;59: 1397–403; discussion 403–4.

48. Yankah AC, Weng Y, Hofmeister J, et al. Freehand subcoronary aortic valve and aortic root replacement with cryopreserved homografts: intermediate term results. J Heart Valve Dis 1996;5:498–504.

49. Prager RL, Fischer CR, Kong B, et al. The aortic homograft: evolution of indications, techniques, and results in 107 patients. Ann Thorac Surg 1997;64:659–63; discussion 63–4.

50. Doty JR, Salazar JD, Liddicoat JR, Flores JH, Doty DB. Aortic valve replacement with cryopreserved aortic allograft: ten-year experience. J Thorac Cardiovasc Surg 1998;115:371–9; discussion 9–80.

51. Kilian E, Oberhoffer M, Gulbins H, Uhlig A, Kreuzer E, Reichart B. Ten years' experience in aortic valve replacement with homografts in 389 cases. J Heart Valve Dis 2004;13:554–9.

52. Konuma T, Devaney EJ, Bove EL, et al. Performance of CryoValve SG decellularized pulmonary allografts compared with standard cryopreserved allografts. Ann Thorac Surg 2009;88:849–54; discussion 554–5.

53. Hopkins RA, Jones AL, Wolfinbarger L, Moore MA, Bert AA, Lofland GK. Decellularization reduces calcification while improving both durability and 1-year functional results of pulmonary homograft valves in juvenile sheep. J Thorac Cardiovasc Surg 2009;137:907–13.

54. Dohmen PM, Konertz W. Can cryopreservation destroy the extracellular matrix of pulmonary allografts? Ann Thorac Surg 2007;83:1921; author reply -2.

55. Dohmen PM, Lembcke A, Holinski S, Kivelitz D, Braun JP, Pruss A, et al. Mid-term clinical results using a tissue-engineered pulmonary valve to reconstruct the right ventricular outflow tract during the Ross procedure. Ann Thorac Surg 2007;84: 729–36.

56. Crescenzo DG, Hilbert SL, Messier RH, Jr., et al. Human cryopreserved homografts: electron microscopic analysis of cellular injury. Ann Thorac Surg 1993;55:25–30; discussion -1.

57. Burkert J, Krs O, Vojacek J, et al. Cryopreserved semilunar heart valve allografts: leaflet surface damage in scanning electron microscopy. Zentralbl Chir 2008;133: 367–73.

58. Domkowski PW, Messier RH, Jr., Crescenzo DG, et al. Preimplantation alteration of adenine nucleotides in cryopreserved heart valves. Ann Thorac Surg 1993;55: 413–9.

59. Abd-Elfattah AS, Messier RH, Jr., Domkowski PW, et al. Inhibition of adenosine deaminase and nucleoside transport. Utility in a model of homograft cardiac valve preimplantation processing. J Thorac Cardiovasc Surg 1993;105:1095–105.

60. Messier RH, Domkowski PW, Aly HM, et al. Adenine nucleotide depletion in cryopreserved human cardiac valves: the "stunned" leaflet interstitial cell population. Cryobiology 1995;32:199–208.

7 The Use of Allografts in Orthopedics

William W. Tomford[1] and Eduardo J. Ortiz-Cruz[2]
[1]Massachusetts General Hospital, Boston, MA, USA
[2]Hospital Universitario La Paz, Madrid, Spain

Introduction

Musculoskeletal tissue transplantation is a worldwide endeavor. Tissue banks are present and active in every major country, and the use of musculoskeletal allografts as transplanted tissues has become a routine procedure. Orthopedic surgeons around the world rely on these tissues to provide their patients with the most reliable substitute for damaged or missing tissues.

Tissue transplantation in orthopedic surgery has classically used bone as an allograft because bone has characteristics that make it an ideal transplant. It can be easily cleansed of any potential donor antigenic tissue including cells without affecting its function. It can be sterilized with minimal damage to its integrity. Best of all, bone can be stored relatively cheaply for long periods without compromising its function.

There are now more than one million deposits of bone in various forms and quantities distributed annually in the USA. Over 27,000 tissue donors provide these transplants, and it is estimated that about a dozen tissue banks process over 90% of these tissues. Likewise, in other countries, there are tissue banks providing most of the bone used by orthopedic surgeons; however, some surgeons run hospital-based bone banks to meet their own surgical needs or for hospital consortia. In the UK, for example, there are some hospital-based bone banks which meet the needs of orthopedic surgeons undertaking hip revision surgery. This is a minority but still a significant activity.

Tissue and Cell Clinical Use: An Essential Guide, First Edition. Edited by Ruth M. Warwick and Scott A. Brubaker.

© 2012 Blackwell Publishing Ltd. Published 2012 by Blackwell Publishing Ltd.

However, bone is only one of several allografts used by orthopedic surgeons. Other musculoskeletal tissues that are being increasingly transplanted include tendons, ligaments, meniscus, and cartilage, both articular and fibrocartilage. Transplantation of these tissues is also becoming routine, particularly in the areas of sports injuries and joint reconstructive surgery.

Tissue banks are also expanding their efforts to include connective tissues and cells that reside inside and around bone. These tissues include bone marrow and adipose tissue, in the form of adult mesenchymal stem cells, and skin. These are the newest transplants being used by orthopedic and now plastic surgeons, and it is clear from the volume of tissues transplanted that this area is the growth area of musculoskeletal tissue transplantation.

This chapter will provide a brief history of orthopedic allograft transplantation, review current usage of various types of musculoskeletal transplants and initiate a look at the types of tissue that may be used as allografts by orthopedic surgeons in the future.

History

Bone is the oldest tissue transplant. Orthopedic allograft transplantation was presaged in the second chapter of the book of Genesis in the Holy Bible. God caused Adam to fall into a deep sleep and created Eve from a rib taken from Adam. Although this story is apocryphal, it illustrates the idea that bone is a tissue that can be easily removed and used in another human.

The second historical use of bone as an allograft was attributed to the Roman saints Cosmas and Damian. A whole lower extremity was removed from a Moor and placed onto a Roman posthumously. This procedure is recorded in Church archives.

The first bone transplant recorded in modern times occurred in Scotland in 1878. Sir William Macewen (1848–1926) removed an infected humerus from a 12-year-old boy and replaced it with three allografts [1]. Donors were amputees, the transplants were cylinders of bone that were stacked on top of one another, and the three cylinders reportedly healed over four years.

Following Macewen's approach, early procedures involving bone transplantation relied upon fresh bone from amputees as a source of allograft. For example, in the early 1900s, Lexer in Berlin developed a procedure to remove a long bone from an amputee in one operating room and transport the graft to an adjacent operating room to be transplanted immediately into a recipient [2].

In 1912, the Nobel laureate Alexis Carrel predicted the storage of tissues for future transplantation, and from about that time tissue transplantation became easier and thus more popular [3]. In most instances, the surgeons who used the bone in clinical situations were the tissue bankers. These surgeon-bankers included Inclan working in Cuba, Bush, Wilson, and Hibbs working in New York, Hult working in Sweden, and Judet working in France. Most of their banks were simply refrigerators.

The advance in tissue storage that had the most effect on transplantation of bone was the development of freeze-drying as a process for storage of bone. In the 1950s, the US Navy Tissue Bank in Bethesda, Maryland adapted methods of lyophilization from the food preservation industry and applied the process to preservation of bone. This method of preservation and storage allows bone to be easily stored, transported, and transplanted without any electrical or mechanical requirements.

The Navy Tissue Bank was the first major tissue bank capable of supplying more than a few surgeons at one medical center. It was originally designed to serve military surgeons in wartime to be able to easily transplant bone in a battle zone. However, it soon became an invaluable source of bone graft for civilian surgeons. It was the prototype and forerunner of all major tissue banks today, and many of the founders of these banks trained in, or were associated with, the Navy Tissue Bank.

Current use of allograft transplants

Bone

During the 1970s, bone allograft usage in orthopedics consisted mainly of supplementing autograft bone taken from the iliac crest in the treatment of scoliosis and other childhood orthopedic conditions. The use of small deposits or packages of freeze-dried bone, mostly 40–50 cm^3, were used because autograft bone from the iliac crest is insufficient for large spine fusions. The Navy Tissue Bank along with The University of Miami Tissue Bank supplied almost all of these grafts in the US during this time.

The increasing use of bone allograft of all types began with the popular use of frozen-stored, long bone allografts. As noted above, Lexer popularized the use of fresh long bone allografts in the early 1900s but it was a procedure seldom performed. However, once long-term freezer storage of long bones became feasible, limb-sparing surgery using this type of bone allograft to avoid amputations in the treatment of malignant skeletal tumors became popular. Parrish in Houston, Texas, and Mankin in Boston, Massachusetts, began use of this type of bone allograft and published their results [4, 5]. The realization occurred to the orthopedic profession that if very large segments of bone could be transplanted successfully, smaller segments could also be used. This intuitive observation resulted in a very large increase in the use of bone allograft.

Although adult spine surgeons had been using posterior lumbar interbody fusion grafts for many years, an increasing use of spine fusion procedures

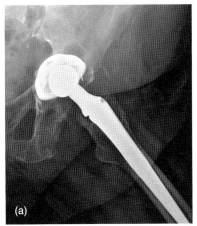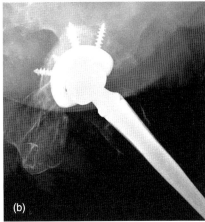

Figure 7.1 Left hip, 68-year-old female, un-cemented left total hip revision performed 18 years ago. (a) Preoperative radiograph of left hip (frog lateral) showing protrusion of acetabular shell through medial wall eroding into pelvis owing to osteolysis; (b) postoperative radiograph of left hip (frog lateral) taken 4 months after surgery showing bone graft consisting of cancellous chips milled to approximately 3–5 mm^3 that fill the space behind the cup and is beginning to incorporate into host bone.

for the treatment of back pain created a large demand for these types of grafts. Because posterior lumbar interbody fusion grafts in most instances had to be shaped in the operating room by the surgeon, which consumed valuable operating room time, computerized cutting of femoral rings by tissue banks, and the advent of special instrumentation developed specifically for lumbar segment fusions became very popular. Once results showed that the use of these special grafts resulted in improved surgery in the lumbar spine, there was a natural extension of the approach to cervical fusions. Currently bone allograft used in spine fusions accounts for most of the use of bone allografts.

Revision joint replacement surgeons also began to experience the need for large amounts of bone allograft for replacement of bone loss due to osteolysis (Figure 7.1a,b). This surgery created a demand for bone that could not be met with storage of surgical bone femoral heads from living donors by multiple medical centers. To meet this demand in the USA, tissue-processing facilities were started to develop methods of preparation of bone chips and other allograft configurations using advanced processing technologies and bone.

Soft tissues

Simultaneously with the development of large-scale processing and provision of bone chips and wedges for transplantation during the late 1970s and early 1980s, soft tissue allografts of the musculoskeletal system experienced an increase in popularity. As sports medicine specialists began to report good results with anterior cruciate ligament reconstruction, problems associated with the procurement and use of autograft tendon for these operations began to be noted. In addition, revisions in circumstances in which the autograft failed were difficult. To avoid these issues, sports medicine surgeons began to use allograft Achilles tendons with bone blocks, anterior and posterior tibial tendons, and bone–patellar tendon–bone blocks as allograft transplants for a torn anterior cruciate ligament.

One of the major concerns in using allograft anterior cruciate ligament transplants was the transmission of disease. Bone chips and wedges can be easily cleaned of all antigenic donor tissue or even sterilized by irradiation or other means to reduce the possibility of disease transmission to practically zero. However, if not properly controlled, similar treatment of soft tissue grafts such as Achilles tendons can change the structure of the graft to the degree that it is no longer acceptable as a substitute tissue.

The solution to this problem has been twofold. First, the infectious disease tests for relevant transmissible diseases in donors have been developed to the point where they are extremely sensitive. Nucleic acid testing, for human immunodeficiency virus type 1 (HIV-1) and for hepatitis C, has an extremely low probability of giving false-negative results and greatly enhances the ability to detect active disease. Second, new methods of processing that involve chemicals to kill bacteria and viruses, but which do not harm the soft tissues, have been developed.

Articular cartilage

One of the growth areas in musculoskeletal transplantation is articular cartilage transplantation. Most of the over 80 million Americans who suffer from some form of arthritis, most commonly osteoarthritis, will do fine with a complete joint replacement performed in their later years of life. However, these devices are not applicable in young active individuals who have cartilage lesions, which do not warrant full replacement.

Several approaches using autologous cartilage as replacement tissue are currently being used clinically. One approach involves retrieval of autograft cartilage, isolation, and expansion of the cells in this tissue and replacement of these cells into the defect. Another approach involves the insertion of plugs of autograft cartilage taken as osteochondral pieces from a non-weight-bearing area in the same knee.

Transplants of allograft cartilage have been performed, using both fresh and frozen grafts, and both as large and small pieces. For the treatment of very large defects, such as might occur in a bone or cartilage tumor,

Enneking showed that transplants of frozen cryopreserved and non-cryopreserved cartilage on osteoarticular transplants such as proximal and distal femurs do not last more than a few years [6]. Gross showed that transplants of fresh living cartilage in areas as large as a hemi-condyle may last several years before requiring further surgery [7]. Both of these authors also showed that malalignment of the transplanted joint results in early deterioration of these grafts. This finding is particularly true where there is an incongruity with the opposing joint surface and where there is any degree of malalignment with abnormal forces sustained by the cartilage transplant.

For the treatment of small osteochondral lesions up to about two centimeters in diameter, tissue banks supply hemi-condyles of femurs stored by refrigeration or freezing. Special instrumentation allows surgeons to core out the area of cartilage degeneration on the host condyle and replace it with a core or dowel of bone and cartilage taken from the allograft condyle. This method provides a smooth condylar surface which serves the biomechanical goal of restoration of normal joint mechanics, but where the articular cartilage is unlikely to thrive and hence will require replacement in the future.

No approach to cartilage replacement has proven to be consistently successful. Most have relieved pain, which has been the goal of surgeons up to this point, but the ideal replacement is living hyaline cartilage, a goal that has proven, thus far, to be elusive.

One of the driving forces behind current research in cartilage transplantation is the arthroscopic finding that many people in the 30–60 year age range have small but painful cartilage lesions. In these patients, alignment is normal or not sufficiently abnormal to warrant correction. These lesions are amenable to some kind of local treatment to relieve pain, and it is believed that successful treatment will prevent further deterioration of the joint and delay or possibly prevent the need for joint replacement.

Treatment of these Outerbridge II or III lesions [8] – either with the deepest layers of cartilage exposed or down to subchondral bone and measuring about one centimeter or less in diameter – may be beneficial in providing pain relief and may possibly prevent progression to more significant and widespread damage. The most common current approach is to fracture the bony bed of the osteochondral lesion in an attempt to allow host stem cells to penetrate the bone and grow and fill in the area. By filling in the defect, pain is at least partly relieved, but the fibrocartilage will breakdown within a few years and further treatment will be required.

Structural allografts: orthopedic oncology surgery

We present four cases. In these, we favor the use of an allograft bone transplant for the reconstruction of the skeletal defect after bone tumor resection:

use of osteoarticular allograft after intra-articular proximal tibia resection; intercalary allograft after intercalary resection; hemicortical allograft subsequent to periosteal osteosarcoma resection; and intracavitary cortical allograft in a fibrous dysplasia. For these structural reconstructions, we prefer to use non-irradiated allografts that are deep frozen. All the graft data and X-rays of the graft are reviewed by the surgeon, before acceptance of the allograft.

CASE STUDY 7.1

Benign bone tumor: fibrous dysplasia of the femoral neck (cortical allogeneic graft)

A 26-year-old female, who had no history of acute trauma and an unremarkable past medical history, presented with a well-known geographic osteolytic lesion located on the proximal femur. It was radiologically shown to consist of fibrous dysplasia that was incidentally diagnosed 7 years ago. She was referred because she suffered moderate pain of the left hip of spontaneous onset, which was related to increased activity. At examination, exquisite tenderness was noted in the left hip and hip motion was diminished in the last degrees.

The radiograph demonstrated a well-delimited osteolytic lesion on the proximal femur and a fatigue pathologic fracture in the medial cortex. The bone scan showed unique increased level of uptake in the area of left proximal femur. The clinical and radiological characteristics were consistent with a monostotic fibrous dysplasia. An intralesional resection was performed and the intraoperative histological examination of the frozen section confirmed the fibrous dysplasia. The cavity was filled with autologous iliac crest cancellous grafts, so a 15-cm long deep-frozen fibular allogeneic graft was used to reinforce the femoral neck. The fibular graft was cut in two parts (7.5 cm each), trimmed to allow apposition, and impacted into the femoral neck (Figure 7.2a). At 4 years postoperatively, she was experiencing normal life without restriction and there was good bone healing (Figure 7.2b).

Discussion. Many different methods of treatment are reported in the literature about fibrous dysplasia when surgery is indicated. These methods vary from simple curettage to curettage and bone grafting. The choice of internal fixation and type of grafting varies among surgeons and for different cases. When curetted fibrous dysplasia cavities are filled with autologous cancellous bone grafts, the grafts are initially revascularized and rapidly unite; however, as internal repair and remodeling begin, the grafts of normal bone are gradually replaced by dysplastic bone. Cortical autologous or allogeneic grafts inserted through dysplastic lesions persist longer than cancellous grafts and strengthen the bone against fracture. Fibrous dysplasia is one of the few instances in which allogeneic grafts are biologically and mechanically more desirable than autologous grafts [9].

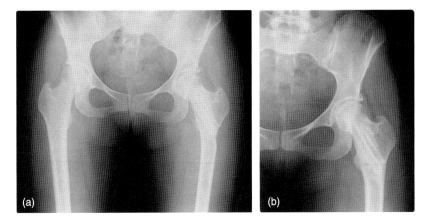

Figure 7.2 Left femoral neck, 26-year-old female, fibrous dysplasia, cortical allogeneic graft. (a) Postoperative radiograph showing the allogeneic cortical fibular grafts that were inserted after resection of the lesion and filling of the cavity with autologous cancellous bone grafts; (b) two-year postoperative radiograph showing complete healing and incorporation of the cortical grafts and significant intralesional ossification with no further fractures.

CASE STUDY 7.2

Malignant bone tumor: chondrosarcoma of the distal femoral diaphysis (intercalary allograft reconstruction)

A 53-year-old female had suffered continuous pain in her right thigh for 6 months. The pain had a spontaneous onset and was not related to activity. The radiograph demonstrated an osteolytic, poorly marginated lesion on the right distal diaphysis of the femur, associated with a punctate and arc-like mineralization. Magnetic resonance imaging (MRI) demonstrated a soft tissue mass and cortical disruption (Figure 7.3a). The biopsy confirmed chondrosarcoma grade 2. The staging did not demonstrate metastases.

A wide resection and reconstruction with intercalary allograft was indicated. After one year, the distal osteotomy was united, but the proximal osteotomy had non-union (Figure 7.3b). Consequently, autografting using iliac crest bone to adjust osteosynthesis was performed and a new plate was added. Proximal union was successfully achieved after 6 months. The patient had no restrictions of activity after 4 years (Figure 7.3c).

Discussion. Intercalary allograft reconstruction has a long-term success rate of about 84% [9]. We believe that an intercalary allograft transplant is a safe, effective treatment for an intercalary defect resulting from resection of a tumor. There is considerable controversy among surgeons as to whether metal implants or osteoarticular allografts are best suited for the treatment of lesions when a joint must be resected, but there is far less doubt about the use of intercalary segments, in which a joint plays no role.

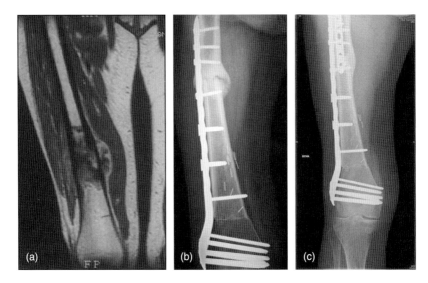

Figure 7.3 Right femoral diaphysis, 53-year-old female, chondrosarcoma, intercalary allograft. (a) Coronal view of the MRI showing the extent of the neoplasm in the distal femur with a small soft tissue mass and cortical disruption; (b) anteroposterior radiograph show a reconstruction with intercalary allograft with the distal osteotomy united, but the proximal osteotomy without union; (c) anteroposterior radiograph demonstrating complete union of both osteotomy sites after autografting with iliac crest bone.

CASE STUDY 7.3

Malignant bone tumor: osteosarcoma of the proximal tibia (osteoarticular allograft reconstruction)

An 18-year-old female, who had discontinuous pain over her right knee for 3 months, presented with pain that had spontaneous onset. She did not remember previous trauma. Plain radiographs revealed a bone-forming osteolytic and poorly marginated lesion on the right proximal tibia (Figure 7.4a). The MRI demonstrated a small, soft-tissue mass. A core needle biopsy confirmed a high-grade osteosarcoma. The staging did not demonstrate metastases.

Neoadjuvant chemotherapy was indicated, after which she had surgery that consisted of a wide intra-articular resection of the proximal tibia and reconstruction with osteoarticular allograft (Figure 7.4b). Concurrently, rotation of a medial gastrocnemius flap was used with the intention of placing viable muscle over the allograft to improve coverage of the reconstruction; however, she required two additional operative procedures. The first surgery was indicated because of

(Continued)

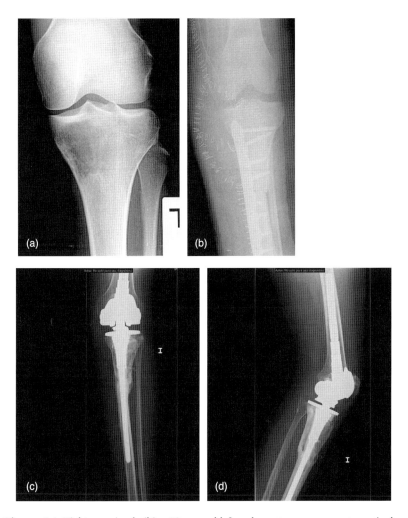

Figure 7.4 Right proximal tibia, 18-year-old female, osteosarcoma, osteoarticular allograft. (a) Anteroposterior radiograph showing an osteolytic, poorly marginated lesion on the right proximal tibia; (b) immediate anteroposterior radiograph showing insertion of a proximal tibial osteoarticular allograft, with good congruence of the joint; (c, d) anteroposterior and lateral radiographs of the allograft–prosthesis composite that has functioned successfully after resurfacing the allograft. Note that the graft is united with host bone and the stem of the prosthesis completely spans and supports the allograft.

non-union of the osteosynthesis site after 1 year. Additionally, the internal fixation was adjusted using autologous bone graft, and union was achieved. The second surgical procedure was done after 4 years when the patient noted instability of the knee and pain, which were interpreted as symptomatic degeneration of the joint. This was confirmed by radiographs; resurfacing, using a knee prosthesis, was indicated and performed (Figure 7.4c,d).

Discussion. The use of proximal tibia osteoarticular allografts after tumor resection may restore bone stock and reconstruct the extensor mechanism. Limb salvage surgery of the proximal tibia is one of the most demanding reconstructions owing to difficulties with soft tissue coverage, a high rate of infection, and the necessity of restoring the knee extensor mechanism. The osteoarticular reconstruction has more reconstructive options than intercalary reconstruction. Three types of reconstruction are currently used: megaprosthesis; an osteoarticular allograft; and an allo-prosthetic composite. Each method has advantages and disadvantages, but none has been found to be the best for every situation. One advantage of selecting an osteoarticular allograft procedure is that it has the potential to restore bone stock, and the stump of the allograft patellar ligament allows extensor mechanism repair. Conversion of a massive osteoarticular allograft to a total knee arthroplasty can extend the functional life of the original limb salvage procedure [10–12].

CASE STUDY 7.4

Malignant bone tumor: parosteal osteosarcoma distal femur (hemicortical intercalary allograft)

A 36-year-old male was evaluated in the emergency room for a knee sprain. X-rays incidentally discovered a bone-forming tumor on the posterior aspect of the right distal femur. Later, radiographs and computed tomography demonstrated a surface tumor with the appearance of dense bone formation pasted onto the cortex (Figure 7.5a). An MRI scan demonstrated that the medullary space was not involved. A biopsy confirmed low-grade parosteal osteosarcoma; staging did not demonstrate metastases. Surgery was indicated and consisted of wide hemicortical intercalary resection of the distal femur and reconstruction with hemicortical allograft (Figure 7.5b). In time, the allograft incorporated with the host bone and the patient returned to his normal life (Figure 7.5c).

Discussion. A wide hemi-resection of the cortical bone with a hemicortical bone allograft reconstruction is indicated in low-grade periosteal osteosarcoma without medullary involvement. Graft union is achieved owing to the large contact area between the allograft and host bone, which facilitates union and remodeling. Although the hemicortical resection is technically demanding, clinical results make it clearly worthwhile for selected patients [13].

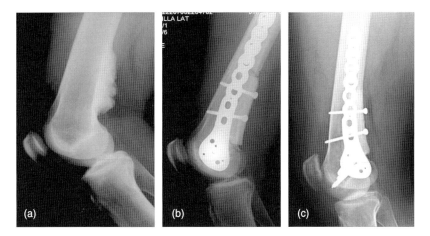

Figure 7.5 Right distal femur, 36-year-old male, parosteal osteosarcoma, hemicortical intercalary allograft. (a) Preoperative lateral view radiography showed a relatively dense and well-demarcated ossified mass arising on the posterior surface of the distal femur; (b) immediate postoperative lateral view radiography showing the hemicortical allograft; (c) postoperative lateral view radiography showing the hemicortical allograft incorporated to the host bone.

Mesenchymal stem cell transplants

The realization that mesenchymal stem cells could be transplanted relatively innocuously has resulted in the ability of tissue banks to provide small amounts of grafting material that contains these cells which are used to promote bone growth. Orthopedists have, of course, been using adult stem cells retrieved from the patient's iliac crest and other sites for over a century as sources of autologous stem cells. Although these cells meet the three criteria of an ideal bone graft – osteoconductive, osteoinductive and osteogenic – there are few stem cells per unit area in adults, and retrieval, particularly from the iliac crest, results in pain and prolongs operative time. Therefore, the ability to use an "off-the-shelf" package of stem cells is extremely attractive.

Although allograft mesenchymal stem cells are available to surgeons, no studies have been performed that conclusively show that they promote bone growth in humans. Animal studies strongly suggest that this is the case, but even though several hundred patients have received mesenchymal stem cell transplants, these cases have not been collected or analyzed.

There are other concerns about use of mesenchymal stem cell transplants, which raise questions. First, are they truly non-immunogenic? Second, how long do the transplanted cells survive? Third, what is the minimum number of cells required for effective promotion of bone growth? Fourth, although the safety of the transplant is similar to that of any fresh graft such as a fresh articular cartilage transplant, is there the possibility of graft versus host disease in immunosuppressed patients? All of these questions need to be answered through analysis of well-controlled studies. Some of these issues are discussed in Chapter 16.

Demineralized bone, bone matrix, and osteobiologics

Urist showed that minerals can be removed from bone with resultant exposure of collagen, a process that also exposes growth factors [14]. These growth factors are mostly a form of a bone morphogenic protein (BMP). There is no doubt that BMPs are important in the formation of bone, and the development of demineralized bone tissue forms by tissue banks has been an attempt to provide growth factors in a relatively inexpensive tissue.

There are two major types of demineralized bone available from tissue banks. The first is small segments of demineralized bone provided as chips or cubes. These have not been very popular because they have no structural integrity. The second type is demineralized bone matrix, which has been extremely popular and is used frequently by orthopedists and other surgical specialties.

Demineralized bone matrix can be prepared in several forms: paste, powder, putty, gels, ribbons, and a mixture of two or three of these. The most popular form is the paste and usually is available in 1, 5, and $10\,cm^3$ amounts. The paste is provided in a syringe and directed into the area in which the graft is needed.

Demineralized bone matrix was first developed as a means of making use of the shards and shreds of cortical bone remaining from preparation of cortical bone allografts such as wedges, strips, struts, or dowels. By morselizing these remnant pieces of bone and subjecting them to exposure to acid soaks followed by washes in buffered solution, a demineralized powder can result. In subsequent years, this successful grafting material was partly liquefied and became formable by the addition of a carrier component such as glycerol or hyaluronic acid. These grafts became known as "osteobiologics." With this approach, the active constituents of bone can be concentrated and formable to fill defects better, which represented a significant advance in the science of bone grafting.

Adjuvants and alternatives to bone grafts

BMP

In the 1960s Urist researched and described a protein found in bone that promotes bone formation. This protein did not become feasible for practitioner use until it was produced by recombinant means in 2003. Although this product, as currently available, is obviously not an allograft, the first isolates used by Urist were xenografts and allografts in the sense that they were isolated from the bones of cows and of humans.

Two forms of BMP are commercially available: OP-1™ (BMP-7) and Infuse™ (BMP-2). Both are human recombinant products and each has been shown to be very effective in stimulating and promoting bone formation.

The disadvantages of using commercially available BMPs are numerous. First, they are very expensive, ranging up to US$5000 for a single application. Second, if used in certain areas of the body, for example, in the cervical spine, they may cause an inflammatory response with adverse consequences. Third, the US Food and Drug Administration has limited the applications of these powerful drugs to specific indications such as single-level spine fusion or long bone non-union. Despite these limitations, the use of these products has expanded to the point where up to 90% of use is off-label (used in indications for which they were not originally approved by the Food and Drug Administration).

Bone substitutes (synthetics)

Bone substitutes are chemical concoctions that can be used as substitutes for allograft bone. They are osteoconductive because they provide a scaffold on which new bone can be deposited by the recipient's osteoblasts. Also known as synthetic bone, the three main categories of these products are calcium sulfate, calcium phosphate, and tricalcium phosphate [15]. Although there are also combinations of these chemicals available, all synthetics on the market to date are osteoconductive.

Bone substitutes were developed in part to avoid the possible risk of disease transmission from human bone allografts. However, the risk of disease transmission in allografts is very low today given the sensitivity of the tests available to screen human donors and improved donor risk-assessment screening techniques. In addition, processors of allograft bone have developed reliable methods of treating and sterilizing bone with minimal, if any, compromise of the graft's biomechanical structure.

The most attractive feature of synthetic bone substitutes is their capability to be formed into various shapes and sizes. This characteristic allows surgeons to pack the bone into spaces in which cancellous bone chips or cubes cannot be packed.

To improve the osteogenic potential of these osteoconductive products, many manufacturers recommend adding autograft bone to the product at the time of placement. Using trephines, bone slurry can be obtained from the iliac crest or distal femur or proximal femur and added to the synthetic bone when packing it. Although procurement of autograft is not a benign procedure, this method only requires a small incision over the bone from which the autograft is taken, which minimizes trauma and subsequent pain.

Organization of tissue banking

Bone transplantation is most frequently performed in the USA, but the use of allograft bone is becoming more common in Europe and Asia. In each of these areas, tissue bank organizations exist to provide exchange of ideas, development of standards, guidance for best practice, educational programs and broad representation of tissue bank constituents in the formation of national politics.

The American Association of Tissue Banks (AATB) was founded in 1976 by a group of orthopedic and transplant surgeons along with individuals who were managing the few tissue banks that existed in the USA at that time. Most of these individuals had served in the US Navy and were involved in the direction of the US Navy Tissue Bank.

Initially, the AATB was founded to be a member organization of tissue banks only. However, because there were less than a dozen tissue banks at the time that could provide tissues to surgeons throughout the USA, the AATB elected to grow by opening the organization to individual members, a decision that was strategic in its development. Currently, the AATB has over 1000 individuals and over 100 accredited tissue banks as members.

Regional tissue banks were established in Europe, first in the former Czechoslovakia (Hradec Kralove) in 1952, the former German Democratic Republic (Berlin) in 1956, in the UK (Leeds, Yorkshire) 1955, and in Poland (Warsaw) in 1962.

The European Association of Tissue Banks (EATB) was founded in 1991 at a meeting in Berlin, which was the 1st European Conference on Tissue Banking. Over 250 participants met and developed the idea that European banks should gather annually to discuss issues facing tissue banks in Europe that were different than those faced by US tissue banks. In Europe, compared with the USA, national governments were much more involved in the development of regulation of tissue banks. Hence, standards varied from country to country. The EATB has worked successfully toward standardizing the regulations to which European banks should adhere and the issuance of the European Directives for cells and tissues is another attempt at harmonization within the European Union.

There are additional tissue-bank organizations that have been started to address the need to bring interested parties together to review tissue-banking issues. Some of these include the Latin American, British, Spanish, and Australasian associations, as well as the Asia Pacific Association of Surgical Tissue Banking. Most of these organizations have developed relationships with the AATB and EATB.

Future use of allograft in orthopedics

One of the current issues in tissue banking is the lack of differentiation among allograft provided by various tissue banks. For example, bone chips and bone–tendon–bone allograft from one tissue bank are basically the same as similar allografts sourced from a different tissue bank. The donors are tested in the same manner, are screened for the same diseases and the grafts are prepared in similar ways. The final preparations often achieve a sterile product that works in a reliable and predictable fashion.

This situation is due in large part to the laudable efforts by the AATB to ensure that tissue banks follow the highest standards when preparing allografts. The result of the AATB efforts is that surgeons and patients can be confident that tissue allografts are safe and effective.

However, this situation also implies that the most commonly used bone and soft tissue allografts have become commodities rather than specialty items. In the future, because these allografts have become commodities, the major differentiation among grafts provided by tissue banks will be cost or price to the medical center purchasing the allografts.

In this circumstance, in which the major difference among the most commonly used orthopedic allografts is cost, several implications arise. First, the orthopedic surgeon becomes superfluous to the choice of allograft supplier because the low bidder will generally be the supplier. Contracts signed by a medical center will diminish or even eliminate the influence of the orthopedic surgeon. Second, tissue banks will become financially constrained and could find it difficult to pursue any capital-intensive projects involving research. This lack of funds will mean that fewer advances in tissue banking such as improved preparations of allografts will be developed in the future. Third, there may be a contraction among tissue banks as some are unable to meet the demands of competition.

Epilogue

In the early days of tissue banking, there were very few large tissue banks because there was little demand for allograft tissues. Early major banks in the USA included the Navy Tissue Bank and the University of Miami Tissue Bank. In the 1970s, as patients having spine surgery, revision arthroplasty surgery, and sports medicine surgery began to increase, the use of allografts in orthopedic surgery expanded rapidly. To meet the demand for allografts, several large tissue banks began operation. Now, however, with the standardization of tissue banking practices and the expansion of logistics that allow for rapid and easy movement of preserved tissues, the need for many tissue banks no longer exists. In the future, allografts for a country the size of the USA may be provided by less than half a dozen banks.

This does not mean, however, that there will be a need for fewer people in the field of tissue banking. The number of allograft transplants will continue to expand as orthopedists find new uses for tissues, and tissue banks will hopefully be able to respond to their needs.

KEY LEARNING POINTS

- Musculoskeletal allografts have been used for more than 100 years.
- Orthopedic surgeons use over 1 million orthopedic allografts annually.
- Tissue banks provide safe and effective allografts.
- Transplantation of musculoskeletal allografts provides the ability for recipients to return to normal activities after injury or disease.

References

1. Macewen W. Observations concerning transplantation of bone. Proc R Soc Lond 1881;32:232–47.
2. Lexer E. Substitution of whole or half joints from freshly amputated extremities by free plastic operation. Surg Gynecol Obstet 1908;6:601–7.
3. Carrel A. The preservation of tissues and its application in surgery. JAMA 1912;59:523–7.
4. Parrish FF. Allograft replacement of all or part of the end of a long bone following excision of a tumor: report of twenty-one cases. J Bone Joint Surg Am 1973; 55A:1–22.
5. Mankin HJ, Fogelson FS, Thrasher AZ. Massive resection and allograft replacement in the treatment of malignant bone tumors. N Engl J Med 1976;294:1247–55.
6. Enneking WF, Mindell ER. Observations on massive retrieved human allografts. J Bone Joint Surg Am 1991;73A:1123–31.
7. Gross AE, Beaver RJ, Zukor DJ, et al. The use of fresh osteochondral allografts to replace traumatic joint defects. In Orthopaedic Allograft Surgery Czitrom AA, Winkler H (eds.) Springer-Verlag, Vienna and New York, 1996; pp. 280–292.
8. Outerbridge RE. The etiology of chondromalacia patellae. J Bone Joint Surg 1961;43B:752–7.
9. DiCaprio MR, Enneking WF. Fibrous dysplasia. Pathophysiology, evaluation, and treatment. J Bone Joint Surg Am 2005;87:1848–64.
10. Ortiz-Cruz E, Gebhardt MC, Jennings LC, Springfield DS, Mankin HJ. The results of transplantation of intercalary allografts after resection of tumors. A long-term follow-up study. J Bone Joint Surg Am 1997;79:97–106.
11. Muscolo DL, Ayerza MA, Farfalli G, Aponte-Tinao LA. Proximal tibia osteoarticular allografts in tumor limb salvage surgery: Clin Orthop Relat Res. 2010;468: 1396–404.
12. DeGroot H 3rd, Mankin H. Total knee arthroplasty in patients who have massive osteoarticular allografts. Clin Orthop Relat Res 2000;373:62–72.

13. Deijkers RL, Bloem RM, Hogendoorn PC, Verlaan JJ, Kroon HM, Taminiau AH. Hemicortical allograft reconstruction after resection of low-grade malignant bone tumours. J Bone Joint Surg Br 2002;84:1009–14.
14. Urist MR, Mikolski AJ, Boyd SD. A chemosterilized antigen extracted bone morphogenetic alloimplant. Arch Surg 1975;110:416–420.
15. Neel MD. Bone grafting and bone graft substitutes. In Orthopaedic Knowledge Update: Musculoskeletal Tumors 2. Schwartz, HS (ed.) American Academy of Orthopaedic Surgeons, Chicago, 2009; pp. 41–53.

8 Neurosurgical Use of Bone Allografts and Dural Substitutes

Jau-Ching Wu[1] and Praveen V. Mummaneni[2]
[1]Taipei Veterans General Hospital, Taiwan
[2]University of California, San Francisco, CA, USA

Introduction

Neurosurgeons (and orthopedic surgeons) often need to replace the patient's intervertebral disc, bone, or dura with substitute materials. The underlying etiology can be owing to a spinal abnormality through degenerative disease or trauma, or patients can present with intracranial or spinal tumors that require dural replacement.

The scope of this chapter focuses on the most widely encountered grafting material in neurosurgery: grafts derived from bone. Dural grafts, used for the other commonly applied transplantation/repair procedures in neurosurgery, are also briefly discussed to give a complete portrayal of grafting in neurosurgery. The different graft materials are discussed based on their origin and respective advantages and disadvantages in clinical application.

Past

Neurosurgeons have adopted the fundamental strategy of using bone fusion to stabilize damaged spinal segments. Human vertebrae are responsible for maintenance of posture, generation of movement, and protection of critical nerve tissue. This leads to extreme complexity in surgical intervention for this anatomical region. By convention, success of spinal surgery is determined by the achievement of long-term stability, which can be facilitated by short-term instrumentation but requires bone fusion to make it

Tissue and Cell Clinical Use: An Essential Guide, First Edition. Edited by Ruth M. Warwick and Scott A. Brubaker.
© 2012 Blackwell Publishing Ltd. Published 2012 by Blackwell Publishing Ltd.

sustainable. Fusion inevitably depends on the materials applied and the methods of grafting. Thanks to great strides made in biomedical science, many approaches have emerged for applying and choosing bone, and various forms of bone, as graft material.

Anterior cervical spine surgery is one of the most common procedures in spinal surgery that requires the use of bone grafts. The history of the development of bone-grafting materials perfectly parallels evolution of bone graft applications in spinal surgery. A brief history of the evolution of development of graft material assists with understanding progression of procedures that use new grafts in neurosurgery. To minimize and control the variables in this discussion, most of the clinical evidence described pertains to anterior cervical interbody fusion, which is supported by an abundance of data in the medical literature. Although not directly described, analogies can be made with surgical repair of the lumbar spine (posterior lumbar interbody fusion).

History of anterior cervical interbody bone grafting

Anterior cervical spine surgery was not widely performed until the 1950s. In 1952 when Bailey and Bagley [1] first performed anterior cervical stabilization with an onlay autograft fusion harvested from the iliac crest. In 1955, Robinson and Smith [2] published their operative techniques of anterior discectomy with interbody grafting. In 1958, Cloward [3] also described a technique to treat herniated cervical discs using cylindrical bone autograft or allograft, for fusion. It seemed fortuitous that outstanding surgeons from different institutions in various parts of the world developed surgical techniques in the same era. Over the past few decades, anterior cervical discectomy and fusion (ACDF) has quickly gained popularity amongst spine surgeons to treat herniated discs and stenosis. ACDF is amongst the most successful procedures in contemporary spine surgery with excellent long-term results.

Initially, bone fusion in ACDF was performed using autograft, harvested from the patient's iliac crest, to fill the discectomy space. To obtain a piece of bone, another 3–5 cm incision has to be made parallel to the anterior superior iliac crest and 1 inch (≈ 2.5 cm) distal to the crest prominence to minimize the risk of injury to the lateral femoral cutaneous nerve. After sub-periosteal dissection for exposure of the crest, an oscillating saw is used to cut the desired size of tricortical autograft. Wound closure follows standard procedures. The middle third of the fibula can be used for autograft harvesting if a longer strut is required, as in corpectomy cases, when resection of the entire vertebrae is necessary. These two autograft sources have been used for many years. The quality of these grafts is usually optimal for fusion, but donor site morbidity is a problem that has never been completely overcome. Thus allograft has been widely used and is preferred.

Cloward [3–5] pioneered the use of allograft in cervical interbody fusion with reports of excellent fusion results. However, allografting has the inherent potential problem of disease transmission and localized immunogenic reactions. Tremendous effort has been devoted to searching for the best material that offers the fastest incorporation of graft into the neighboring vertebral bodies with the least morbidity and complications. Autografts collected from different anatomic sites, allografts that undergo a variety of processing treatments, and emergence of synthetic materials are the current options for fusion substrate. None of these options is perfect and each has its own merits and drawbacks.

Principles and processes of bone fusion

Bone itself, in vivo, is a biologically dynamic tissue continuously undergoing deposition, resorption, and remodeling. Bone fusion can be considered a process of healing in which metabolically active cells, matrices, and minerals are integrated into a rigid framework. The process is greatly influenced by hormonal, biochemical, biomechanical, anatomic, pathological, as well as genetic functions in each individual. For example, it is a well known clinical observation that bone fusion in spinal surgery is adversely affected in those patients who smoke cigarettes [6, 7]. Osteoporosis, a common and insidious disease, may lead to fusion failure owing to unbalanced bone resorption and metabolism.

Alternatively, patients with ankylosing spondylitis often have spontaneously fused spines as a consequence of over-reactive inflammation and healing, resulting in brittle kyphotic deformities. In neurosurgery and orthopedics, experience has shown that the biological activities of bone healing must be maximized to treat spinal diseases by stabilization (or fusion) of motion segments presenting with abnormal pathology. Three major physiologic properties directly influence the quality and rapidness of graft incorporation: osteogenesis, osteoinduction, and osteoconduction.

Osteogenesis is new bone formation through cellular proliferation by osteoblastic activity, which requires the presence of bone-forming cells, osteoprogenitor cells or osteogenic precursor cells. Osteogenesis potential is mostly found in fresh autologous bone grafts or bone marrow cells because they contain viable cells. Osteoinduction is the stimulation of precursor cells to differentiate into mature bone cells. Usually, the graft itself contains materials with such properties, or supplements can be added. The most well-known osteoinduction effects come from molecules like bone morphogenetic proteins (BMPs) and demineralized bone matrix (DBM). Osteoconduction refers to three-dimensional scaffolds into which viable bone cell growth and neovascularization can take place. This process is dependent on the physical properties of the material, such as porosity and pore size, architecture, and structural stiffness.

Biomechanical concerns

Wolff's law, a theory proposed in the nineteenth century by the German surgeon Julius Wolff, describes that mechanical stress is responsible for determining the architecture of bone [8]. In other words, bone adapts to the load it is placed under. In the presence of increased loading, bone remodeling will occur to make the bone stronger over time to resist the loads. To achieve arthrodesis, or interbody spinal fusion, certain amounts of loading must be present to induce remodeling. Because the spine itself serves to share axial loading, as long as the graft is properly manufactured and positioned, there is enough loading stress exerted on the graft-host interface to induce remodeling. Sometimes, in the process of graft incorporation, graft subsidence, a type of graft failure, may be encountered clinically. Subsidence (impaction of one bone surface through the bone–bone interface) can occur in the graft material itself, or in the host endplates above or below. Tailor-made graft materials with appropriate shapes and sizes that best fit individual biomechanical properties will yield the best fusion results.

Present

Today, synthetic bone grafts substitutes are widely available. Some genetically engineered or synthetic biomaterials have the unique advantage of avoiding rejection or biological contamination. Yet, even with the rising consumption of artificial bone fusion materials, the fact is that autograft and allograft bones are inexpensive options and remain widely used for spinal fusion in neurosurgery worldwide. Today, surgeons have four main considerations: (1) clinical efficacy, (2) autograft harvest morbidity, (3) cost, and (4) availability [9]. In addition, cultural and religious considerations may also have a bearing since some cultures do not accept allografts as a fusion option.

Autografts

Autograft bone is transplanted from one part of the body to another so the donor and the recipient are the same. It provides the three properties for successful bone fusion: osteogenesis, osteoinduction, and osteoconduction. Autograft contains viable osteoblasts and osteoprogenitor cells ready for osteogenesis. Endogenous BMPs convey osteoinduction in autografts. Moreover, autografts have similar bone quality and perfect biocompatibility and provide no antigenic insult.

In the clinical setting, the anterior iliac crest, posterior iliac crest, and fibula are among the most common sources of autografts. Cancellous bone allows excellent ingrowth of vasculature and matrix while cortical bone provides structural support, which is readily tailored for individual

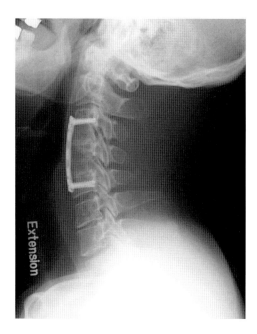

Figure 8.1 Autograft from anterior superior iliac crest used for two-level ACDF, 12 months postoperation.

circumstances. Many clinical studies have shown the superiority of autograft over allograft in graft incorporation and maintenance of disc height in ACDF [10–12] (Figure 8.1). The advantages become even more evident when multiple disc levels are fused. Harvesting autografts for bone fusion is the "gold standard" (Figure 8.2).

Use of autografts, however, can have disadvantages, the most notable being donor graft site morbidity (Table 8.1). In 1998, Menezes et al. [13] reported donor-site morbidity of 3.7% associated with use of rib graft and for iliac crest graft, 25.3%. Complications included pneumonia, persistent atelectasis, wound dehiscence, hematoma requiring evacuation, meralgia paresthetica, iliac spine fracture, and chronic donor-site pain. Other authors [14, 15] also reported various complications and morbidity rates between 26–39% for iliac crest bone harvest. Several series report relatively common morbidity of chronic donor site pain or dysesthesia from 17% to 34% for autograft bone harvested from the iliac crest. Other major complications from iliac crest harvesting in the literature are catastrophic bleeding and deep infection.

Moreover, autograft is of limited supply and requires extra surgical time and procedures to harvest. Patient age, gender, genetic make-up, systemic diseases, and physical wellness may complicate the quantity and quality of

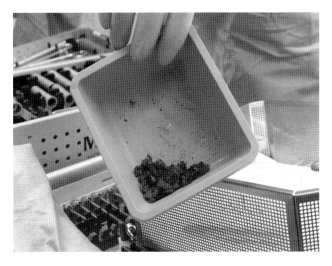

Figure 8.2 Autograft bone harvested from posterior iliac crest during surgery.

Table 8.1 Comparison of bone substitutes

	Clinical efficacy	Procurement morbidity	Potential for disease transmission	Cost
Autograft	+++	+	+++	+++
Allograft	++	+++	+	++
rhBMPs	+++	+++	+++	+
Ceramics	+	+++	+++	++

+, Least favorable; **++,** favorable; **+++,** most favorable.

available autologous bone. The associated cost of use of an autograft compared with other materials is difficult to estimate and lacks comprehensive analysis. Expenses may arise later owing to treating donor site morbidities, plus economic loss from prolonged recuperation.

Allografts

Allograft transplantation is when a graft is used and the donor and recipient are members of the same species. For neurosurgical applications, allograft bone is derived from a deceased donor and the graft is either decontaminated or may undergo a process to sterilize it. Processing methods can influence the rate at which a graft will incorporate in the recipient. Autograft surpasses allograft in terms of bone fusion partly owing to its viable, non-immunogenic cells and abundance of BMPs that optimize osteogenesis and osteoinduction.

Allografts may stimulate localized immune response in the recipient, and can cause delayed fusion [12, 16].

For allografts, balancing clinical efficacy and graft-associated complication is a primary consideration but there are variables in allograft preparation and preservation. Frozen allografts can be readily available and are stored in freezers colder than −20°C, and often as low as −80°C, then simply thawed and washed when prepared for use. Grafts can also be provided as freeze-dried (lyophilized), where preserving the graft entails cooling to −70°C and, under pressure, water is extracted to the point where the residual moisture content of the graft is generally less than 8%. Freeze-dried preparations decrease graft antigenicity, resulting in a reduced incidence of cell-mediated response in the host. Rehydration of lyophilized allografts is recommended before implantation because the low moisture content can result in a brittle graft that should not be subjected to weight bearing loads until properly reconstituted. Access to an inventory of frozen allografts requires that a freezer be purchased and maintained, and the storage temperature continuously monitored, whereas access to an inventory of lyophilized allografts is more easily maintained "on a shelf." Packaging configurations for lyophilized allografts are challenged to maintain a vacuum during their shelf-life while stored. These factors can play a role in which graft type is available for use by the neurosurgeon and in the wider context of whether supporting infrastructure is available in the hospital or country where the procedure takes place.

Fresh-frozen allografts have 10–20% less compression strength but similar bending strength compared with autografts. In contrast, freeze-dried allografts are reduced in bending strength by 50–90% while maintaining their compressive strength. As a consequence, freeze-dried allografts are more susceptible to longitudinal cracks [17]. Some allograft handling processes also involve radiation treatment to sterilize the allograft. Research demonstrates that use of low dose radiation has no adverse effect on graft strength [17].

Various animal and clinical studies compare the clinical efficacy of allograft with autograft. Care must be taken in translating these results into clinical relevance. The fusion environment must be taken into account. For instance, bone grafts used for interbody fusion in anterior cervical discectomy and posterior–lateral lumbar fusion have different requirements. For fresh grafts, cortical bone provides better structural support, but cancellous bone provides a better source of osteoblasts and osteocytes. For spinal column interbody fusion, the cortical component provides resilience to the compression force between two vertebral endplates. However, its limited surface area and stiffness also hinder vascular ingrowth and remodeling. Nevertheless, in circumstances requiring faster new bone formation rather than structural strength, such as with posterior lateral lumbar fusion, use of cancellous bone grafts may yield better results. Clinical studies have compared fusion potential between autografts and allografts in ACDF. High fusion rates are reported in single level cervical arthrodesis in both groups [16, 18]. Floyd and Ohnmeiss [10] report a meta-analysis that includes 310 patients with 379 intervertebral levels of anterior cervical fusion. For both one- and two-level ACDF, there are higher rates of radiographic union and lower incidences of graft collapse with use of autografts versus allografts.

Internal fixation devices can influence fusion rate in ACDF. Zdeblick and Ducker [12] compared the use of freeze-dried allografts and autografts in 87 patients without use of anterior cervical plating. In one-level cervical arthrodesis, there are similar fusion rates of 95% in both groups, but allografts require longer fusion time and have higher incidences (30%) of graft collapse, measured at more than 2 mm compared with autografts (5%). A prospective comparison of 77 patients using autografts versus allografts with demineralized bone matrix composite by An et al. [11] demonstrated that for single-level fusions, 26.3% of patients with autografts had pseudoarthrosis, non-fusion, at one year follow-up versus 47% of patients with allografts; and 11% of autograft patients had graft collapse of more than 3 mm versus 19% in allograft patients. Bishop et al. [6] reported a prospective comparison of 178 fusion levels in 132 patients with freeze-dried tricortical allografts or autografts from the iliac crest. For single-level fusion, higher fusion rate (97% versus 87%) and less graft height collapse (14% versus 24%), which could cause neural foraminal stenosis, were noted in the autograft group. For multiple-level fusion, higher fusion rate was still found in the autograft group (100% versus 89%). Despite high fusion rates reported for both groups at the study endpoint, radiographic non-union was found more in the allograft group in the 12-month follow-up (27% versus 6% in single-level; 47% versus 13% in multi-level fusion), which implied slower fusion for allografts. These fusion results were all obtained without use of any internal fixation devices.

Anterior cervical plating has prevailed because it facilitates fusion and decreases graft subsidence [19, 20]. Kaiser et al. [21] retrospectively reviewed 251 patients who underwent single- or two-level ACDF with cortical allograft. In those who had undergone anterior fixation, fusion rates were 96% and 91% (single- and two-level, respectively) compared with those who did not use anterior plate fixation (90% and 72%, respectively). The favorable effect of plating when combined with allograft becomes more prominent when fusion level increases. Thus the introduction of internal fixation in ACDF, the anterior cervical plate and screw, has made allograft more popular clinically.

The superiority of autograft over allograft in terms of graft incorporation and disc height maintenance is less significant in single-level ACDF using fixation devices and is counter-balanced by the relatively high donor site morbidity. Because allografts offer nearly the same fusion rates as autografts in single-level fusion, attention has been directed towards using autografts for multi-level fusion, or special conditions, such as cigarette smokers [11]. The clinical dilemma of harmonization with fusion ability and comorbidity depends on individualized access-related comorbidity and evaluation of patients.

There is also the issue of availability of allografts since this varies in different cultures and countries, and the supply available in a local inventory can be variable. The shortage of allograft supply can be due to several reasons such as high demand, as sometimes seen in the USA, or the lack of donors due to religious beliefs. For instance, Far Eastern societies may prefer to keep the deceased body intact precluding tissue donation. In other parts of the world, it is still not culturally acceptable for patients to receive implants from the dead. In such cultures and religions, there is a bias towards synthetic materials.

Other bone substitutes for spinal fusion

As technology progresses, many materials have come under trial and some demonstrate great potential as substitutes for bone graft. Demineralized bone matrices (DBMs), ceramics, and spacers of varying kinds have attracted enormous attention.

DBMs are produced by the pulverization and acidic extraction of allograft bone. Collagen and proteins, including growth factors, with capacity for osteoinduction and osteoconduction, are retained after processing. DBMs have no structural strength and their activity for osteoinduction is not consistent. The heterogeneity is caused by the manufacturing process or quality of donor bone.

The use of DBMs for spinal fusion have been studied both in pre-clinical and clinical trials. Some results are positive [22, 23], whereas others are not [11]. Current literature implies that using it as bone graft extender [22, 24] or in conjunction with other structural supporting device is reasonable (Figure 8.3). In practice, the use of DBMs may be overtaken by the trend towards recombinant BMPs in the near future.

Ceramics and synthetic cages or other artificial implantable devices have been marketed for years as bone substitutes and these synthetic devices eliminate the risk of disease transmission from the deceased donor. They are available in unlimited quantity and can be machined into specified sizes and shapes as desired. Ceramics, such as hydroxyapatite and tricalcium phosphate, have the capacity for osteoconduction but are brittle and susceptible to shearing force. Thus, ceramics are better as graft expanders but need to be used in conjunction with internal fixation owing to lack of structural support strength [25].

Some clinical studies have demonstrated results that are not favorable to the use of stand-alone ceramics in anterior interbody fusion both in cervical and lumbar spines [26, 27]. The chemical structure is similar to mineral

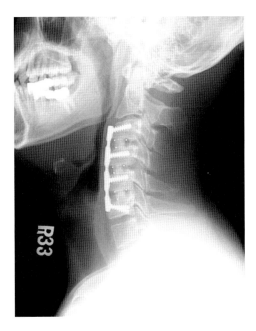

Figure 8.3 Carbon fiber cages containing DBM used for three-level ACDF, 12 months postoperation.

bone, facilitating cellular adhesion and vascular ingrowth for new bone formation but ceramics lack osteogenic and osteoinductive activities, so the local host environment will profoundly affect the efficacy of bone fusion. Therefore, appropriate implant site selection, decortication, and presence of bone marrow or autologous bone grafts as sources of osteogenic progenitor cells are crucial to the successful incorporation of ceramics into newly formed bone. The rate of resorption and remodeling depends on the composition and porosity of the ceramics. Studies disclose that ceramics work well with autologous bone grafts as expanders, so they are potential candidates as vehicles for osteoinductive agents like BMPs [28].

Cages were first developed by Bagby [29] for interbody spinal fusion in horses [30]. The Bagby cage was a stainless steel basket made as a container for autograft bone. Later, its application evolved and expanded, research ensued. Cages are now available in polyetheretherketone (PEEK), carbon fiber, and titanium. Initially, they were cylindrical and used in the lumbar spine by the anterior approach. Now, they can be fabricated into variable shapes and can be placed through several routes into different spinal segments (Figure 8.4).

Cages are used as spacers with capacity for grafting materials of various kinds, sustaining compression-distraction force in the intervertebral disc space. According to the current literature, there is no single type of material

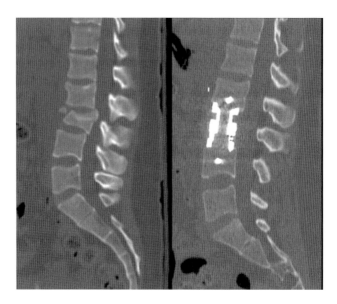

Figure 8.4 Sagittal computed tomography scan demonstrating L3 burst fracture. Left, pre-operation; right, titanium cage filled with autograft bone was used for L2–4 fusion, 6 months postoperation; solid bone growth was identified.

that is superior to others in terms of cervical arthrodesis [31]. Nonetheless, excellent clinical outcomes have been reported using cages in spinal fusion procedures [32–35]. The merits of the devices are structural stiffness and potential to accommodate other graft materials. This type of device is particularly advantageous in selected clinical scenarios, such as for patients who are smokers who need multi-level anterior cervical arthrodesis, where yielded solid fusion using PEEK cages combined with recombinant human (rh)BMPs has been successful [36, 37].

Bone morphogenetic proteins

In 1965, Marshall Urist [38] first discovered that degradation products of dead bone matrix, which was referred to as extracellular matrix, had materials capable of inducing new bone formation when implanted in rabbit connective tissue. In 1971 the effective component was termed bone morphogenetic protein (BMP) [39, 40]. This seminal discovery led to the purification, isolation, and identification of BMP peptides. The term BMPs now refers to a group of growth factors and cytokines that have the capability to induce bone or cartilage formation. Originally, seven such proteins were discovered, and they were therefore termed BMP-1 through BMP-7. Thirteen further BMPs have since been identified.

Initially it took huge amounts of bone to extract a small amount of BMPs because they only comprise a small percentage of bone proteins. Until the development of recombinant DNA technology, BMPs were very rare and extremely expensive. Nowadays, although still costly, rhBMPs are available in high purity and concentration for animal experiments as well as clinical use. Recombinant BMP-2 (rhBMP-2) and recombinant BMP-7 (osteogenic protein-1: OP-1) have been the most studied and have shown the most potency amongst the BMP family.

Clinical application of rhBMPs requires a carrier. rhBMPs are soluble and easily dissolve in vivo, so they must be placed in high concentration within a vehicle to provide controlled release over time. Otherwise, they become inactivated and lose the capacity for osteoinduction. Numerous trials are currently reinvestigating the best vehicle and controlled release of rhBMPs for clinical use. Boden et al. have compared the use of rhBMP-2 in collagen sponge with autograft from the iliac crest filled into threaded cages for lumbar spine interbody fusion. Although there are only a small number of cases, bone fusion is more reliable with rhBMP-2 [41].

Boden et al. also [42] conducted a prospective randomized study for use of rhBMP-2 in posterolateral lumbar fusion. Twenty-five patients were randomized into three groups: autograft with pedicle screw fixation instrumentation, rhBMP-2 with instrumentation, and rhBMP-2 without instrumentation. The rhBMP-2 was applied in the carrier consisting of 60% hydroxyapatite and 40% tricalcium phosphate granules. There was bone fusion in all (100%) of those who received rhBMP-2, with and without instrumentation. On the other hand, only 40% of patients who received autograft had fusion. Several other clinical studies also demonstrated the superiority of rhBMP-2 over autografts or allografts in lumbar spine interbody fusion [43–45], even though a few studies pointed out that rhBMP-2 might cause significant bone resorption of implanted grafts before osteoinduction [46, 47].

In summary, clinical experience has shown that the prudent use of rhBMP-2 in lumbar spinal surgery is more beneficial than allografts or autografts alone. Clinical application of rhBMP-2 has focused on cervical spinal fusion in recent years. Preliminary data have shown early and solid fusion results using rhBMP-2 in anterior cervical fusion [36, 48–50]. Adverse reactions, such as local swelling, dysphagia, and hematoma formation, have been reported as complications of high dose rhBMP-2 use in ACDF and these problems have resulted in a warning from the US FDA to avoid use of rhBMP-2 for anterior cervical surgery [51, 52].

Cahill et al. demonstrated that immediate complication rates comparing the use and non-use of BMPs have no difference in lumbar, thoracic, and posterior cervical fusion [53]. The complication rate is higher in anterior cervical fusion with BMPs in terms of dysphagia, voice, and wound related problems. Whether these complications in anterior cervical fusion are dose dependent remains unclear. Genetic engineering products pose substantial burden on medical expenses, which need analysis for cost-effectiveness. Despite the recent considerable growth in the use of BMPs, more research is needed to determine the indications, optimal dosage, and vehicle to use, as well as resolution of clinical issues including adverse reactions.

Future

State-of-the-art advances in science and technology, including rhBMPs, synthetic fusion devices, and instrumentation, have changed the practice of spinal fusion in neurosurgery. Since the introduction of bone fusion procedures in spine surgery decades ago, many experts in either procurement or processing have refined techniques. However, inherent shortcomings, such as donor site morbidity, limited supply, and risk of disease transmission, related to transplantation of autograft and allograft bone, have never been completely eliminated (Table 8.1). Nowadays, interbody fusion with rhBMPs and cages already demonstrate efficacy in fusion results [48] (especially in patients at high risk for fusion failure such as those with end-stage renal disease, diabetics, or recipients who smoke). Currently, unsolved issues are optimization of controlled local inflammation induced by cytokines, selection of synergistic vehicles, and cost cutting.

Gene therapy also sheds light on future clinical applications. Gene transduction in local host cells for sustainable production of bioactive proteins was originally designed for treatment of some hereditary diseases. In recent studies, successful genetic transduction of genetic codes for bioactive proteins, which facilitate bone fusion, has been performed in animals [54, 55]. Developments in gene therapy show the potential for reducing current requirements of high-dose rhBMPs, which may help minimize local adverse reactions. However, concerns for safety when viral vectors are used in gene transduction need further investigation before clinical application can be realized. Transplantation of mesenchymal stem cells for enhancement of bone fusion has been tried in animal models as well as in the clinical setting [56–58].

As technology rapidly advances, all of the enhancers or alternatives for bone fusion described above have shown promise in revolutionizing bone fusion techniques in spinal surgery. Although there is still a long way to go for the physiologic restoration of complex spinal functions, innovations including intervertebral disc transplantation [59], artificial disc replacement, synthetic fusion devices, gene therapy, and stem cell transplantation are deserving of further investigation. More research in bone biology as well as spinal kinematics is essential to corroborate the safety and efficacy of all these treatment modalities.

Special address on neurosurgical use of dural grafts

Introduction

Neurosurgical procedures very often involve intradural manipulation, and closure of the dural sac to restore the integrity of the central nervous system has been a perpetual challenge. There are circumstances where dural defects are not amenable to reconstruction using sutures, including posterior fossa surgery, skull base tumor resection, and severe craniofacial trauma. Sometimes, neurosurgeons tend to create a generous circulating space for cerebrospinal fluid as well as neural tissue, such as in Chiari malformation correction or decompressive craniectomy, where duraplasty with graft is needed. The ideal dural substitute should offer the following: (1) no risk of disease transmission; (2) minimal inflammation or adhesion; (3) texture and flexibility similar to natural dura; (4) availability in sufficient quantity and low cost; and (5) a watertight closure to prevent cerebrospinal fluid leakage (Table 8.2) [60].

Past

In the history of neurosurgery, over 50 kinds of material have been used as dura substitutes with various results reported in literature. Duraplasty was first proposed in 1890 by Beach using gold foil, but was not performed until two years later and was reported in the literature only in 1897 [61, 62]. Abbe received credit in some literature for performing duraplasty in 1895 using rubber [63]. Numerous kinds of material have been attempted ever since, but only a few have been popularized. These dural grafts can be categorized into biological (i.e., autologous, allogeneic, and xenogeneic) and synthetic materials.

Processed pooled allogeneic dural grafts from deceased donors were used widely worldwide until 1987, when a case report drew great attention from the public health standpoint. A young woman, aged 28, who underwent

Table 8.2 Comparison of dural substitutes

	Biocompatibility (inflammation and adhesion)	Disease transmission	Quantity	Cost	Watertightness
Autologous	+++	+++	+	+++	+++
Allogeneic	++	+	++	++	+++
Xenogeneic	+	++	+++	+	+++
Synthetic	?	+++	+++	+	Varies

+, Least favorable; ++, favorable; +++, most favorable. ?, equivocal.

duraplasty with Lyodura® (B. Braun Melsungen AG, Germany) 19 months previously, presented with gait ataxia, myoclonus, and dementia. Her brain biopsy disclosed spongiform encephalopathy characteristic of Creutzfeldt–Jakob disease (CJD) [64, 65]. Allogeneic dura graft-related CJD has subsequently been reported worldwide [66–68], with the largest numbers in Japan. By 2008, 132 cases of CJD in Japan had been reported through national surveillance, all of whom had received allograft dura mater between 1978 and 1993 [69].

The deadly neurodegenerative disease CJD has been transmitted iatrogenically by corneal transplantation, deep brain electrodes, brain surgery instruments, as well as growth hormones derived from human pituitary glands. It is evident from the Japanese experience that there is an extraordinarily long incubation period between graft receipt and symptom onset, with an average of 11.8 years (range 1.2–24.8 years). It is reasonable to assume that the cases of human transmissible spongiform encephalopathies (TSEs) transmitted by allografts will continue to grow over time.

The actual estimated transmission rate in Japan is very low (less than 0.2%) but the disease has been irreversible and fatal in all reported cases. This has significantly changed neurosurgeons' attitudes toward the use of allograft dura, which is no longer commonly used. On the other hand, well-processed human fascia lata graft has been used as a dural substitute and in urological and orthopedic reconstructive surgery. So far, there is no report of CJD transmission through allogeneic fascia lata transplantation, probably because of its distant location from the central nervous system and because it is not pooled during processing. Allogeneic grafts other than allograft dura are thus still among the choices as dural substitutes for neurosurgeons [62, 70].

Present

Autologous grafting, with pericranium or temporalis fascia, is thought to have the least rejection and risk of disease transmission. These grafts have the best biological behavior and are inexpensive. However, it is not always possible to harvest autografts, particularly when there are skull fractures, as the pericranium is usually damaged. The most widely reported source of autologous material for duraplasty is fascia lata, especially when large areas of graft are needed. As expected, many reports demonstrate better clinical results yielded by autologous grafts [71, 72]. Despite these advantages, autologous dural graft, as with other types of autologous tissue, has not been popular with most neurosurgeons or patients mainly because it often requires a second wound incision, consumes more surgical and anesthesia time, and poses a risk of donor site morbidity. Nonetheless, in selected cases, when there is a small dural defect, local transplantation of autologous pericranium graft or fascia results in excellent clinical results [73, 74].

Xenogeneic grafts come from organisms of different species and are thus theoretically more prone to induce immunologic responses than human donor grafts. Pericardium, dermis, fascia lata, and peritoneum from bovine, ovine, or porcine donors are among the most common sources. Reports in literature demonstrate good clinical outcome with the use of xenogeneic grafts, including fascia, pericardium, and dura mater [75]. A small series of 35 patients reported by Anson and Marchand also demonstrated good clinical results using bovine pericardium graft as a dural substitute [76]. Over the past few decades, the abundance of supply has made its use welcome in many countries. Although bovine pericardium has the merit of uniform thickness, strength, flexibility, possible low immunogenicity, and relatively low cost compared with allogeneic dural grafts, its use has not been demonstrated to be completely free of zoonosis.

Synthetic materials of many kinds have gradually earned popularity as dural substitutes for a variety of reasons. They share common advantages of unlimited supply and little chance of disease transmission. Several clinical series demonstrate the feasibility and efficacy of these materials, including polyester urethane, expanded polytetrafluoroethylene, and biosynthetic cellulose [60, 77, 78]. However, there is still a lack of strong evidence to justify the replacement of biological grafts. The benefit of using synthetic dural substitutes may not outweigh their cost compared with use of bone grafts owing to less donor site morbidity when using autologous fascia.

Future

The development of biotechnology has changed the face of duraplasty in terms of materials used. Sutureless closure and the use of biological sealants have been introduced to facilitate and expedite surgical procedures. Debates on the comparison between all of the substances and techniques neurosurgeons use for duraplasty remain unsettled.

CASE STUDY 8.1

A 66-year-old male with a history of hepatocellular carcinoma presented with progressive mid back pain and right sided weakness for the past 5 days. His hepatic tumor was surgically resected 8 months previously, and he had already undergone chemotherapy. There was asymmetrical decreased sensation in his lower limbs, and on examination his right quadriceps demonstrated grade 4/5 muscle power. Bladder and bowel function was mildly impaired. Computed tomography scan demonstrated

(Continued)

an osteolytic lesion at T5 (Figure 8.5). The thoracic spinal magnetic resonance imaging revealed an enhancing mass lesion at the T5 level with thecal sac compression (Figure 8.6). Findings were compatible with a metastatic tumor causing thoracic myelopathy.

Owing to his debilitating pain and neurological deficit, a surgical decompression and stabilization of the thoracic spine was recommended. He underwent standard thoracic laminectomy for resection of the lesion and internal fixation with pedicle screws (Figure 8.7). Allograft bone was used as a fusion substrate. No autologous bone graft was used for fusion because of the possible contamination of his iliac bone marrow with metastatic neoplasm. His neurological function reached full recovery after surgery.

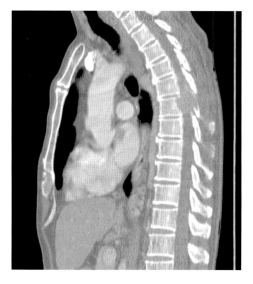

Figure 8.5 Sagittal computed tomography scan demonstrating an osteolytic lesion at T5.

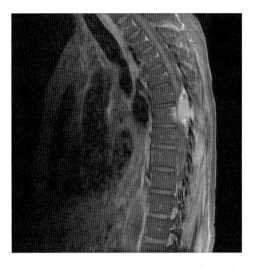

Figure 8.6 Thoracic magnetic resonance imaging revealed an enhancing mass lesion at the T5 level with severe thecal sac compression.

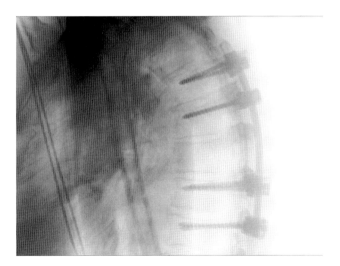

Figure 8.7 Thoracic laminectomy for resection of the lesion and internal fixation with pedicle screws was performed. Allograft bone was used as a fusion substrate.

KEY LEARNING POINTS

- The principles and processes of bone fusion and the main physiological properties – osteogenesis (new bone formation through cellular proliferation by osteoblastic activity), osteoinduction (the stimulation of precursor cells to differentiate into mature bone cells), and osteoconduction (three-dimensional scaffolds into which viable bone cell growth and neovascularization can take place) – are essential for successful bone grafting.

- Features and preparations of each bone substitute are important considerations when selecting the appropriate material to use.

- There are advantages and disadvantages to using various bone substitutes for spinal fusion and repair.

- Historically, use of pooled processed dura allograft was the cause of transmission of disease (CJD) that resulted in deaths.

- There are both advantages and disadvantages to using currently available dural substitutes.

References

1. Bailey RW, Badgley CE. Stabilization of the cervical spine by anterior fusion. J Bone Joint Surg Am 1960;42A:565–94.
2. Robinson R, Smith GW. Anterolateral cervical disc removal and interbody fusion for cervical disc syndrome. Bull Johns Hopkins Hosp 1955;96:223–4.
3. Cloward RB. The anterior approach for removal of ruptured cervical disks. J Neurosurg 1958;15(6):602–17.
4. Cloward RB. Vertebral body fusion for ruptured cervical discs. Am J Surg 1959;98:722–7.
5. Cloward RB. Gas-sterilized cadaver bone grafts for spinal fusion operations. A simplified bone bank. Spine 1980;5:4–10.
6. Bishop RC, Moore KA, Hadley MN. Anterior cervical interbody fusion using autogeneic and allogeneic bone graft substrate: a prospective comparative analysis. J Neurosurg 1996;85:206–10.
7. Glassman SD, Anagnost SC, Parker A, Burke D, Johnson JR, Dimar JR. The effect of cigarette smoking and smoking cessation on spinal fusion. Spine 2000;25:2608–15.
8. Frost HM. A 2003 update of bone physiology and Wolff's Law for clinicians. Angle Orthod 2004;74:3–15.
9. Deutsch H, Haid R, Rodts G, Jr., Mummaneni PV. The decision-making process: allograft versus autograft. Neurosurgery 2007;60(1 Suppl 1):S98–102.
10. Floyd T, Ohnmeiss D. A meta-analysis of autograft versus allograft in anterior cervical fusion. Eur Spine J 2000;9:398–403.

11. An HS, Simpson JM, Glover JM, Stephany J. Comparison between allograft plus demineralized bone matrix versus autograft in anterior cervical fusion. A prospective multicenter study. Spine 1995;20:2211–6.
12. Zdeblick TA, Ducker TB. The use of freeze-dried allograft bone for anterior cervical fusions. Spine 1991;16:726–9.
13. Sawin PD, Traynelis VC, Menezes AH. A comparative analysis of fusion rates and donor-site morbidity for autogeneic rib and iliac crest bone grafts in posterior cervical fusions. J Neurosurg 1998;88:255–65.
14. Heary RF, Schlenk RP, Sacchieri TA, Barone D, Brotea C. Persistent iliac crest donor site pain: independent outcome assessment. Neurosurgery. 2002;50:510–6; discussion 6–7.
15. Silber JS, Anderson DG, Daffner SD, Brislin BT, Leland JM, Hilibrand AS, et al. Donor site morbidity after anterior iliac crest bone harvest for single-level anterior cervical discectomy and fusion. Spine 2003;28:134–9.
16. Malloy KM, Hilibrand AS. Autograft versus allograft in degenerative cervical disease. Clin Orthop Relat Res 2002;394:27–38.
17. Pelker RR, Friedlaender GE. Biomechanical aspects of bone autografts and allografts. Orthop Clin North Am 1987;18:235–9.
18. Brown MD, Malinin TI, Davis PB. A roentgenographic evaluation of frozen allografts versus autografts in anterior cervical spine fusions. Clin Orthop Relat Res 1976;119:231–6.
19. Caspar W, Geisler FH, Pitzen T, Johnson TA. Anterior cervical plate stabilization in one- and two-level degenerative disease: overtreatment or benefit? J Spinal Disord 1998;11:1–11.
20. Wang JC, McDonough PW, Endow KK, Delamarter RB. Increased fusion rates with cervical plating for two-level anterior cervical discectomy and fusion. Spine 2000;25:41–5.
21. Kaiser MG, Haid RW, Jr., Subach BR, Barnes B, Rodts GE, Jr. Anterior cervical plating enhances arthrodesis after discectomy and fusion with cortical allograft. Neurosurgery 2002;50:229–36; discussion 36–8.
22. Girardi FP, Cammisa FP, Jr. The effect of bone graft extenders to enhance the performance of iliac crest bone grafts in instrumented lumbar spine fusion. Orthopedics 2003;26(5 Suppl):s545–8.
23. Vaccaro AR, Stubbs HA, Block JE. Demineralized bone matrix composite grafting for posterolateral spinal fusion. Orthopedics 2007;30:567–70.
24. Cammisa FP, Jr., Lowery G, Garfin SR, Geisler FH, Klara PM, McGuire RA, et al. Two-year fusion rate equivalency between Grafton DBM gel and autograft in posterolateral spine fusion: a prospective controlled trial employing a side-by-side comparison in the same patient. Spine 2004;15;29:660–6.
25. Miyazaki M, Tsumura H, Wang JC, Alanay A. An update on bone substitutes for spinal fusion. Eur Spine J 2009;18:783–99.
26. Thalgott JS, Fritts K, Giuffre JM, Timlin M. Anterior interbody fusion of the cervical spine with coralline hydroxyapatite. Spine 1999;24:1295–9.
27. Thalgott JS, Klezl Z, Timlin M, Giuffre JM. Anterior lumbar interbody fusion with processed sea coral (coralline hydroxyapatite) as part of a circumferential fusion. Spine 2002;27:E518–25; discussion E26–7.
28. Autefage H, Briand-Mesange F, Cazalbou S, et al. Adsorption and release of BMP-2 on nanocrystalline apatite-coated and uncoated hydroxyapatite/beta-tricalcium phosphate porous ceramics. J Biomed Mater Res B 2009;91:706–15.

29. Bagby GW. Arthrodesis by the distraction–compression method using a stainless steel implant. Orthopedics 1988;11:931–4.
30. McAfee PC. Interbody fusion cages in reconstructive operations on the spine. J Bone Joint Surg Am 1999;81:859–80.
31. Ryken TC, Heary RF, Matz PG, et al. Techniques for cervical interbody grafting. J Neurosurg Spine 2009;11:203–20.
32. Hacker RJ. A randomized prospective study of an anterior cervical interbody fusion device with a minimum of 2 years of follow-up results. J Neurosurg 2000;93 (2 Suppl):222–6.
33. Hacker RJ, Cauthen JC, Gilbert TJ, Griffith SL. A prospective randomized multi-center clinical evaluation of an anterior cervical fusion cage. Spine 2000;25:2646–54; discussion 55.
34. Ryu SI, Mitchell M, Kim DH. A prospective randomized study comparing a cervical carbon fiber cage to the Smith–Robinson technique with allograft and plating: up to 24 months follow-up. Eur Spine J 2006;15:157–64.
35. Thome C, Leheta O, Krauss JK, Zevgaridis D. A prospective randomized comparison of rectangular titanium cage fusion and iliac crest autograft fusion in patients undergoing anterior cervical discectomy. J Neurosurg Spine 2006;4:1–9.
36. Boakye M, Mummaneni PV, Garrett M, Rodts G, Haid R. Anterior cervical discectomy and fusion involving a polyetheretherketone spacer and bone morphogenetic protein. J Neurosurg Spine 2005;2:521–5.
37. Tumialan LM, Pan J, Rodts GE, Mummaneni PV. The safety and efficacy of anterior cervical discectomy and fusion with polyetheretherketone spacer and recombinant human bone morphogenetic protein-2: a review of 200 patients. J Neurosurg Spine 2008;8:529–35.
38. Urist MR. Bone: formation by autoinduction. Science 1965;150:893–9.
39. Urist MR. Bone histogenesis and morphogenesis in implants of demineralized enamel and dentin. J Oral Surg. 1971;29:88–102.
40. Urist MR, Strates BS. Bone morphogenetic protein. J Dent Res 1971;50:1392–406.
41. Boden SD, Zdeblick TA, Sandhu HS, Heim SE. The use of rhBMP-2 in interbody fusion cages. Definitive evidence of osteoinduction in humans: a preliminary report. Spine 2000;25:376–81.
42. Boden SD, Kang J, Sandhu H, Heller JG. Use of recombinant human bone morphogenetic protein-2 to achieve posterolateral lumbar spine fusion in humans: a prospective, randomized clinical pilot trial: 2002 Volvo Award in clinical studies. Spine 2002;27:2662–73.
43. Burkus JK, Dorchak JD, Sanders DL. Radiographic assessment of interbody fusion using recombinant human bone morphogenetic protein type 2. Spine 2003;28:372–7.
44. Burkus JK, Transfeldt EE, Kitchel SH, Watkins RG, Balderston RA. Clinical and radiographic outcomes of anterior lumbar interbody fusion using recombinant human bone morphogenetic protein-2. Spine 2002;27:2396–408.
45. Slosar PJ, Josey R, Reynolds J. Accelerating lumbar fusions by combining rhBMP-2 with allograft bone: a prospective analysis of interbody fusion rates and clinical outcomes. Spine J 2007;7:301–7.
46. McClellan JW, Mulconrey DS, Forbes RJ, Fullmer N. Vertebral bone resorption after transforaminal lumbar interbody fusion with bone morphogenetic protein (rhBMP-2). J Spinal Disord Tech 2006;19:483–6.

47. Pradhan BB, Bae HW, Dawson EG, Patel VV, Delamarter RB. Graft resorption with the use of bone morphogenetic protein: lessons from anterior lumbar interbody fusion using femoral ring allografts and recombinant human bone morphogenetic protein-2. Spine 2006;31:E277–84.

48. Baskin DS, Ryan P, Sonntag V, Westmark R, Widmayer MA. A prospective, randomized, controlled cervical fusion study using recombinant human bone morphogenetic protein-2 with the CORNERSTONE-SR allograft ring and the ATLANTIS anterior cervical plate. Spine 2003;28:1219–24; discussion 25.

49. Takahashi T, Tominaga T, Watabe N, Yokobori AT, Jr., Sasada H, Yoshimoto T. Use of porous hydroxyapatite graft containing recombinant human bone morphogenetic protein-2 for cervical fusion in a caprine model. J Neurosurg 1999;90(2 Suppl): 224–30.

50. Lanman TH, Hopkins TJ. Early findings in a pilot study of anterior cervical interbody fusion in which recombinant human bone morphogenetic protein-2 was used with poly(L-lactide-co-D,L-lactide) bioabsorbable implants. Neurosurg Focus 2004;16: E6.

51. Shields LB, Raque GH, Glassman SD, et al. Adverse effects associated with high-dose recombinant human bone morphogenetic protein-2 use in anterior cervical spine fusion. Spine 2006;31:542–7.

52. Vaidya R, Carp J, Sethi A, Bartol S, Craig J, Les CM. Complications of anterior cervical discectomy and fusion using recombinant human bone morphogenetic protein-2. Eur Spine J 2007;16:1257–65.

53. Cahill KS, Chi JH, Day A, Claus EB. Prevalence, complications, and hospital charges associated with use of bone-morphogenetic proteins in spinal fusion procedures. JAMA 2009;302:58–66.

54. Boden SD, Titus L, Hair G, et al. Lumbar spine fusion by local gene therapy with a cDNA encoding a novel osteoinductive protein (LMP-1). Spine 1998;23: 2486–92.

55. Helm GA, Alden TD, Beres EJ, et al. Use of bone morphogenetic protein-9 gene therapy to induce spinal arthrodesis in the rodent. J Neurosurg 2000;92(2 Suppl): 191–6.

56. Gan Y, Dai K, Zhang P, Tang T, Zhu Z, Lu J. The clinical use of enriched bone marrow stem cells combined with porous beta-tricalcium phosphate in posterior spinal fusion. Biomaterials 2008;29:3973–82.

57. Minamide A, Yoshida M, Kawakami M, et al. The use of cultured bone marrow cells in type I collagen gel and porous hydroxyapatite for posterolateral lumbar spine fusion. Spine 2005;30:1134–8.

58. Wang T, Dang G, Guo Z, Yang M. Evaluation of autologous bone marrow mesenchymal stem cell-calcium phosphate ceramic composite for lumbar fusion in rhesus monkey interbody fusion model. Tissue Eng 2005;11:1159–67.

59. Ruan D, He Q, Ding Y, Hou L, Li J, Luk KD. Intervertebral disc transplantation in the treatment of degenerative spine disease: a preliminary study. Lancet 2007;369: 993–9.

60. Danish SF, Samdani A, Hanna A, Storm P, Sutton L. Experience with acellular human dura and bovine collagen matrix for duraplasty after posterior fossa decompression for Chiari malformations. J Neurosurg 2006;104(1 Suppl):16–20.

61. Caroli E, Rocchi G, Salvati M, Delfini R. Duraplasty: our current experience. Surg Neurol 2004;61:55–9; discussion 9.

62. Costantino PD, Wolpoe ME, Govindaraj S, et al. Human dural replacement with acellular dermis: clinical results and a review of the literature. Head Neck 2000; 22:765–71.

63. Bejjani GK, Zabramski J. Safety and efficacy of the porcine small intestinal submucosa dural substitute: results of a prospective multicenter study and literature review. J Neurosurg 2007;106:1028–33.

64. Update: Creutzfeldt-Jakob disease in a patient receiving a cadaveric dura mater graft. MMWR Morb Mortal Wkly Rep 1987;36:324–5.

65. Thadani V, Penar PL, Partington J, Kalb R, Ssen R, Schonberger LB, et al. Creutzfeldt-Jakob disease probably acquired from a cadaveric dura mater graft. Case report. J Neurosurg 1988;69:766–9.

66. Brooke FJ, Boyd A, Klug GM, Masters CL, Collins SJ. Lyodura use and the risk of iatrogenic Creutzfeldt-Jakob disease in Australia. Med J Aust 2004;180:177–81.

67. Will RG. Acquired prion disease: iatrogenic CJD, variant CJD, kuru. Br Med Bull 2003;66:255–65.

68. Brown P, Preece M, Brandel JP, et al. Iatrogenic Creutzfeldt-Jakob disease at the millennium. Neurology 2000;55:1075–81.

69. Update: Creutzfeldt-Jakob disease associated with cadaveric dura mater grafts – Japan, 1978–2008. MMWR Morb Mortal Wkly Rep 2008;57:1152–4.

70. Dufrane D, Marchal C, Cornu O, Raftopoulos C, Delloye C. Clinical application of a physically and chemically processed human substitute for dura mater. J Neurosurg 2003;98:1198–202.

71. Martínez-Lage JF, Perez-Espejo MA, Palazon JH, Lopez Hernandez F, Puerta P. Autologous tissues for dural grafting in children: a report of 56 cases. Childs Nerv Syst 2006;22:139–44.

72. Malliti M, Page P, Gury C, Chomette E, Nataf F, Roux FX. Comparison of deep wound infection rates using a synthetic dural substitute (neuro-patch) or pericranium graft for dural closure: a clinical review of 1 year. Neurosurgery 2004;54: 599–603; discussion 4.

73. Stevens EA, Powers AK, Sweasey TA, Tatter SB, Ojemann RG. Simplified harvest of autologous pericranium for duraplasty in Chiari malformation Type I. Technical note. J Neurosurg Spine 2009;11:80–3.

74. Rosen DS, Wollman R, Frim DM. Recurrence of symptoms after Chiari decompression and duraplasty with nonautologous graft material. Pediatr Neurosurg 2003;38:186–90.

75. Parizek J, Mericka P, Husek Z, et al. Detailed evaluation of 2959 allogeneic and xenogeneic dense connective tissue grafts (fascia lata, pericardium, and dura mater) used in the course of 20 years for duraplasty in neurosurgery. Acta Neurochir 1997;139:827–38.

76. Anson JA, Marchand EP. Bovine pericardium for dural grafts: clinical results in 35 patients. Neurosurgery 1996;39:764–8.

77. Yamada K, Miyamoto S, Takayama M, et al. Clinical application of a new bioabsorbable artificial dura mater. J Neurosurg 2002;96:731–5.

78. Narotam PK, van Dellen JR, Bhoola KD. A clinicopathological study of collagen sponge as a dural graft in neurosurgery. J Neurosurg 1995;82:406–12.

9 The Use of Allografts in Sports Medicine

Scott A. Rodeo[1], Alexander E. Weber[2], René Verdonk[3], Joan C. Monllau[4], and Eva-Lisa Heinrichs[5]

[1]The Hospital for Special Surgery, New York, NY, USA
[2]University of Michigan, Ann Arbor, MI, USA
[3]Ghent University Hospital, Ghent, Belgium
[4]Universitat Autònoma de Barcelona, Barcelona, Spain
[5]Orteq Ltd, London, UK

A brief history of allograft use in sports medicine

Orthopedic transplantation scholars refer to the origin of their discipline in 1668 when Job van Meekeren reported on grafting a defect in a soldier's cranium with bone from a dog's skull. Bone grafting ideas evolved through scientists like Van Leeuwenhoek, Duhamel, De Heyde, and Ollier, describing the structure of bone and callus formation as well as ontogenesis in the late seventeenth and the early eighteenth centuries [1]. The term "creeping substitution" as developed by Barth, Curtis, and Phemister at the turn of the nineteenth century seemed to be the most important contribution setting the stage for clinical bone transplantation. Indeed, the first allograft procedure in orthopedic practice was performed by Sir William Macewen in 1880 for treatment of an infected humerus in a young boy. In 1915, Dr Fred H. Albee's work was published and widened the use of allograft tissue.

More recently, soft tissue allografts have been used in sports medicine for replacement of meniscus, ligament, and osteochondral defects. Ligament reconstruction using tendon allografts has become a popular choice in surgery. The advantages of allograft include increased versatility of the graft, elimination of the time needed for collecting autograft tissue and autograft morbidity, and an easier postoperative recovery. In complex procedures, autograft harvesting may not be possible because of the need for multiple grafts.

The use of musculoskeletal allograft tissue has been rising extensively since the end of the century, increasing from estimates of 350,000 in 1990

Tissue and Cell Clinical Use: An Essential Guide, First Edition. Edited by Ruth M. Warwick and Scott A. Brubaker.
© 2012 Blackwell Publishing Ltd. Published 2012 by Blackwell Publishing Ltd.

to more than 850,000 in 2001 in the USA [2]. Despite this dramatic increase in efficient use of allografts, most surgeons (73%) report concern about safety regarding graft sterility and potential for disease transmission. Contemporary sterilization processes may adversely affect tissue quality and long-term efficacy [3].

No autograft alternative exists when the clinician is confronted with sequelae arising from total meniscectomy. Meniscal allograft represents a viable clinical alternative.

Milachowski and Wirth in 1984 first described meniscal allografting when confronted with a meniscus-deficient knee. They considered meniscal replacement as an addition to extensive ligament repair to stabilize the knee joint effectively [4]. Only later did isolated meniscal allografting become an indication in painful meniscectomized knee joints. Initially, lyophilized menisci were used. However, these grafts were found to undergo shrinkage and some degree of resorption. Thus, other techniques have developed using cryopreservation and fresh-frozen preservation [4–6].

Gross et al. developed fresh osteochondral allografts for reconstruction of osteoarticular defects. They found osteochondral allograft survival at 25 years based on retrieval studies [7]. Freezing osteochondral tissue adversely affects chondrocyte viability [8], which has led to the use of cryopreserved allografts with increased cell viability. However, cryopreservation still has limitations, as only the surface cells are preserved [9, 10]. This has led to the use of fresh tissue, which can contain viable chondrocytes.

Present status of allograft use in sports medicine

Allograft tissues are currently used in sports medicine applications for treatment of ligament, meniscus, and cartilage injuries. Although the most common applications are in the knee, allograft tissue is being used increasingly for reconstruction of injury in the shoulder, elbow, hip, and ankle. This chapter reviews the risks associated with the use of connective tissue allografts and potential adverse outcomes of allograft use (such as disease transmission and immunologic reaction), current protocols for tissue treatment and processing, current indications for allograft use, issues related to size matching, and current outcome data.

General risks associated with connective tissue allografts

Despite advances in allograft tissue recovery and preparation, there is potential risk of transmitting disease. In modern times, the major viral infectious agents to be considered are human immunodeficiency virus (HIV) and hepatitis B and C viruses (HBV and HCV). Recently, concern has shifted also to consider new pathogens such as Chagas' disease, West Nile virus, Cruetzfeldt–Jakob disease, Q fever, and other emerging or re-emerging infections. Currently, the estimated probability of a tissue donor in the USA having HIV at the time of donation is 1 in 173,000 [11]. The first case of HIV infection through allograft tissue occurred in 1984, before HIV screening of donors began [12]. The most recent case of HIV infection through allograft tissue occurred from a donor recovered in 1985, which was long ago when screening techniques and testing requirements lacked the sophistication of risk reduction measures used today. There have been no reported cases of HIV transmission using allograft during the past 25 years, in large part because of the implementation of more stringent donor screening and testing protocols that include the use of nucleic acid testing. This methodology has markedly decreased the window period for the detection of HIV and HCV [11, 13].

In the USA, the probability that a tissue donor has HCV is estimated at 1 in 421,000 [11]. In 2003 the US Centers for Disease Control and Prevention (CDC) reported a patient was infected with HCV after an anterior cruciate ligament (ACL) reconstruction using allograft tissue. Further investigation concluded that this particular graft was procured from a donor that had tested negative for HCV antibody upon original serologic testing but was found to be HCV positive during subsequent testing using HCV nucleic acid testing [14]. This case illustrated the difficulty of detecting HCV infection in a donor when using only a standard enzyme immunoassay serology test. This type of donor screening test can detect antibody produced after exposure to the hepatitis C virus but only when antibody production is at a detectable level by the test being used, and when a qualified (undiluted) blood sample is collected and tested. As of August 2007, the US Food and Drug Administration has required tissue banks in the USA to test all tissue donors using a nucleic acid testing assay for HIV-1 and HCV [15, 16]. American Association of Tissue Banks (AATB)-accredited tissue banks were required to implement these more sensitive tests over two years earlier, by March 9, 2005.

The risk of bacterial infection from musculoskeletal allograft tissue is increased compared with the risk of viral transmission. The estimated incidence of allograft associated bacterial infection is 1 in 250,000 cases [16]. In 2002 the CDC released a report of 26 cases of allograft-associated bacterial infection [17]. Half of the 26 cases resulted in clostridial infections, and eight of those infections involved allograft used in ACL reconstructions. In each case the processor of the tissue failed to detect contamination in the allograft. Delay in procurement of allograft tissue can allow hematogenous spread of bacterial flora into musculoskeletal tissues to be recovered [18]. In response to the CDC report, the American Academy of Orthopaedic Surgeons formed a Tissue Banking Project Team to collaborate with both the US Food and

Drug Administration and CDC with hopes of further regulating donor tissue recovery. Allografts that are minimally processed to support the maintenance of cell viability may pose the highest risk of bacterial contamination because some chemical and detergent treatment methods cannot be used to greatly reduce or eliminate contaminants that may be present.

Despite reports of allograft-associated infections, there are few studies comparing infection rates of knee surgery with allograft tissue and those with autograft tissue. In 2005, Crawford and colleagues reviewed 331 ACL reconstructions (290 allograft and 41 autograft) and found 11 infections in their allograft group compared with 0 infections in their autograft group. Owing to the generally small numbers in their two treatment groups this difference was not statistically significant [19]. Another study reviewed 170 autograft and 628 allograft reconstructions and found no difference in infection rates [20].

Immunologic response to connective tissue allografts

In general, a clinically evident immune response does not occur after implantation of connective tissue allografts. The dense matrix of these tissues shields the resident cells from immunoreactive cells in the host. Furthermore, the freezing process (used routinely for tendon and meniscus allografts) is said in the literature from the 1980s to reduce immunogenicity [21, 22]. However, the molecular structure of cell-surface histocompatibility antigens is preserved even after freeze–thaw cycles. For example, a generalized expression of class I and class II human leukocyte antigen (HLA) antigens was found in the endothelial and synovial cells of meniscus tissue even after two freeze–thaw cycles [23]. Also, matrix proteins themselves may be immunogenic. Thus, an immune response does seem likely to occur at the microscopic level. Indeed, a microscopic immune response has been documented after implantation of allograft meniscus and tendon [24, 25]. This response may affect graft revascularization and graft incorporation, but there is little evidence to suggest that an immune response plays an important role in the clinical outcome of soft tissue grafts. At this time, the use of immunosuppressive agents or matching for HLA antigens is not recommended.

Current protocols for tissue treatment and processing

After procurement and testing for infectious diseases, musculoskeletal allograft tissues must be processed and preserved or prepared for storage and later shipment to the end user. Traditionally, many tissues used in sports medicine applications are frozen. The freezing process generally maintains biomechanical properties (i.e., strength) but can kill many cells. Gamma irradiation has been used to decrease bacterial contamination but the levels of irradiation required to eradicate viral DNA (such as HIV) can adversely affect the tissue material properties [26]. As a result, new proprietary techniques have been developed that allow sterilization while protecting the tissue during the treatment process. These proprietary techniques use novel chemicals, oxygen free-radical scavengers, low oxygen tension environments (such as in a vacuum), or very low temperatures to minimize the adverse effects of gamma irradiation. Alterations in matrix proteins caused by tissue processing may adversely affect eventual graft healing and incorporation; thus, further study is required to evaluate the effect of these new graft processing techniques on graft function and clinical outcome.

Indications for soft tissue allografts in sports medicine

Meniscus

Meniscus allograft tissue is used to replace absent meniscal tissue in order to restore the important functions of the meniscus. The primary function of the meniscus is to transmit load across the tibiofemoral joint and thus decrease contact stress on the articular cartilage. It is well established that meniscus deficiency accelerates the onset of osteoarthritis. Thus, it is reasonable to assume that meniscus replacement may forestall or possibly prevent the progressive degenerative changes that occur in the meniscus-deficient knee. The typical indication for meniscus transplantation is a patient who has undergone previous meniscectomy and who has developed symptoms of early arthrosis (pain and joint swelling) (Figure 9.1 and Plate 9.1). Meniscus transplantation is indicated for knees with only minimal articular cartilage degeneration, as clinical experience has demonstrated poorer results in knees with more advanced arthrosis. Meniscus transplantation as an isolated procedure is also contraindicated in knees with malalignment. For example, a medial meniscus transplant should not be done in a knee with uncorrected varus alignment. Concomitant ligamentous instability and chondral damage are not absolute contraindications as it is possible to correct instability with ligament reconstruction or chondrosis with a cartilage resurfacing procedure. These corrective procedures are described in the literature as being performed before, or in conjunction with, meniscal transplantation [27–30]. Figure 9.2 provides an illustrative case example where meniscus transplantation was combined with other procedures for joint reconstruction.

The menisci also play a role in joint stability, as the medial meniscus serves as a secondary stabilizer to anterior–posterior translation. Absence of the medial meniscus leads to increased stress on an ACL reconstruction graft and can lead to increased failure rates [31]. Medial meniscus replacement

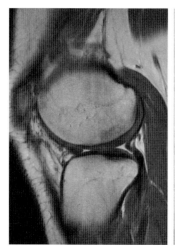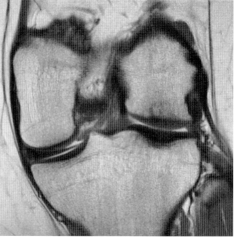

Figure 9.1 A 15-year-old female status after resection of a discoid lateral meniscus, resulting in complete absence of the lateral meniscus. This was treated with a lateral meniscus allograft transplant. Preoperative MRI demonstrating absence of the lateral meniscus with intact articular cartilage on the femur and tibia.

is thus considered in the setting of ACL reconstruction where previous meniscectomy has been performed, which is a rather common clinical situation.

Osteochondral allograft

Osteochondral allograft tissue is used to replace an injured or deficient segment of a joint surface. Several options exist for treatment of smaller chondral lesions, such as microfracture, autologous chondrocyte implantation, or osteochondral autograft tissue implantation. Autograft osteochondral transplantation is an option for smaller defects; however, this technique has size restrictions given that the donor cartilage must be collected from another zone of the affected knee. Therefore, the current indications for autograft osteoarticular transplantation are for defects less than 2–3 cm [32, 33]. In defects larger than 2–3 cm, osteochondral allograft transplantation has become a viable and successful treatment option [34–37] (Figure 9.2). Allograft tissue is also indicated if there is significant bone loss. The most common location where osteochondral tissue is used is for one of the femoral condyles in the knee. Other anatomic locations include the talus and humeral head.

Osteochondral grafts may be provided fresh, fresh frozen, cryopreserved, or cold-stored (refrigerated) in culture medium. The freezing process renders most of the cells in the graft non-viable, so most surgeons no longer use

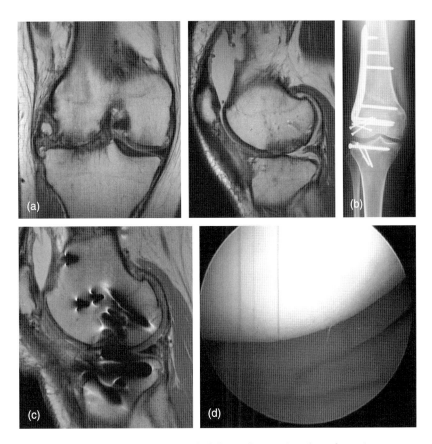

Figure 9.2 A 25-year-old female with failure of a previous lateral meniscus transplantation and osteochondral autograft procedure. There is cartilage loss on the lateral femoral condyle and architectural deformity of the lateral tibial plateau, with absence of the lateral meniscus, and valgus malalignment. This was addressed with a combined procedure consisting of (1) lateral tibial hemi-plateau allograft with an attached lateral meniscus, (2) cold-stored viable osteochondral allograft to lateral femoral condyle, and (3) varus-producing distal femoral osteotomy. (a) Preoperative MRI showing lateral compartment arthrosis; (b) postoperative radiograph following the above procedure; (c) postoperative MRI showing reconstructed lateral compartment; (d) Arthroscopic view of lateral compartment one year after allograft reconstruction.

fresh frozen tissue. The value of maintaining cell viability is that these cells are required to maintain cartilage matrix homeostasis, thus providing potentially better long-term graft structure and function. Fresh osteochondral allografts have viable chondrocytes but are also more immunogenic, which may adversely affect graft incorporation [3]. Fresh allografts also must be implanted within several days of procurement, which for the surgeon creates difficult logistics as far as scheduling a patient for surgery and for the tissue bank in ensuring all the safety checks are completed within a tight time frame. The cryopreservation process involves controlled-rate freezing of the graft in the presence of chemicals (large molecules such as glycerol) to preserve cell viability. However, the cryopreservation process typically only preserves viability of cells in the superficial cartilage layer owing to poor penetration of the cryoprotectant. Cold-stored grafts can have viable cells in the cartilage matrix. Cold-stored osteochondral allografts allow preservation of viable chondrocytes while easing the logistical challenges attendant to the use of fresh tissue. These allografts are currently stored at refrigerator temperature for a minimum of 14 days to allow for serologic and microbiologic testing before implantation. Chondrocyte viability in refrigerated grafts has been shown to decrease gradually over time, so implantation within 28 days is recommended. Further studies are required to substantiate the long-term benefits of implanting grafts with viable cells.

Allogeneic chondrocytes for articular cartilage repair

Chondrocyte implantation has been used for treatment of articular cartilage defects in the knee. The standard technique uses autologous cells that are harvested from an unaffected area of the joint. These cells are then cultured for several weeks before re-implantation into a cartilage defect. A significant limitation of this technique is the need for a separate procedure to harvest the cartilage biopsy. Allograft chondrocytes would allow an "off-the-shelf" source of chondrocytes. A recent study demonstrated promising results using allogeneic chondrocytes suspended in alginate beads to treat a chondral defect in the knee in 21 patients [38]. Human chondrocytes maintain their phenotype in alginate, as evidenced by continued synthesis of the important cartilage matrix molecules collagen II and aggrecan. More recently, allograft chondrocytes from juvenile donors (under 13 years of age) has become commercially available. The rationale for the use of juvenile chondrocytes is the higher synthetic capacity of juvenile tissue [39].

Ligament reconstruction

Tendon allografts are commonly used for ligament reconstruction in the knee. The most common indication for allograft use is anterior cruciate ligament reconstruction. Ruptures of the ACL are the most commonly reported complete ligamentous injury in the knee. It is estimated that more than 250,000 Americans elect to undergo ACL reconstruction each year [40]. Allograft is used, in particular, for revision ligament reconstruction and for older patients. Allograft tendon is also used for reconstruction of other knee ligaments, such as the posterior cruciate ligament, collateral ligaments, and medial patellofemoral ligament.

Another relatively common indication for allograft use is multiple ligament reconstruction, where it is essentially impossible to collect adequate autologous tissue. In the case of a multiligamentous injury to the knee, where there is injury to one or both cruciate ligaments as well as a collateral ligament, the need for multiple tissue grafts makes allograft tissue an attractive option. Allograft in this case can provide tissue of sufficient size, strength, and length for complex reconstructions of the knee. Allograft tissue also affords the benefits of decreased operative time with no donor-site morbidity in an already traumatized knee [41].

Allograft tendon is also used for soft tissue reconstruction in other anatomic locations. Some examples include reconstruction of the lateral ligaments in the ankle, coracoclavicular ligaments in the shoulder, and lateral collateral ligament in the elbow. Soft tissue allografts have also been used to replace or augment deficient/weakened shoulder capsule in patients with recurrent shoulder instability who have failed previous surgical repair (Figure 9.3 and Plate 9.2).

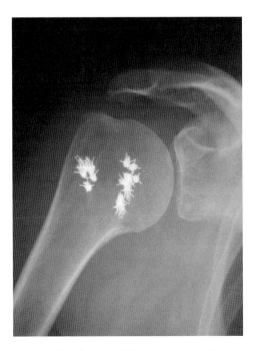

Figure 9.3 A 30-year-old female with Ehlers–Danlos syndrome (connective tissue abnormality leading to tissue laxity and weakness), with recurrent shoulder instability after several previous surgical repairs. There was deficiency of the shoulder capsule. This was treated with Achilles tendon allograft to reconstruct both the anterior and posterior shoulder capsule. Postoperative radiograph showing suture anchors in the glenoid margin and proximal humerus that were used to secure the allograft tissue.

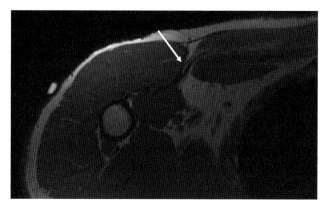

Figure 9.4 A 40-year-old patient with a failed pectoralis major tendon repair with tissue deficiency. This was treated with revision repair and use of an Achilles tendon allograft to augment the repair. Preoperative MRI showing pectoralis major tendon rupture and deficiency of the distal tendon (arrow).

Tendon repair

Allograft tendon tissue can be used to augment repair of poor quality or attenuated tendon, such as for patellar tendon, quadriceps tendon, or pectoralis major tendon repair (Figure 9.4 and Plate 9.3). This is often required in the setting of revision surgery or in situations where there is tissue loss, such as after previous infection. Allograft tissue has special application for extensor mechanism reconstruction in the knee and is often the only viable treatment option for chronic tendon ruptures with tissue deficiency.

Allograft sizing

Meniscus

Appropriate size matching of osteochondral and meniscus allograft tissue is critical. A meniscus must match the size of the recipient's tibial plateau. Size matching for meniscal transplants is typically done using plain radiographs to measure the width (medial–lateral dimension) and length (anterior–posterior) of the recipient tibial plateau. Magnetic resonance imaging (MRI) may also be used to make these measurements. Most tissue banks supply the allograft meniscus with the attached tibial plateau, so the sizing is done by simply matching the bone dimensions of the graft to the patient. However, if the tissue bank only supplies the meniscus with no bone attached, as some banks do, it is necessary to use direct measurements of meniscus dimensions, such as height and width. The meniscus dimensions in the contralateral knee can be used as a guide, but the contralateral meniscus may not be an identical "mirror image" of the involved meniscus. At this time the tolerance of the joint to size mismatch is not known, but it is recommended that the transplanted meniscus be within 2–3 mm of the length and width of the native meniscus.

Osteochondral allograft

Osteochondral allograft tissue consists of a segment of bone and overlying cartilage that is used to replace an injured area of the joint surface. The critical issue related to sizing of osteochondral allograft tissue is the need to match the radius of curvature of the joint surface. The grafts are matched based on measurements of bone dimensions. The tissue bank typically provides the whole joint segment, i.e., the entire medial or lateral femoral condyle. Thus, the surgeon chooses the site from which to harvest the graft intra-operatively based on the exact location of the cartilage lesion that requires treatment. As such, the ability to resurface exactly the joint depends to some degree on surgeon experience and judgment. In the future, computer navigation approaches may improve accuracy in choosing the best site on an osteochondral allograft to reproduce most accurately the architecture and radius of curvature of a joint surface.

Ligament/tendon

No specific sizing is required for tendon allografts that are used for ligament reconstruction or for augmentation of tendon repair. The most commonly used tendons include patellar tendon, Achilles tendon, and posterior tibial tendon. The only concern is graft length, which is typically not a concern as there is usually adequate length available.

Clinical outcomes

Meniscus

Most outcome data are from retrospective studies. These studies demonstrate predictable improvement in symptoms of pain and swelling in properly selected patients. Since the original description of meniscal allograft transplantation, outcome studies have demonstrated that meniscus transplantation can result in improved knee joint function and good to excellent subjective outcomes in the medium term [42–46]. The current literature describes good or excellent subjective results in approximately 85% of meniscal allograft transplantations [47]. The overall success of meniscus transplantation is directly correlated to the degree of degenerative joint disease, such that knees with more advanced arthritis have less predictable results. Despite generally good clinical outcomes as far as symptom improvement, direct evaluation of the transplanted meniscus by arthroscopic inspection and MRI often demonstrates gradually progressive degenerative changes in the transplant. These changes include fragmentation, tears, and extrusion of the meniscus. These adverse changes are likely caused by the harsh biomechanical environment in the degenerative knee. We have found a direct correlation between the MRI appearance of the meniscus transplant and the degree of degenerative change in the respective tibio-femoral compartment [48]. In particular, gradual changes in the morphology of the joint surface as evidenced by flattening of the condyle is associated with a higher failure rate of meniscus transplantation.

There are currently very few data to suggest that meniscus transplantation can change the natural history once there is degenerative joint disease present. Although it is reasonable to postulate that meniscus transplantation can prevent or delay progressive articular cartilage degeneration, there is currently very little data available to answer this question. Further long-term studies are required to define better the role of meniscus transplantation in preventing progressive degenerative changes after meniscectomy.

Osteochondral allograft

Recent work by several authors suggests two factors are crucial for long-term success after osteochondral allograft transplantation. The first is that the long-term durability of the allograft is dependent on the ability of the chondrocytes to synthesize cartilage extracellular matrix [49–51]. The second is that to prevent bony collapse, the allograft bone must be remodeled by host cell repopulation of the allograft bone [52, 53].

Current clinical studies demonstrate generally favorable outcomes after transplantation of osteochondral allograft tissue. These grafts can restore joint surface architecture by replacing both bone and cartilage. Clinical results are generally good as far as improvements in symptoms of pain and swelling. Long-term follow-up of fresh osteochondral allograft transplantation has resulted in good to excellent subjective results with a mean survival of 12 years [7]. Clinical experience with cold-stored and cryopreserved osteochondral allografts is less extensive and long-term results are not currently available. However, mid-term clinical outcome studies of cryopreserved osteochondral allografts have shown comparable patient-centered results [54, 55]. A recent report of 23 patients treated with a refrigerated osteochondral allograft found good clinical results at average three-year follow-up. Radiographic evaluation at final follow-up revealed that 22 of the 23 grafts were in stable position with good osseous incorporation into host bone, with no graft failures [56].

Ligament grafts

Allograft tendon has been used for ligament reconstruction in the knee for many years, in particular for ACL reconstruction. The results of allograft ligament reconstruction have been generally comparable to reconstructions using autograft tissue. Although there is still debate about the clinical success of allograft compared with autograft, two recent systematic reviews of the literature suggest that when evaluating the general population undergoing ACL reconstruction, clinical outcomes are equivalent when either autograft or allograft tissue is used [57, 58].

Of interest to many sports medicine surgeons is the performance of ACL reconstructions in the young, highly active, or elite athlete patient population. This cohort of patients has different needs and desires for rehabilitation and return to play. Recent studies have reported higher failure rates in young, highly active patients undergoing ACL reconstruction with fresh-frozen allograft. Age less than 25 years was found to be a significant risk factor for graft failure in a cohort of patients treated with Achilles allograft ACL reconstructions [59]. Similar results were reported from the Multi-center Orthopedic Outcomes Network prospective cohort database [60]. These authors controlled for age and gender while using logistic regression analysis to determine the role of activity level after reconstruction and/or graft type (allograft tibialis tendon versus autograft hamstring tendon) on the rate of graft failure. They found that higher activity level after ACL reconstruction and allograft use were both independent risk factors for graft failure and that when coupled together (i.e., a highly active patient undergoes ACL reconstruction with allograft tissue) there is a multiplicative increase in the likelihood of ACL graft failure [60].

Other tendon and ligament reconstructions

There is very little rigorous data on the outcomes of allograft use for less common indications such as medial patellofemoral ligament reconstruction or for augmentation of chronic tendon ruptures. In the case of medial patel-lofemoral ligament reconstruction allograft usage has shown 90% good to excellent results in a recent case series of 20 patients treated for recurrent patella dislocations [61]. For chronic proximal hamstring ruptures in which the tendon is retracted from its origin, Folsom and Larson have described augmenting the repair with Achilles tendon allograft with results compara-ble to primary repair of acute proximal hamstring ruptures [62]. In similar fashion to the proximal hamstring, the patellar tendon is primarily repaired in acute cases; however, in chronic patellar tendon rupture reconstruction with allograft tissue may be required and has shown good to excellent clini-cal outcomes [63].

Future applications in sports medicine

New approaches to partial meniscus replacement

The treatment of irreparable meniscal tears remains a major challenge for the orthopedic community today. Removal of all or part of the meniscus eventually leads to degenerative changes of the articular cartilage and subsequent clinical symptoms [64] The current treatment of choice for irreparable meniscus tears is partial meniscectomy, which aims to remove only the pathologic or torn tissue thereby minimizing risk to the articular cartilage. Total meniscectomy is now almost completely obsolete; however, it still remains necessary for large irreparable tears [64]. The use of meniscal allografts has proved promising in patients with meniscus tissue loss; however, it is generally only used in patients who have undergone total or subtotal meniscectomy. [64]

Until recently, for young, active adults who desire a return to pre-injury functionality and who have many productive years ahead of them, no satisfactory solution has been available to replace or regenerate meniscal tissue. For such patients, provided they have correct alignment and normal ligament status, partial meniscal tissue regeneration is an emerging possibility. The use of meniscal scaffolds to regenerate the lost tissue has become a valid treatment option. Two are described next.

Menaflex™

The Menaflex, former collagen meniscus implant (CMI), was developed from bovine collagen in the early 1990s to promote meniscal regeneration in segmental defects of meniscal tissue [65]. Experimental and clinical experience with the medial CMI, so far, have shown promising results [66–68] and a lateral CMI has recently been developed. Evidence supporting CMI-promoted regrowth of meniscal-like tissue has been provided [66]. This prospective randomized trial included more than 300 patients with an irreparable medial meniscus injury or previous partial medial meniscectomy. The patients were divided into two study arms: an acute group with no previous surgery to the medial meniscus and a chronic group with up to three previous surgeries to the involved meniscus. The patients were randomized either to undergo CMI treatment or partial medial meniscectomy (controls). Second-look arthroscopies and biopsies performed in the CMI patients one year postoperatively showed that the implant was able to produce new meniscus-like tissue. Furthermore, after an average follow-up of five years, the patients in the chronic group regained significantly more of their lost activity than did the control patients, and they underwent significantly fewer operations.

The device is placed in the space where a damaged meniscus has been removed, and is anchored to the surrounding tissue. After implantation, the matrix is invaded by cells and undergoes a process of remodelling. The CMI has already been applied clinically for partial meniscus replacement. Subsequently, the formation of a newly formed meniscus was observed in over two thirds of cases. Selecting the suitable candidate is one of the key factors in achieving a successful outcome. The knee must be stable and well aligned. Technically, a secure intra-articular attachment is probably the most critical factor in achieving implant stability and function. Therefore, the surgeon should be familiar with current meniscus repair and reconstruction techniques and skilled in performing them.

Actifit™ implant

Research has demonstrated that a biocompatible, degradable polyurethane scaffold (Actifit developed by Orteq Ltd.), with proven cellular ingrowth potential in animal models (ovine and canine models) [69–71], is safe and effective for the treatment of irreparable meniscal tears or meniscal tissue loss. Tailored to the meniscal defect, the scaffold provides a three-dimensional matrix enabling vascular ingrowth, thereby facilitating tissue regeneration to replace the surgically removed tissue. The primary aim of this treatment is to provide pain relief and restore functionality.

It is intended for use in the treatment of irreparable, partial meniscal tissue defects to reduce pain and restore compromised functionality by restoring the load-bearing and shock-absorbing capacity of the meniscus. Actifit™ is available in two configurations, medial and lateral, to fit the corresponding defect.

Candidates suitable for implantation must have an intact meniscal rim and sufficient tissue present both in the anterior and the posterior horns to allow for secure fixation. In addition, the candidates should have a well-aligned stable knee, a body mass index (BMI) below 35kg/m^2, and must be free from systemic disease or infection sequelae. Cartilage damage should not exceed an International Cartilage Repair Society classification of grade 3. Long-term data showing chondroprotection postimplantation of Actifit are not yet available. Once such data become available, Actifit could also be indicated for acute partial meniscectomies not yet affected by chronic disability.

Safety, performance, and efficacy results to support the use of Actifit in the treatment of irreparable meniscal tears or meniscus tissue loss were obtained from a prospective, non-randomized, single-arm, clinical investigation conducted at several orthopedic centers of excellence located throughout Europe. Subjects recruited (n = 52) had an irreparable medial or lateral meniscus tear or partial meniscus loss, intact rim, presence of both horns, and a stable well-aligned knee.

Between March 2007 and April 2008, 52 patients were enrolled into the study described above. At the time of preparation of this chapter, preliminary 12-month efficacy data were available for 46 patients, with full safety data available for all 52 patients. Of the enrolled subjects, 34 received a medial meniscal implant and 18 received a lateral implant. The demographics and baseline characteristics were representative of the population for which Actifit is intended. The mean age of the subjects was 30.8 ± 9.4 years and the majority were male (75%). The longitudinal length of the meniscus defects ranged from 30 to 70 mm (mean, 47.1 ± 10.0 mm). Baseline values were for visual analog scale (VAS) 45.7 (±26.2), International Knee

Documentation Committee (IKDC) 46.2 (±17.5), and Lysholm knee scale 58.9 (±20.6).

No safety issues related to the scaffold, including cartilage damage or inflammatory reactions to the scaffold or its degradation products, were observed during gross examination at 12 months. MRI findings at 12 months postimplantation showed successful tissue ingrowth and stable or improved cartilage scores in the index compartment compared with baseline. Statistically significant improvements compared with baseline ($p < 0.05$) were reported for functionality on the IKDC and Lysholm scoring scales, as well as for knee pain on VAS, at 3, 6, and 12 months postimplantation. For the five subcomponents of the Knee Injury and Osteoarthritis Outcome Score (KOOS) questionnaire, statistically significant improvements ($p < 0.05$) were reported in pain, daily living and quality of life at 3, 6, and 12 months postimplantation, and in sports/recreation and symptoms at 6 and 12 months postimplantation.

Summary

Ongoing research into improved methods of allograft tissue processing and preservation, basic biology of soft tissue healing and regeneration, stem cell technology, tissue engineering, and biomaterials has tremendous potential to lead to new methods to treat orthopedic soft tissue injuries. Continued progress in these fields is likely to lead to novel solutions to meniscus, ligament, tendon, and articular cartilage injuries.

KEY LEARNING POINTS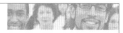

- Musculoskeletal allografts have been used successfully for many years; today, allograft tissues are currently used in sports medicine applications for treatment of ligament, tendon, meniscus, and cartilage injuries.

- Processing and preservation methods continue to evolve and must be formally evaluated to understand better the parameters that lead to the best outcomes for patients.

- The risk for viral or bacterial transmission of disease via use of allografts for sports medicine applications is very low today; however, allografts that are minimally processed can pose the highest risk (fresh, frozen, cryopreserved).

- The sports medicine surgeon must be cognizant of specific indications and contraindications involving the recipient's status when deciding whether to use allograft meniscus.

- Osteochondral allograft, allogeneic chondrocytes, meniscus, ligaments, and tendons are commonly used in sports medicine surgery.
- Appropriate size matching of osteochondral and meniscus allograft tissue with the recipient is critical.
- Ongoing research into allograft tissue processing and preservation, basic biology of soft tissue healing and regeneration, stem cell technology, tissue engineering, and biomaterials has tremendous potential to lead to new methods to treat orthopedic soft tissue injuries.

References

1. Czitrom AA, Gross AE. Allografts in Orthopaedic Practice. Baltimore: Williams and Wilkins, 1992.
2. U.S Census Bureau. Statistical abstract of the United States 2001, No. 168, organ transplants and grafts, 1990–2000. Available at: http://www.census.gov/prod/2002pubs/01statab/health.pdf. (accessed July 2010).
3. Harner CD, Lo MY. Future of Allografts in Sports Medicine. Clin Sports Med 2009;28:327–340.
4. Milachowski KA, Weismeier K, Wirth CJ. Homologous meniscus transplantation: experimental and clinical results. Int Orthop 1989;13:1.
5. Verdonk R. Alternative treatments for meniscal injuries. J Bone Joint Surg Br 1997;79:866.
6. Van Arkel ER, De Boer HH. Human meniscal transplantation. Preliminary results at 2–5 year follow-up. J Bone Joint Surg Br 1995;77:589.
7. Gross AE, Kim OO, Kim W, et al. Fresh osteochondral allografts for posttraumatic knee defects: long term follow-up. Clin Orthop Relat Res 2008;466:1863.
8. Pearsall AW 4th, Tucker JA, Hester RB, Heitman RJ. Chondrocyte viability in refrigerated osteochondrale allografts used for transplantation within the knee. Am J Sports Med 2004:32:125.
9. Malinin TI, Mnaymneh W, Lo HK, Hinkle DK. Cryopreservation of articular cartilage. Ultrastructural observations and long-term results of experimental distal femoral transplantation. Clin Orthop Relat Res 1994;303:18.
10. Ohlendorf C, Tomford W, Mankin HJ. Chondrocyte survival in cryopreserved osteochondrale articular cartilage. J Orthop Res 1996;14:413.
11. Zou S, Dodd RY, Stramer SL et al. Probability of viremia with HBV, HCV, HIV, and HTLV among tissue donors in the United States. N Engl J Med 2004;351:751–9.
12. CDC. Transmission of HIV through bone transplantation: case report and public health recommendations. MMWR 1988;37:597–9.
13. Dodd RY, Notari EP 4th, Stramer SL. Current prevalence and incidence of infectious disease markers and estimated window-period risk in the American Red Cross blood donor population. Transfusion 2002;42:975–9.
14. CDC. Hepatitis C virus transmission from an antibody-negative organ and tissue donor – United States, 2000–2002. MMWR 2003;52:273–6.

15. McAllister DR, Joyce MJ, Barton JM et al. Allograft update: the current status of tissue regulation, procurement, processing, and sterilization. Am J Sport Med 2007;35:2148–58.
16. CDC. (2005) Workshop on preventing organ and tissue allograft-transmitted infection: priorities for public health intervention. http://www.cdc.gov/ncidod/dhqp/pdf/bbp/organ_tissueWorkshop_June2005.pdf.
17. CDC. Update: allograft-associated bacterial infection – United States, 2002. MMWR 2002;51:207–10.
18. Kainer MA, Linden JV, Whaley DN et al. *Clostridium* infections associated with musculoskeletal-tissue allografts. N Engl J Med 2004;350:2564–71.
19. Crawford C, Kainer M, Jernigan D et al. Investigation of postoperative allograft-associated infections in patients who underwent musculoskeletal allograft implantation. Clin Infect Dis 2005;41:195–200.
20. Katz LM, Battaglia TC, Patino P et al. A retrospective comparison of the incidence of bacterial infection following anterior cruciate ligament reconstruction with autograft versus allograft. Arthroscopy 2008;24:1330–5.
21. Stevenson S. The immune response to osteochondral allografts in dogs. J Bone Joint Surg Am 1987;69:573–82.
22. Stevenson S, Dannucci GA, Sharkey NA et al. The fate of articular cartilage after transplantation of fresh and cryopreserved tissue-antigen-matched and mismatched osteochondral allografts in dogs. J Bone Joint Surg Am 1989;71:1297–307.
23. Khoury MA, Goldberg VM, Stevenson S. Demonstration of HLA and ABH antigens in fresh and frozen human menisci by immunohistochemistry. J Orthop Res 1994;12:751–7.
24. Rodeo SA, Seneviratne A, Suzuki K et al. Histological analysis of human meniscal allografts. A preliminary report. J Bone Joint Surg Am 2000;82A:1071–82.
25. Pinkowski JL, Rodrigo JJ, Sharkey NA et al. Immune response to nonspecific and altered tissue antigens in soft tissue allografts. Clin Orthop Relat Res 1996;326:80–5.
26. Fideler BM, Vangsness CT Jr, Moore T et al. Effects of gamma irradiation on the human immunodeficiency virus. A study in frozen human bone-patellar ligament-bone grafts obtained from infected cadaver. J Bone Joint Surg Am 1994;76:1032–5.
27. Rue JP, Yanke AB, Busam ML et al. Prospective evaluation of concurrent meniscus transplantation and articular cartilage repair: minimum 2-year follow-up. Am J Sports Med 2008;36:1770–8.
28. Verdonk PC, Demurie A, Almqvist KF et al. Transplantation of viable meniscal allograft. Survivorship analysis and clinical outcome of one hundred cases. J Bone Joint Surg Am 2005;87:715–24.
29. Noyes FR, Barber-Westin SD, Hewett TE. High tibial osteotomy and ligament reconstruction for varus angulated anterior cruciate ligament-deficient knees. Am J Sports Med 2000;28:282–96.
30. Rueff D, Nyland J, Kocabey Y et al. Self-reported patient outcomes at a minimum of 5 years after allograft anterior cruciate ligament reconstruction with or without medial meniscus transplantation: an age-, sex-, and activity level-matched comparison in patients aged approximately 50 years. Arthroscopy 2006;22:1053–62.

31. Allaire R, Muriuki M, Gilbertson L et al. Biomechanical consequences of a tear of the posterior root of the medial meniscus. Similar to total meniscectomy. J Bone Joint Surg Am 2008;90:1922–31.
32. Rihn JA, Harner CD. The use of musculoskeletal allograft tissue in knee surgery. Arthroscopy 2003;19 (Suppl 1):51–66.
33. Gross AE. Repair of cartilage defects in the knee. J Knee Surg 2002;15:167–9.
34. Volkov M. Allotransplantation of joints. J Bone Joint Surg Am 1970;52:49–53.
35. Gross AE, Silverstein EA, Falk J et al. The allo-transplantation of partial joints in the treatment of osteoarthritis of the knee. Clin Orthopaed Relat Res 1975;108: 7–14.
36. Gross AE, McKee NH, Pritzker KP et al. Reconstruction of skeletal deficits at the knee: a comprehensive osteochondral transplant program. Clin Orthopaed Relat Res 1983;174:96–106.
37. McDermott AG, Langer F, Pritzker KP et al. Fresh small-fragment osteochondral allografts. Long-term follow-up study on first 100 cases. Clin Orthopaed Relat Res 1985;197:96–102.
38. Almqvist KF, Dhollander AA, Verdonk PC et al. Treatment of cartilage defects in the knee using alginate beads containing human mature allogenic chondrocytes. Am J Sports Med 2009;37:1920–9.
39. McCormick F, Yanke A, Provencher MT et al. Minced articular cartilage – basic science, surgical technique, and clinical application. Sports Med Arthrosc Rev 2008;16:217–20.
40. Baer GS, Harner CD. Clinical outcomes of allograft versus autograft in anterior cruciate ligament reconstruction. Clin Sports Med 2007;26:661–81.
41. Shelton WR. Collateral ligament augmentation versus reconstruction using allograft tissue. Clin Sports Med 2009;28:303–10.
42. Stollsteimer GT, Shelton WR, Dukes A et al. Meniscal allograft transplantation: a 1- to 5-year follow-up of 22 patients. Arthroscopy 2010;20:129–40.
43. Rath E, Richmond JC, Yassir W et al. Meniscal allograft transplantation. Two- to eight-year results. Am J Sports Med 2010;29:410–4.
44. Yoldas EA, Sekiya JK, Irrgang JJ et al. Arthroscopically assisted meniscal allograft transplantation with and without combined anterior cruciate ligament reconstruction. Knee Surg, Sports Traumatol, Arthrosc 2003;11:173–82.
45. Graf KW Jr, Sekiya JK, Wojtys EM. Long-term results after combined medial meniscal allograft transplantation and anterior cruciate ligament reconstruction: minimum 8.5 year follow-up study. Arthroscopy 2004;20:129–40.
46. Sekiya JK, West RV, Groff YJ et al. Clinical outcomes following isolated lateral meniscal allograft transplantation. Arthroscopy 2006;22:771–80.
47. Alford W, Cole BJ. The indications and technique for meniscal transplant. Orthoped Clin North Am 2005;36:469–84.
48. Rodeo SA. Meniscal allografts – where do we stand? Am J Sports Med 2001;29:246–61.
49. Allen RT, Robertson CM, Pennock AT et al. Analysis of stored osteochondral allografts at the time of surgical implantation. Am J Sports Med 2005;33: 1479–84.
50. Rohde RS, Studer RK, Chu CR. Mini-pig fresh osteochondral allografts deteriorate after 1 week of cold storage. Clin Orthopaed Relat Res 2004;427:226–33.

51. Williams RJ 3rd, Dreese JC, Chen CT. Chondrocyte survival and material properties of hypothermically stored cartilage: an evaluation of tissue used for osteochondral allograft transplantation. Am J Sports Med 2004;32:132–9.
52. Langer F, Gross AE. Immunogenicity of allograft articular cartilage. J Bone Joint Surg Am 1974;56:297–304.
53. Oakeshott RD, Farine I, Pritzker KP et al. A clinical and histologic analysis of failed fresh osteochondral allografts. Clin Orthopaed Relat Res 1988;233:283–94.
54. Flynn JM, Springfield DS, Mankin HJ. Osteoarticular allografts to treat distal femoral osteonecrosis. Clin Orthopaed Relat Res 1994;303:38–43.
55. Bakay A, Csonge L, Papp G et al. Osteochondral resurfacing of the knee joint with allograft: clinical analysis of 33 cases. Int Orthopaed 1998;22:277–81.
56. LaPrade RF, Botker J, Herzog M et al. Refrigerated osteoarticular allografts to treat articular cartilage defects of the femoral condyles. J Bone Joint Surg Am 2009;91:805–11.
57. Carey JL, Dunn WR, Dahm DL et al. A systematic review of anterior cruciate ligament reconstruction with autograft compared with allograft. J Bone Joint Surg Am 2009;91:2242–50.
58. Foster TE, Wolfe BL, Ryan S et al. Does the graft source really matter in the outcome of patients undergoing anterior cruciate ligament reconstruction? An evaluation of autograft versus allograft reconstruction results. Am J Sports Med 2010;38: 189–99.
59. Singhal MC, Gardiner JR, Johnson DL. Failure of primary anterior cruciate ligament surgery using anterior tibialis allograft. Arthroscopy 2007;23:469–75.
60. Borchers JR, Pedroza A, Kaeding C. Activity level and graft type as risk factors for anterior cruciate ligament graft failure. Am J Sports Med 2009;37:2362–7.
61. Zhang L, Li Z, Liu J et al. Anatomical double bundle reconstruction of the medial patellofemoral ligament with allograft tendon in patellar dislocations. Chin J Reparat Reconstruct Surg 2010;24:100–3.
62. Folsom GJ, Larson CM. Surgical treatment of acute versus chronic complete proximal hamstring ruptures: results of a new allograft technique for chronic reconstructions. Am J Sports Med 2008;36:104–9.
63. Nazarian DG, Booth Jr RE. Extensor mechanism allografts in total knee arthroplasty. Clin Orthopaed Relat Res 1999;367:123–9.
64. Verdonk PCM, Van Laer MEE, Verdonk R. Meniscus replacement: from allograft to tissue engineering. Sports Orthopaed Traumatol 2008;24:78–82.
65. Stone KR, Rodkey WG, Webber RJ et al. Future directions. Collagen-based prostheses for meniscal regeneration. Clin Orthop 1990;252:129–35.
66. Rodkey WG, DeHaven KE, Montgomery WH et al. Comparison of the collagen meniscus implant with partial meniscectomy. a prospective randomized trial. J Bone Joint Surg 2008;90A:1413–26.
67. Steadman JR and Rodkey WG. Tissue-engineered collagen meniscus implants: 5- to 6-year feasibility study results. Arthroscopy 2005;21:515–25.
68. Zaffagnini S, Giordano G, Vascellari A et al. Arthroscopic collagen meniscus implant results at 6 to 8 years follow up. Knee Surg Sports Traumatol Arthrosc 2007;15: 175–83.
69. Maher SA, Doty SB, Rosenblatt L, et al. Evaluation of a meniscal repair scaffold in an ovine model. Poster presented at the 55th Annual Meeting of the Orthopaedic Research Society, Las Vegas, Nevada, USA, February 22–25, 2009.

70. Tienen TG, Heijkants RG, de Groot JH, et al. Replacement of the knee meniscus by a porous polymer implant: a study in dogs. Am J Sports Med 2006;34: 64–71.

71. Welsing RT, van Tienen TG, Ramrattan N, et al Effect on tissue differentiation and articular cartilage degradation of a polymer meniscus implant: a 2-year follow-up study in dogs. Am J Sports Med 2008;36:1978–89.

10 Allograft Tissue Used for the Practice of Dentistry

Danny Holtzclaw[1] and Tolga Fikret Tözüm[2]
[1]Private Practice, Periodontics, Austin, TX, USA
[2]Hacettepe University, Ankara, Turkey

Introduction

To comprehend the applications of allografts in the field of dentistry, a basic understanding of the oral cavity is essential. The major components of the oral cavity include the tongue, teeth, and periodontium. The tongue is a complex muscular organ whose major functions include speech, taste, and deglutination (swallowing). Teeth are highly mineralized structures used for mastication, specifically the chewing of food. Basic anatomy of teeth includes the clinical crown and the root. The clinical crown is the part of the tooth one can see when looking in the mouth and is used for piercing, tearing, and grinding food. Under healthy conditions, the root of the tooth is not visible as it is hidden beneath tissues known collectively as the "periodontium." The periodontium is composed of gingiva (gums), periodontal ligament, cementum, and bone. The periodontium protects the root of the tooth and serves as a complex support and attachment apparatus uniting the teeth with the body.

Periodontitis is defined as "inflammation of the supporting tissues of the teeth (periodontium); usually a progressively destructive change leading to loss of bone and periodontal ligament" [1]. Periodontitis is a near ubiquitous condition. Depending on the parameters measured and thresholds used, the prevalence of periodontitis is as high as 87.4% in specific population groups [2]. There are several different forms of periodontitis. Although chronic periodontitis is the most common form of the periodontal disease, other more destructive variations of the condition exist. Localized aggressive

Tissue and Cell Clinical Use: An Essential Guide, First Edition. Edited by Ruth M. Warwick and Scott A. Brubaker.
© 2012 Blackwell Publishing Ltd. Published 2012 by Blackwell Publishing Ltd.

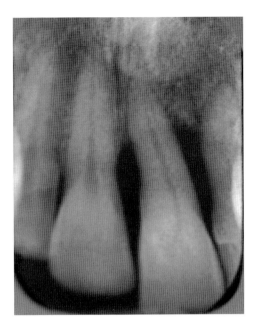

Figure 10.1 Severe bone loss affecting the central incisor in a patient with localized aggressive periodontitis.

periodontal disease, formerly known as localized juvenile periodontitis, is a rapidly destructive form of periodontitis with an age at onset close to puberty. Localized aggressive periodontitis typically presents with a classic pattern of advanced bone and attachment loss on at least two permanent teeth, one of which is a first molar and involving no more than two teeth other than the first molars and incisors (Figure 10.1) [3]. This condition progresses rapidly with evidence suggesting a rate of bone loss up to four times faster than that seen in chronic periodontal disease [4]. Fortunately, the prevalence of localized aggressive periodontitis is less than 1%, although certain population groups are affected somewhat more frequently than others [5]. Another even more destructive form of periodontal disease exists in the form of generalized aggressive periodontitis. Although localized aggressive periodontitis is typically limited to a few specific teeth, the generalized aggressive form of the disease may result in severe bone loss affecting most of the teeth in the dentition. This condition is seen even more infrequently than localized aggressive periodontitis, with a prevalence of 0.13% [6].

The loss of attachment and destruction of bone associated with periodontal disease tends to follow particular patterns. Two of the most common defects seen in periodontal disease include dehiscences and fenestrations. Dehiscence denotes a lack of bone on the upper extent of the tooth closest

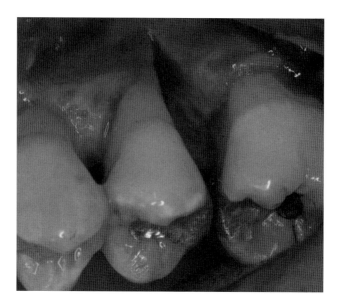

Figure 10.2 Intrabony defect affecting maxillary premolar.

to the clinical crown (coronal), whereas a fenestration is a "window-like" aperture or opening in the bone covering the lower aspects of the tooth (apical) [7]. Anatomic studies of skulls from various population groups have found the prevalence of dehiscences and fenestrations to range anywhere from 7.5 to 20% [8, 9]. Fenestrations were most commonly found in the maxilla (upper jaw) while findings in the mandible were mixed. Another pattern of bone loss typically seen with periodontal disease is the intrabony defect. Unlike dehiscences and fenestrations which are located on the facial (exterior) and lingual (interior) surfaces of bone supporting teeth, intrabony defects are located within the bone (Figure 10.2). In a classic study that evaluated patterns of bone loss in human patients receiving periodontal surgery, interdental craters (Figure 10.3) were the most frequent type of intrabony defect seen [10]. Such defects are confined between the outer (buccal) and inner (lingual) bone. They represented 35.2% of all defects recorded and 62% of all mandibular defects. The prevalence of these defects was much higher in posterior teeth versus anterior teeth. Another much larger study radiographically evaluated nearly 9000 teeth for the frequency and location of interproximal intrabony defects [11]. Like the Manson study [10], the most frequent location for intrabony defects were posterior teeth, although their prevalence was slightly lower at only 23%. When intrabony defects extend to the lingual or buccal cortical plates of bone, they may convert to one, two, or three walled defects, depending on how many walls of bone remain in the defect. Such defects are more commonly found in the

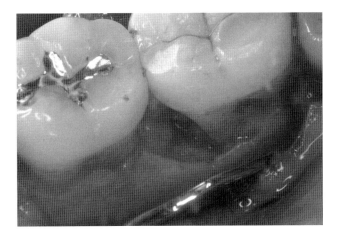

Figure 10.3 Interdental crater affecting mandibular molar.

maxilla whereas interdental craters are more commonly found in the mandible [10–13]. The preferential development of these defects in different areas of the mouth may be explained by anatomic features of bone specific to certain locations. Bone in the mandible tends to have thicker buccal and lingual walls [14]. As such, the development of interdental craters is more frequent here because the soft inner trabecular bone resorbs faster than the dense cortical outer bone. In the maxilla, less dense bone with thinner outer walls results in a higher prevalence of multi-walled defects, typically involving the buccal plate of bone.

Although periodontal disease is a major cause of bone loss in the oral cavity, another cause of significant bone resorption is the simple act of losing a tooth. The extent of intraoral alveolar resorption after tooth loss was quantitatively assessed by Schropp in 2003 [15]. In this prospective study, 46 human patients had a variety of different teeth extracted and changes in the bone surrounding the extraction sites were monitored for 12 months. During this period of healing, bone width was reduced by approximately 50% (Figure 10.4), with most loss occurring within the first three months after tooth extraction. Changes in the height of bone were minimal. Bone loss after tooth extraction holds particular significance in modern dentistry. Over the past 20 years, the dental implant has become one of the most popular treatment options for missing teeth. To treat a patient with dental implants, a sufficient quantity of bone must exist at the site of the former tooth. Recommendations for minimum dental implant alveolar housings range from 5 to 6 mm of residual bone width before implant placement [16, 17] or from 1 to 1.5 mm of bone width around all lateral aspects of the implant following its delivery [18, 19]. In cases of inadequate bone width or height, which is often seen in edentulous alveolar ridges, augmentation

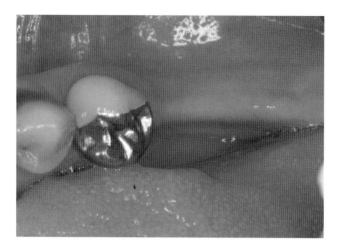

Figure 10.4 Significant loss of ridge width following tooth loss.

procedures are frequently required to facilitate the placement of dental implants.

The past use of allografts in dentistry

Contemporary use of allografts in the practice of dentistry was initiated nearly 40 years ago as clinicians sought an alternative to autologous bone in the treatment of periodontal defects [20]. Although autologous bone had proven effective in the treatment of oral intrabony defects, procurement of this graft material was time consuming and increased patient morbidity through the requirement of secondary surgical sites [20]. Limited intraoral supplies of autologous grafts, and extraoral autologous sources such as the iliac crest which were often associated with root resorption, compounded the problem [21].

In the early 1970s several studies produced the first clinical and histologic reports about use of human bone allografts (Figure 10.5) for the treatment of periodontal defects. In these early studies, which used cryopreserved human allografts of iliac cancellous bone and marrow, graft rejection was a major concern and great efforts were made to ensure proper cross-matching of human lymphocyte antigens (HLAs) [20]. Clinical results of these studies compared favorably with those of autografts in terms of osseous defect fill and pocket depth reduction. More importantly, these studies demonstrated that bone allografts used for the treatment of dental defects were well tolerated by the body. In nearly all cases, postoperative sequelae were uneventful and there was a complete lack of immune rejection phenomenon. The lack of graft rejection was significant because although no grafts were rejected, antigenic differences were present in all grafted patients and none were

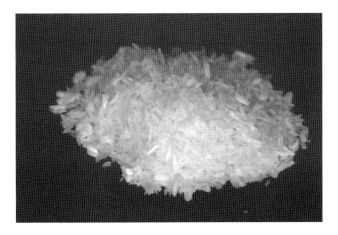

Figure 10.5 Bone allograft.

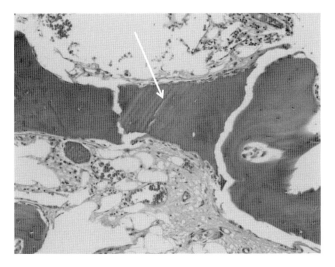

Figure 10.6 Low powered hemotoxylin and eosin (H&E) stain of a bone allograft particle (arrow) incorporated with live bone.

treated with immunosuppressive therapy. These findings showed that dental patients could be treated with bone allografts in an outpatient setting without immunosuppressive medication. Additionally, these studies demonstrated that allografts could produce positive results in a contaminated environment such as the oral cavity.

With questions about graft compatibility, safety, and clinical efficacy initially satisfied, the ultimate fate of the allograft in the healing milieu was examined. Histologically, allograft incorporation (Figure 10.6) within bone was noted with eventual complete replacement of the graft. Allograft parti-cles were determined to be inert and generally exhibited a complete lack of inflammatory infiltrate.

Although treatment of periodontal defects with bone allografts yielded results commensurate to those achieved with autologous grafts, the exact mechanism by which these results were achieved was not known. Did allo-grafts possess the potential to induce/enhance active bone formation (osteo-genesis) or did they simply augment the innate reparative capacity of the periodontium? To determine the regenerative capacity of bone allografts, several studies evaluated allograft healing in ectopic sites. Repeatedly, find-ings from these controlled studies demonstrated that decalcified freeze-dried bone allograft (DFDBA) possessed high osteogenic potential, whereas freeze-dried bone allograft (FDBA) did so to a lesser extent [22]. The higher osteo-genic potential of DFDBA was attributed to greater ease of access to bone morphogenetic proteins (BMPs). Unlike FDBA, which is mineralized and must undergo partial resorption to release its BMPs, DFDBA is demineralized by design, which allows faster release of its BMPs into the healing milieu. Controlled studies strongly supported this concept by demonstrating that commercially prepared DFDBA retained a variety of proteins including BMP-2, BMP-4, and BMP-7 [23]. Additional studies examining allograft particle size determined that smaller particle sizes (typically 250–1000 μm) enhanced osteogenesis, possibly because of an overall increase in graft surface area and easier resorption for release of BMPs [24].

The classic histologic evaluation of new attachment studies by Bowers et al. [25] provided proof of principle for the regeneration of a new attachment apparatus (bone, cementum, and periodontal ligament) when allografts were used to treat periodontal intrabony defects [25]. Accordingly, many studies in the 1980s and 1990s focused on this very subject and helped usher the concept of guided tissue regeneration (GTR). GTR is exclusively used for the treatment of defects that affect the dentition (Figure 10.7).

Although the concept of GTR was gaining acceptance, another treatment modality which would eventually require extensive use of bone allografts was rapidly taking hold: the dental implant. Dental implants are titanium fixtures that replace the root of a tooth (Figure 10.8) and are restored with a crown to replace the clinical crown of the tooth. Dental implants are a popular option for the replacement of missing teeth because, unlike fixed partial dentures, which require adjacent teeth to be irreversibly altered, treatment with dental implants does not involve other teeth. Dental implants require an adequate volume of bone for placement and, as such, bone allo-grafts were increasingly used to reconstruct deficient alveolar ridges. This led to the concept of guided bone regeneration (GBR) and is now one of the main uses for bone allografts in modern dental practice.

Whereas bone allografts constitute most allograft use in the practice of dentistry, another application for dental allografts developed in the mid to

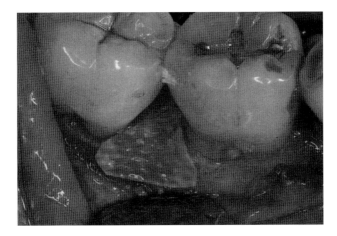

Figure 10.7 Resorbable collagen membrane used for guided tissue regeneration (GTR) between two mandibular molars.

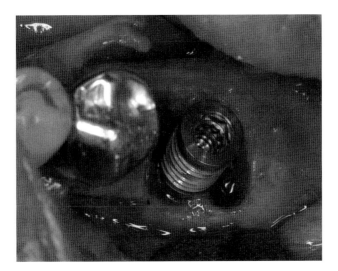

Figure 10.8 Dental implant used to replace immediately an extracted mandibular molar.

late 1990s. In 1996, the first reports documenting use of soft tissue allografts such as an acellular dermal allograft for treating mucogingival defects began to appear [26]. Mucogingival defects encompass a variety of gingival maladies, ranging from inadequate amounts of keratinized gingiva to excessive gum loss, which exposes underlying portions of the tooth such as the root and cementum (Figure 10.9). Although treatment of mucogingival defects

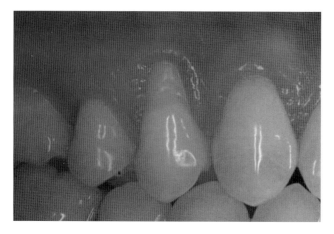

Figure 10.9 Gingival recession affecting the maxillary first premolar.

with autologous tissue had gained mainstream acceptance less than 10 years previously, allograft alternatives for mucogingival procedures were desired owing to the limited availability of host palatal tissue and patient resistance to this treatment. When treating mucogingival defects with autologous sources, connective tissue is procured from the hard palate, typically in a region limited to an area between the canine and first molar. In addition to producing secondary donor site patient morbidity (Plate 10.1), anatomic features such as the greater palatine artery produce risks which may be avoided with allograft tissue.

The present use of allografts in dentistry

With GTR and GBR procedures constituting most bone allograft use in contemporary dentistry, selection of candidate patients for these procedures is of paramount importance. In general, all patients may be considered candidates for dental procedures involving bone allografts. Although a variety of conditions may affect decisions about the general surgical suitability of a patient (i.e., hemophilia, AIDS, history of recent intravenous bisphosphonate use, etc.) no single condition, medication, or other physical parameter precludes the use of bone allografts for dental procedures. Other factors, however, such as religious beliefs and personal preferences must be considered before allograft use and all patients should be fully informed and give informed consent, i.e., relating to source of the allograft and associated risks. When consenting the patient for use of such material, it is wise to know all aspects of the allograft such as history, safety, donor screening procedures, general processing steps, and success rates. Patients may ask questions about any of these topics and if the treatment provider cannot answer these queries, the patient may relent in their acceptance of the proposed treatment.

When considering a patient for GTR and bone allograft procedures to treat periodontal defects, several clinical parameters should be evaluated before treatment. Bony defect depth, width, location, and the number of walls housing the defect are essential determinants of successful outcomes when using bone allografts and GTR. In general, deep narrow intrabony defects with a maximum number of surrounding walls produce the most successful outcomes. Additionally, a classic, well-respected study determined that treating patients with systemic antibiotics produced better surgical outcomes when combined with bone allograft use [27]. Many clinicians combine allografts with antibiotics such as tetracycline to harness the anti-collagenase properties of this specific antibiotic, but the efficacy of this protocol is anecdotal. Factors to consider that may impair or reduce the success of bone allografts include active tobacco smoking, poor plaque control, and inadequately controlled systemic conditions such as diabetes.

With proper patient selection and treatment protocols, use of bone allografts is very successful in the treatment of periodontal defects. In a review of the literature comprising nearly 1000 sites treated with bone allografts, Mellonig noted complete or greater than 50% bony defect fill (Figures 10.10 and 10.11) in 67% of sites [28]. Other controlled studies have corroborated these findings [29] and when bone allografts are combined with occlusive barriers for GTR in a submerged environment, regeneration of bone, cementum, and periodontal ligament has been achieved [25].

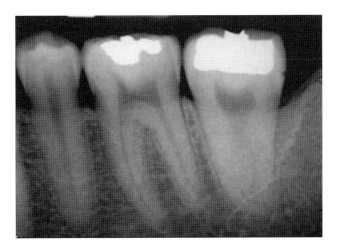

Figure 10.10 Vertical bone loss of approximately 60% affecting the distal root of the mandibular second molar.

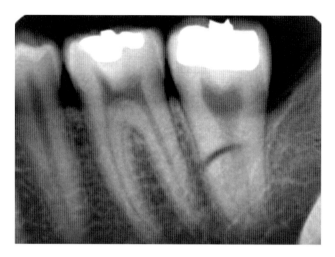

Figure 10.11 The case from Figure 10.10, one year after treatment with bone allograft and GTR. Note significant improvement of vertical intrabony defect.

As bone allografts proved successful in the treatment of periodontal defects, it was only natural that they were eventually used to treat alveolar ridge deficiencies to facilitate the placement of dental implants. Beginning in the late 1980s, dental implants became an increasingly popular option for the treatment of missing teeth. One of the absolute requirements for the placement of dental implants is an adequate volume of host bone to house the implant fixture circumferentially. Unfortunately, such situations do not exist at many edentulous sites. With tooth extraction or loss, it is well documented that resorption of the alveolar ridge will occur. Most resorption of horizontal and vertical ridge volume occurs during the first three months after tooth loss and may continue for up to a total of 12 months. An average of 6.1 mm of horizontal ridge loss (approximately 50% of the original ridge width) and 1.2 mm of vertical loss can be expected in most situations [30]. Ridge reduction may be even greater in molar regions and mandibular resorption tends to be greater than that seen in the maxilla.

Beginning in the late 1990s, bone allografts were used for "site preservation," a new concept to counteract the effects of ridge resorption following tooth extraction. With this concept, particulate bone allograft is used as an intrasocket graft (case 2 is shown in Plates 10.2 and 10.3) to stabilize blood clots and act as a scaffold for future bone formation. The benefits of site preservation were clearly shown in a well-designed, controlled, randomized, and blinded study where extraction sites were either left empty or grafted with FDBA and covered with a resorbable collagen membrane. Up to 125% more loss of ridge width was seen in the absence of site preservation (approximately 1.2 mm of horizontal ridge loss with site preservation compared with approximately 2.6 mm of horizontal ridge loss without site preservation). Concerning vertical ridge height, the results were even more dramatic. Without site preservation, up to 244% more loss of ridge height was realized (approximately 1.3 mm gain in vertical height with site preservation versus approximately 0.9 mm loss of vertical ridge height without site preservation) [30]. Knowing that it is much easier to prevent complications than to treat them, the concept of site preservation has gained rapid acceptance and is now practically ubiquitous in modern dental implant practices.

Although site preservation has proven effective in maintaining adequate ridge width/height following tooth loss, it is unfortunately not always used and there are circumstances where alveolar ridges must be reconstructed to facilitate the placement of dental implants. In such cases, GBR may be accomplished with bone allografts. When GBR was initially used in the mid-1990s, questions revolved around how implants would react with regenerated bone. Several studies both in animals and humans repeatedly confirmed that implant success rates in regenerated bone were similar to those achieved with native bone. With the knowledge that implants could successfully be supported by regenerated bone formed as the result of GBR and use of allograft, the limits of horizontal and vertical bone formation needed to be determined. Numerous clinical trials found that horizontal GBR with particulate bone allograft (case 3 is shown in Plates 10.4–10.6) is fairly predictable with average gains of just over 3 mm. When larger gains are desired, freeze-dried block allografts may be used (case 4 is shown in Figures 10.12–10.14), but with somewhat less predictability in certain areas of the oral cavity. Concerning vertical GBR with particulate bone allograft,

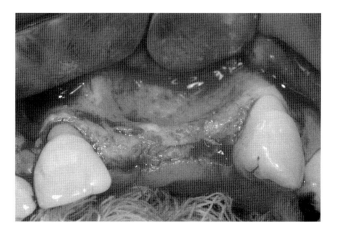

Figure 10.12 Significantly resorbed maxillary ridge at the site of the central and lateral incisors.

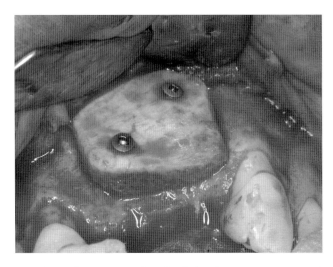

Figure 10.13 Block allograft secured to the defect from Figure 10.12 with a pair of screws.

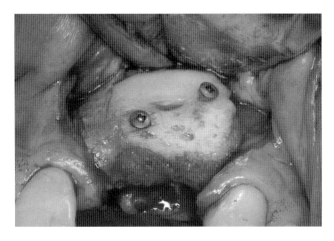

Figure 10.14 Maxillary ridge from Figures 10.12 and 10.13 after four months of healing from GBR treatment. Note the significant improvement in ridge width.

lack of predictability is also a concern, even more so than with block allografts.

Although bone grafts constitute most allografts used in modern dentistry, soft tissue allografts (a case study is shown in Figure 10.15) are gaining some acceptance. Allograft materials currently used for soft tissue dental grafting include acellular dermal matrix, pericardium, amnion, and fascia. Unlike bone allografts, however, contemporary soft tissue allografts have not

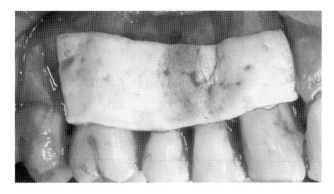

Figure 10.15 Soft tissue allograft used to treat multiple mucogingival defects affecting maxillary teeth.

demonstrated the same levels of success as autografts. Compared with autologous palatal connective tissue and free gingival grafts, soft tissue allografts have yet to achieve commensurate gains in long-term defect coverage, gingival thickness, or keratinization [31]. When not being used for root coverage procedures, soft tissue allografts have been used as GTR membranes with varying levels of success.

The future use of allografts in dentistry

The future of allograft use in the practice of dentistry is currently following two distinct paths: (1) combining allografts with biologic growth factors; and, (2) the new and rapidly growing practice of tissue engineering.

Allograft combination with biologic growth factors

When used alone or combined with GTR, bone allografts have proven successful in the treatment of periodontal and other intraoral defects. Likewise, soft tissue allografts have demonstrated relative levels of success in certain applications of dental reconstruction. Although these allografts have proven successful in their current applications, new ways of enhancing the performance of these grafts are constantly being evaluated. Recently, numerous in vitro and in vivo studies have shown evidence regarding the significant positive effects of highly concentrated growth factors in biologics such as platelet-rich plasma (PRP) [32], recombinant human platelet-derived growth factor (rhPDGF) [33], enamel matrix derivative (EMD) [34], and rhBMP [35] when combined with allografts.

Studies evaluating the combination of DFDBA with rhBMP have shown improved bone densities and faster allograft replacement with native bone versus non-rhBMP controls. Additionally, when rhBMP is used in combination with dental implants, the speed of osseointergration is significantly enhanced and the quantity/quality of bone formation around the implants is improved as well [35]. Similar results hold true for rhPDGF [33]. Multiple studies have shown greater gains in bone formation and improved densities when allografts were combined with rhPDGF. rhPDGF has also been used in the successful treatment of gingival recession defects [36]. Like rhPDGF, combining EMD with bone allografts has resulted in significant improvements versus allograft alone [34]. Although initially promising, long-term evaluation of these results must be accomplished to appreciate fully the value of these biologics. Use of PRP, for example, in multiple early studies provided very promising results for improved hard and soft tissue healing. Over time, however, several studies have found negligible results for PRP and many now question the true efficacy of PRP [37]. To avoid premature and overzealous expectations about growth factor use with allografts, further research and long-term monitoring are needed to corroborate initial positive findings.

Tissue engineering

Like growth factor applications, tissue engineering is a field that has recently received considerable attention in dental research. Tissue engineering is the functional restoration of tissue structure and physiology for damaged tissues through biologic mediators and matrices. Soft and hard tissue engineering for dental applications is in the developmental phase and focuses on key elements including living progenitor cells, morphogens, and suitable extracellular matrix scaffolds. With tissue engineering, these key elements are placed in an appropriate environment to reproduce a developmental sequence of events that finally ends with the formation of functional tissue. Progenitor cells (adult stem cells) are undifferentiated cells that have the ability to maintain their characteristics until they are exposed to appropriate signals. Progenitor cells may also maintain their multipotent differentiation capacity and differentiate into a variety of specialized cells. Morphogens are extracellularly secreted signals that include entities such as BMPs, fibroblast growth factors (FGFs), and tumor necrosis factor (TNF) families. These biological factors functionally direct multipotent stem cells to morph into a variety of specialized cell types such as osteoblasts or keratinocytes. Scaffolds are biologic or artificial structures that provide a biological and physicochemical three-dimensional environment, which houses cells for adhesion, differentiation, and migration. With tissue engineering, scaffolds are often the vehicles through which progenitor cells or morphogens can be delivered to the desired site of treatment [38–40].

Tissue engineering procedures

Recombinant protein therapy is the delivery of appropriate growth factors to an ectopic or orthotropic environment. With this therapy, selected growth factors are delivered on a suitable scaffold, such as collagen sponge or beta-tricalcium-sulfate, and together act to induce and guide cellular growth. One of the most popular recombinant proteins in contemporary dentistry is rhBMP-2. rHBMP-2 has shown great promise in dental regenerative procedures and appears to be a simple and safe procedure [33, 39]. Accordingly, products using rhBMP such as INFUSE® (Medtronic, Minneapolis, Minnesota, USA) have recently been introduced to the field of dentistry for mainstream therapeutic use. With this being said, however, the ideal dose of recombinant protein, its degradation timeframe, the ideal scaffold, and knowledge of other proteins that interact at the surgical site have not been completely clarified.

Gene therapy, considered a more complex method than recombinant protein therapy, uses the gene of the delivered growth factor to induce cells to secrete gene product with an acceptable level of protein production. After procuring stem cells from the patient in a clinical setting, the cells are genetically modified by viruses, loaded on a suitable scaffold, and transplanted back to the patient. This technology is still in its infancy in dentistry and has currently been limited to use with treatment of oral cancers [41].

Cell-based therapy is the delivery of specific cells to the surgical site. After transplantation of cells, growth factors are expressed and induction of the regeneration process ensues. Choosing the correct cell and tissue types are one of the most critical decisions for cell therapy applications. Mechanisms occurring after the transplantation of specific cells for use in a different anatomic location than where it is found is still unclear and includes a wide spectrum of cells (i.e., adult stem cell, undifferentiated stem cell) and tissues (i.e., bone marrow, adipose, muscle, skin) to be studied.

It should be noted that these therapies are still in the developmental phase and need extensive basic research supported by evidence-based clinical applications before full-scale therapeutic use. Some estimates conclude that it may take up to 20 years or more before these applications are regularly used in the practice of dentistry.

Dental applications of tissue engineering

The use of allogeneic soft and/or hard tissue engineering has a wide spectrum in clinical dentistry including oral biology, periodontics, oral and maxillofacial surgery, and endodontics. The most likely use for dental tissue engineering in the near future, however, will be enhanced reconstruction of osseous and soft tissue intraoral defects. Essentially, tissue engineering will augment or ultimately replace the current practices of GTR/bone grafting, GBR, and mucogingival grafting.

Concerning reconstruction of periodontal or osseous defects, tissue engineering seeks to achieve the three beneficial properties of native tissue: osteoconduction, osteoinduction, and osteogenesis. Realization of this goal will allow for the rapid reconstruction of dental defects while eliminating the morbidity associated with secondary autograft harvests. Because these procedures will improve comfort and reduce potential complications associated with secondary surgical sites, patients may be more readily accepting of these procedures. As such, so long as costs can be maintained to a reasonable level, the number of patients seeking this treatment can be expected to increase over current levels. Additionally, an increasingly aging population may swell the number of patients seeking treatment. For example, according to the US Department of Health and Human Services' Administration on Aging, shifts in birth rates and declines in death rates will result in very significant increases in the number of elderly persons in the population during the next two to three decades. As a large portion of the US population reaches its fifth decade and older, aging "baby boomers" will likely face progressive dental deterioration and disease [42]. The same can be said for the repair of mucogingival defects. Although there is relatively minimal risk in the autologous harvest of palatal connective tissue for the treatment of periodontal gingival defects, many patients reject this treatment because of fear and perceptions of pain. Use of tissue engineering may eliminate these fears and will likely lead to an increase in the number of patients seeking treatment for such problems. Ultimately, these treatments will improve the overall oral health of patients and allow for restoration of comfort, function, and esthetics.

Although treatment of osseous and soft tissue defects is certainly a goal of dental tissue engineering, one of the ultimate goals of this field is the repair of damaged teeth and the replacement of missing teeth. Recent research suggests that immature tooth bud may be one of the pivotal tissues in oral biology for the restoration of damaged tooth structures (both hard and soft tissues), in which very complex mechanisms are involved during the formation of enamel, dentin, and dental pulp. For example, tooth bud cells can be seeded in a biodegradable scaffold and implanted into the host, which may result in the formation of significant amounts of enamel, dentin, and dental pulp [43]. Another example involves dental pulp stem cells which are transduced with rhBMP gene and transferred to a scaffold to differentiate into odontoblasts. These osteoblasts, in turn, result in the formation of the dentin-pulp system. The allogeneic dentin–pulp complex may be transferred into a damaged pulp for nerve and vascular regeneration. Molecular determination of epithelial and mesenchymal dental stem cells, including genes involved in the control of dental cell differentiation, is likely to be a continued focus of dental allograft research for years to come [39].

In clinical dentistry, autologous tooth transplantation is a viable and relatively successful option for the replacement of missing dentition if the patient has available teeth. If no autologous teeth are available, tooth allografts may be used, but this has led to irreversible root resorption followed by the loss of the transplanted tooth. Root resorption depends on the rejection of the allogeneic tissue by the host, where periodontal ligament is the main initiator of inflammation with final results of root resorption. Gene therapy may one day offer improved success for tooth allografts. Transgenic animal models in which specific genes were knocked out can be used alternatively to understand the mechanisms involved in the rejection of allogeneic tooth transplantation. Teeth of lacZ transgenic mice transplanted to a wild-type animal have provided early success, with dental pulp and periodontal tissues being replaced and regenerated by host cells after allograft transplantation if the vascular supply into the surgical area is sufficient [44].

Conclusions

Since their mainstream introduction to dentistry just over 40 years ago, allografts have significantly changed and improved the manner in which dental care is provided to patients. The evolution of this treatment option has led to continually improving outcomes and has certainly achieved the goals of improving patient comfort, function, and esthetics. Over the next 40 years, advancements in this field will continue with the hope that one day, dentists may treat patients in the least invasive manner possible.

CASE 1

A 34-year-old male presented with an 8 mm probing depth at the distal of the left mandibular second molar. The preoperative radiograph suggested a deep vertical bony defect affecting 60% of the distal surface of the tooth (Figure 10.10). The defect was surgically cleaned and grafted with demineralized freeze dried bone allograft (DFDBA). Guided tissue regeneration (GTR) was accomplished with a resorbable collagen membrane placed over the DFDBA. One year later, the 8 mm probing depth was reduced to 3 mm and there was significant improvement in the radiographic bone fill of the defect (Figure 10.11).

CASE 2

A 27-year-old male presented with a fractured right maxillary lateral incisor. The tooth was carefully removed to preserve the facial plate of bone (Plate 10.2). After removal of the tooth, the socket was grafted with freeze dried bone allograft (FDBA) for site preservation (Plate 10.3).

CASE 3

A 44-year-old female presented with a severely resorbed posterior right mandibular ridge (Plate 10.4). The site was grafted with titanium screws and FDBA (Plate 10.5). GTR was accomplished with a resorbable collagen membrane. Four months after the initial surgery, the width of the alveolar ridge improved significantly to a point acceptable for dental implant placement (Plate 10.6).

CASE 4

A 43-year-old male presented with a significant defect at the site of the maxillary left central and lateral incisors (Figure 10.12). A block allograft was trimmed to intimately adapt to the defect site and secured with a pair of titanium screws (Figure 10.13). GTR was accomplished with a resorbable collagen membrane. Four months after the initial surgery, the width of the alveolar ridge improved significantly to a point acceptable for dental implant placement (Figure 10.14).

KEY LEARNING POINTS

- Allografts provide a safe and less invasive alternative to autologous tissue for the reconstruction of hard and soft tissue intraoral deficiencies. Without this option, certain patients would likely opt for no treatment.

- Bone allografts have been safely used in the practice of dentistry for nearly 40 years, whereas soft tissue allografts have been safely used for nearly 20 years.

- Past use of allografts in the practice of dentistry were typically limited to minor bone defects affecting periodontally compromised teeth.

- Current uses of allografts in the practice of dentistry have greatly expanded with the explosive growth of dental implants. In addition to the traditional use of bone allografts for the repair of periodontally related bony defects, current uses of bone allografts are heavily weighted toward the facilitation of dental implant placement. Additionally, use of soft tissue allografts for the treatment of mucogingival defects is gaining acceptance.

- Future uses of allografts in the practice of dentistry are closely intertwined with the development of growth factors and tissue engineering.
  Such advances are likely to enhance the efficacy of allografts in the future.

References

1. Glossary of Periodontal Terms (4th Edition). Chicago. American Academy of Periodontology. 2001. Page 42.
2. Holtfreter B, Kocher T, Hoffmann T, Desvarieux M, Micheelis W. Prevalence of periodontal disease and treatment demands based on a German dental survey (DMS IV). J Clin Periodontol 2010;37:211–9.
3. Lang N, Bartold PM, Cullinan M, et al. Consensus report: aggressive periodontitis. Ann Periodontol 1999;4:53.
4. Baer PN. The case for periodontosis as a clinical entity. J Periodontol 1971; 42:516–20.
5. Melvin WL, Sandifer JB, Gray JL. The prevalence and sex ratio of juvenile periodontitis in a young racially mixed population. J Periodontol 1991;62:330–4.
6. Löe H, Brown LJ. Early onset periodontitis in the United States of America. J Periodontol 1991;62:608–16.
7. Glossary of Periodontal Terms (4th Edition). Chicago. American Academy of Periodontology, 2001; p.118.
8. Elliot G, Bowers G. Alveolar dehiscences and fenestrations. Periodontics 1963; 1:245–8.
9. Edel A. Alveolar bone fenestrations and dehiscences in dry Bedouin jaws. J Clin Periodontol 1981;8:491–9.
10. Manson JD. Bone morphology and bone loss in periodontal disease. J Clin Periodontol 1976;3:14–22.
11. Dundar N, Ilgenli T, Kal BI, Boyacioglu H. The frequency of periodontal infrabony defects on panoramic radiographs of an adult population seeking dental care. Community Dent Health 2008;25:226–30.
12. Saari JT, Hurt WC, Biggs NL. Periodontal bony defects on the dry skull. J Periodontol 1968;39:278–83.
13. Larato DC. Intrabony defects in the dry human skull. J Periodontol 1970;41: 496–8.
14. Flanagan D. A comparison of facial and lingual cortical thicknesses in edentulous maxillary and mandibular sites measured on computerized tomograms. J Oral Implantol 2008;34:256–8.
15. Schropp L, Wenzel A, Kostopoulos L, Karring T. Bone healing and soft tissue contour changes following single-tooth extraction: a clinical and radiographic 12-month prospective study. Int J Periodontics Restorative Dent 2003;23:313–23.
16. Misch CM, Misch CE, Resnik RR, Ismail YH. Reconstruction of maxillary alveolar defects with mandibular symphysis grafts for dental implants: a preliminary procedural report. Int J Oral Maxillofac Implants 1992;7:360–6.
17. de Wijs FL, Cune MS. Immediate labial contour restoration for improved esthetics: a radiographic study on bone splitting in anterior single-tooth replacement. Int J Oral Maxillofac Implants 1997;12:686–96.
18. Albrektsson T, Jansson T, Lekholm U. Osseointegrated dental implants. Dent Clin North Am 1986;30:151–74.
19. Shulman LB. Surgical considerations in implant dentistry. Int J Oral Implantol 1988;5:37–41.

20. Schallhorn RG, Hiatt WH. Human allografts of iliac cancellous bone and marrow in periodontal osseous defects. II. Clinical observations. J Periodontol 1972;43: 67–81.

21. Dragoo MR, Sullivan HC. A clinical and histological evaluation of autogenous iliac bone grafts in humans. II. External root resorption. J Periodontol 1973;44: 614–625.

22. Mellonig JT, Bowers GM, Bailey RC. Comparison of bone graft materials. Part I. New bone formation with autografts and allografts determined by Strontium-85. J Periodontol 1981;52:291–6.

23. Shigeyama Y, D'Errico JA, Stone R, Somerman MJ. Commercially-prepared allograft material has biological activity in vitro. J Periodontol 1995;66:478–87.

24. Shapoff CA, Bowers GM, Levy B, Mellonig JT, Yukna RA. The effect of particle size on the osteogenic activity of composite grafts of allogeneic freeze-dried bone and autogenous marrow. J Periodontol 1980;51:625–30.

25. Bowers G, Chadroff B, Canevalle R, et al. Histologic evaluation of new attachment apparatus formation in humans – part 1. J Periodontol 1989;60:664–74.

26. Shulman J. Clinical evaluation of an acellular dermal allograft for increasing the zone of attached gingiva. Pract Periodontics Aesthet Dent 1996;8:201–8.

27. Sanders JJ, Sepe WW, Bowers GM, et al. Clinical evaluation of freeze-dried bone allografts in periodontal osseous defects. Part III. Composite freeze-dried bone allografts with and without autogenous bone grafts. J Periodontol 1983;54:1–8.

28. Mellonig JT. Freeze-dried bone allografts in periodontal reconstructive surgery. Dent Clin North Am 1991;35:505–20.

29. Quintero G, Mellonig JT, Gambill VM, Pelleu GB Jr. A six-month clinical evaluation of decalcified freeze-dried bone allografts in periodontal osseous defects. J Periodontol 1982;53:726–30.

30. Iasella JM, Greenwell H, Miller RL, Hill M, Drisko C, Bohra AA, Scheetz JP. Ridge preservation with freeze-dried bone allograft and a collagen membrane compared to extraction alone for implant site development: a clinical and histologic study in humans. J Periodontol 2003;74:990–9.

31. Harris RJ. A short-term and long-term comparison of root coverage with an acellular dermal matrix and a subepithelial graft. J Periodontol 2004;75:734–43.

32. Marx RE, Carlson ER, Eichstaedt RM, Schimmele SR, Strauss JE, Georgeff KR. Platelet-rich plasma: Growth factor enhancement for bone grafts. Oral Surg Oral Med Oral Pathol Oral Radiol Endod 1998;85:638–46.

33. Nevins M, Camelo M, Nevins ML, Schenk RK, Lynch SE. Periodontal regeneration in humans using recombinant human platelet-derived growth factor-BB (rhPDGF-BB) and allogenic bone. J Periodontol 2003;74:1282–92.

34. Aspriello SD, Ferrante L, Rubini C, Piemontese M. Comparative study of DFDBA in combination with enamel matrix derivative versus DFDBA alone for treatment of periodontal intrabony defects at 12 months post-surgery. Clin Oral Investig 2011;15:225–32.

35. Wikesjö UM, Qahash M, Polimeni G, et al. Alveolar ridge augmentation using implants coated with recombinant human bone morphogenetic protein-2: histologic observations. J Clin Periodontol. 2008;35:1001–10.

36. McGuire MK, Scheyer T, Nevins M, Schupbach P. Evaluation of human recession defects treated with coronally advanced flaps and either purified recombinant human platelet-derived growth factor-BB with beta tricalcium phosphate or

connective tissue: a histologic and microcomputed tomographic examination. Int J Periodontics Restorative Dent 2009;29:7–21.

37. Esposito M, Grusovin MG, Coulthard P, Worthington HV. The efficacy of various bone augmentation procedures for dental implants: a Cochrane systematic review of randomized controlled clinical trials. Int J Oral Maxillofac Implants 2006; 21:696–710.

38. Nussenbaum B, Krebsbach PH. The role of gene therapy for craniofacial and dental tissue engineering. Adv Drug Deliv Rev 2006;58:577–91.

39. Nakashima M, Akamine A. The application of tissue engineering to regeneration of pulp and dentin in endodontics. J Endod 2005;31:711–8.

40. Kleinman HK, Philp D, Hoffman MP. Role of the extracellular matrix in morphogenesis. Curr Opin Biotechnol 2003;14:526–32.

41. Lavorini-Doyle C, Gebremedhin S, Konopka K, Düzgüneş N. Gene delivery to oral cancer cells by nonviral vectors: why some cells are resistant to transfection. J Calif Dent Assoc 2009;37:855–8.

42. Department of Health and Human Services. Administration on Aging. Statistics: Aging into the 21st century. Washington, DC: HHS, 2004. http://www.aoa.gov

43. Yelick PC, Vacanti JP. Bioengineered teeth from tooth bud cells. Dent Clin North Am 2006;50:191–203.

44. Kim E, Cho SW, Yang JY, et al. Tooth survival and periodontal tissues healing of allogenic-transplanted teeth in the mice. Oral Dis 2006;12:395–401.

11 The Use of Allograft Skin in Burn Surgery

Peter Dziewulski[1] and Steven E. Wolf[2]
[1]St Andrews Centre for Plastic Surgery and Burns, Chelmsford, UK
[2]University of Texas Health Science Center at San Antonio, San Antonio, TX, USA

Introduction

The skin is the largest organ in the human body and has several vital protective and homeostatic functions. A burn can be defined as coagulative destruction of the surface layers of the body. Burn injury to the skin can range from being relatively trivial to one of the most severe injuries the human body can sustain and survive. Major burn injury often requires multidisciplinary care in an intensive care setting, multiple surgical procedures to achieve wound healing followed by prolonged rehabilitation, and possibly a lifetime of reconstructive procedures to achieve psychosocial, esthetic, and functional recovery.

The management of a burn depends on many variables including the age of the patient, comorbid factors, the size, depth, and anatomical location of the injury. In general the aims of burn care are to restore form, function, and feeling. This involves early esthetic wound closure, optimal rehabilitation to pre-injury activities and psychosocial recovery. The removal of dead or devitalized tissue saves lives, improves form, and optimizes function. Once the devitalized tissue is removed, wound closure must be achieved either with autologous skin or a temporary or permanent skin substitute.

Tissue and Cell Clinical Use: An Essential Guide, First Edition. Edited by Ruth M. Warwick and Scott A. Brubaker.
© 2012 Blackwell Publishing Ltd. Published 2012 by Blackwell Publishing Ltd.

The past

History of skin grafting and use of human deceased donor allograft skin

The technique of skin procurement and transplantation was initially described approximately 2500–3000 years ago with the Hindu Tilemaker caste in the reconstruction of amputated noses. Reverdin in 1869 reported the first reliable technique of skin grafting, with Pollock (1870) being the first to describe the successful use of skin grafting in the treatment of a burn. At this time the use of allograft from amputated extremities and preputial skin was reported.

Girdner in 1881 was the first to report the successful use of allograft in the treatment of a burnt child. In 1886 Thiersch formulated requirements for skin grafting, popularizing the clinical use of split thickness skin grafts.

Wentscher described the storage of human skin in 1903 but tissue banking did not become developed in clinical practice until the 1930s. The benefit of allograft in the closure of more extensive burn wounds was described by Bettman in 1938 who reported its use in a series of children with extensive burns. Further work on skin storage led to the development of modern tissue banking. Billingham and Medawar demonstrated effective cryopreservation of skin with glycerol. In the 1950s Brown in the USA and Jackson in the UK popularized the use of human deceased donor allografts as temporary biological dressings for burn wounds. Zaroff reported a 10-year experience in the use of human deceased donor skin in burn care and other authors reported the use in other types of wounds.

Since the 1950s, the use of human deceased donor skin in burn care has increased with regular reporting. An increasingly aggressive surgical approach to major full-thickness burn injury developed throughout the 1970s and refined the use of human deceased donor skin during the 1980s. This has become the standard of care to assist with wound closure [1].

The present

Burn wound healing

The skin is comprised of the epidermis and dermis with the adnexal structures such as the hair follicles, sweat glands, and sebaceous glands residing in the deeper parts of the dermis. These adnexal structures are important as they are the source of proliferating epithelial cells (keratinocytes), which resurface wounds when the skin has been injured. Loss of the barrier function of the skin allows invasion of microorganisms and systemic sepsis. Increased fluid losses from the injured skin also occur until re-epithelialization occurs.

Burn injury to the skin can be classified as partial or full thickness. If the epidermis and the superficial part of the dermis have been injured (superficial partial thickness injury), most adnexal structures are preserved, epithelialization is rapid (10–14 days) and the risk of hypertrophic scarring is low. If the burn extends down into the deeper parts of the dermis, more adnexal structures are destroyed, epithelialization is slower (three to six weeks), and there is a high incidence of hypertrophic scarring. Full-thickness burns involve destruction of all constituents of the skin and usually will require surgical intervention to achieve timely wound healing.

In general, the pursuit of early aggressive surgical intervention in deeper injury limits the duration of burn illness and reduces associated morbidity and mortality. Treatment planning depends on the assessment of the following factors: the patient's general condition and comorbid factors, patient age, burn depth, burn size, and anatomical distribution of the injury.

Principles of burn wound management

The aim of management of superficial partial thickness wounds is to promote rapid spontaneous re-epithelialization with a minimum number of painful dressing changes and to prevent infection, which can convert the injury to a deeper one that requires skin grafting.

The partial thickness wound needs cleaning and removal of loose epidermis and blisters. The wound can then be covered with a semi-biological dressing or conventional dressings. A topical antimicrobial such as Flamazine® (silver sulphadiazine 1%) can be used with the conventional dressing to try to limit bacterial colonization.

Deep partial thickness injury has a significant morbidity in terms of time to healing, infective complications, and subsequent scarring. Conservative management leading to spontaneous healing usually involves prolonged and painful dressing changes and the resultant scar is invariably hypertrophic leading to cosmetic and functional debility. Thus an early surgical approach that tries to preserve dermis and achieve prompt wound healing is preferred.

Full-thickness burns will not heal spontaneously unless very small and invariably require skin grafting. The necrotic tissue usually requires excision and the resultant wound requires closure to reduce the risks of invasive infection and systemic sepsis. Prompt excision and wound closure reduces morbidity and mortality in patients with such injuries [2].

Modern surgical approach

Burns that are deemed deep are best excised and the wounds covered with autologous split skin grafts. The grafts usually require meshing and the amount of wound that can be closed with autograft depends on the donor sites available and the mesh ratio used.

Cosmetically and functionally sensitive areas such as the face and hands need thicker sheet autograft for wound closure. In general it is preferable to use sheet grafts in children as they give a better aesthetic result, but this

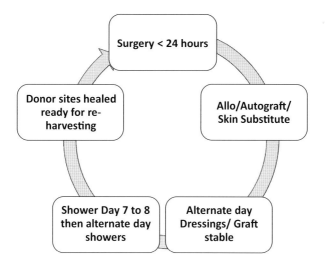

Figure 11.1 Surgical wound treatment program for major burn injury.

decision must be made in balance with the need for rapid wound closure. If the burn size is large or if there is a lack of donor sites then temporary wound closure with allograft, xenograft, other biological or semi-biological dressings and/or synthetic skin substitutes may be required while the donor sites heal. Patients with larger burns need to return to the operating room for further grafting when their donor sites are healed. This is usually done on a weekly basis (Figure 11.1).

Serial wound excision and grafting is commonly practiced. This method is used for larger burns where donor sites are scarce. The surgical technique is similar to that described above but the amount of burn wound excised is the amount that can be covered by meshed split skin grafts from available donor sites. Un-excised areas are treated with topical antimicrobials until autograft donor sites have healed and can be re-harvested, usually 7–14 days later. The un-excised, un-healed areas of burn wound are susceptible to invasive wound infection and this treatment method has a higher morbidity and mortality compared to early excision. The use of the topical antimicrobial flamacerium (silver sulphadiazine and cerium nitrate) has been reported to decrease episodes of invasive wound infection, morbidity and mortality [3].

An early aggressive surgical approach has been shown to improve mortality in patients with large full-thickness burns. In addition, patients treated with early excision were shown to have a shorter time to wound healing and shorter inpatient stay [2].

After wound excision it is vital to obtain wound closure. Wound closure is permanent with autologous split skin grafts or temporary using allograft

---

Box 11.1 Indications for human deceased donor skin
(Adapted from Kagan R, Robb E, Plessinger R. The skin bank. In: Herndon D, editor. Total burn care. 3rd edition. Philadelphia: 2007. p. 229–381.)

- Physiological wound closure where autograft donor sites not available.
- Intermingling autograft/allograft techniques: "sandwich" grafting.
- Physiological wound closure in large partial thickness burns.
- Physiological wound closure in desquamating skin conditions (Stevens–Johnson syndrome, toxic epidermal necrolysis, staphylococcal scalded skin syndrome).
- Wound bed testing and preparation before autografting.
- Dermal replacement for cultured epithelial autograft.

---

or skin substitutes. Physiological closure of the burn wound reduces invasive infection, evaporative water loss, heat loss, pain, and promotes wound healing (see Box 11.1).

The ideal skin replacement
The skin consists of two basic layers: the epidermis attached by a basement membrane to the dermis. Skin is incredibly complex and has a multitude of functions including protection, sensation, homeostasis, endocrine, immune, and cosmetic. The epidermis provides most of the protective barrier functions. The dermis provides the durable and pliable structure that allows function and cosmesis but also contains the adnexal structures that are important in the other functions of the skin.

The perfect skin substitute will have the properties listed in Box 11.2. It should be a barrier to bacteria, prevent water and electrolyte losses from the wound, be inexpensive and readily available, easy to store, use, and secure, be flexible and contour well, be pliable and durable in the long term, be available "off the shelf" with a long shelf life, not transmit any infectious diseases, not stimulate an inflammatory response, minimize scarring, be capable of "growth", and ideally have other important skin structures such as hair follicles, sweat glands, and sebaceous glands, and neurosensory receptors to allow sensation [4].

Autograft
The current "gold standard" in skin replacement after burn injury remains autologous split thickness skin graft. This is harvested from available donor sites and then is applied and secured to the excised wound surface. The choice of donor site varies according to availability, amount required and specific recipient site.

A donor site is, in essence, a superficial partial thickness skin wound and should heal within seven days depending on the thickness of the graft

> **Box 11.2 Characteristics of the ideal skin substitute**
> (Adapted from Sheridan RL, Tompkins RG. Skin substitutes in burns. Burns 1999;25(2):97–103.)
>
> • Inexpensive
> • Off the shelf
> • Long shelf life
> • Non-antigenic
> • Durable
> • Flexible
> • Prevents water loss
> • Barrier to bacteria
> • Conforms to irregular surfaces
> • Easy to secure
> • Grows with children
> • Applied in one operation
> • Does not become hypertrophic

harvested. Care of the donor site is equally as important as the grafted area. Most donor sites will invariably heal, but slow healing or subsequent hypertrophic scarring can be a major problem.

Split thickness donor sites heal by epithelialization from epithelial appendages such as the hair follicles, sweat, and sebaceous glands. The thicker the graft taken or if the same site is harvested repeatedly then the number of epidermal appendages is reduced with slower healing and a higher rate of hypertrophic scar formation. Donor site healing is also dependent on other factors such as age, depth of harvest, wound management, and blood supply to the donor site. In larger burns with limited donor sites that require repeated harvesting, recombinant human growth hormone (0.2 mg/kg/day) has been shown to increase donor site healing by up to 25% [5]. Choice of donor site is important especially in patients with smaller burns where scarring and deformity should be minimized. In young females with small burns requiring grafting, donor sites should be hidden and skin should be harvested from either the buttock or the upper inner aspect of the thighs. In young males the upper outer aspect of the thigh can be used in addition to the above. The scalp is also an attractive donor site, as subsequent hair growth completely hides the scars. In patients with larger burns, choice of donor sites is limited and skin grafts should be harvested from any available site.

Grafts are meshed using machines which cut holes in the skin allowing it to be stretched to cover a larger area than that harvested. The grafts can be meshed at varying ratios, 1:1, 1.5:1, 2:1, 3:1, 4:1, 6:1, and 9:1, using different machine parts. In practice, grafts meshed with an expansion ratio more than 3:1 need additional protection as the wound bed that lies in the interstices (holes) of the graft is prone to desiccation. The wound bed can undergo desiccation and necrosis with subsequent graft loss and deepening of the underlying wound. Therefore special techniques are used to protect widely meshed grafts. Once the graft has taken and the interstices re-epithelialize, hypertrophic scarring in the interstices can be significant with a "crocodile skin" appearance. This is more pronounced with widely meshed grafts; thus they are reserved for large burns. Mesh ratios of greater than 4:1 are not frequently used. In addition to expanding the area covered by a graft, meshing allows drainage of any underlying hematoma or seroma. Sheet grafts give a better cosmetic appearance but are more susceptible to loss secondary to hematoma or seroma. Sheet grafts are used in cosmetically and functionally important areas such as the face and hands.

Points about use of skin from deceased donors
Loss of barrier function of the skin leads to several significant adverse physiological effects. These include increased evaporative and direct fluid losses, protein loss, increased risk of microbial colonization and invasive infection, desiccation of the wound leading to progressive cell death and deepening of the wound. If the wound cannot be closed using autograft skin then other strategies for physiological wound closure must be sought.

Physiological wound closure will help with protection from mechanical trauma, reduction of pain, increased compliance with physiotherapy, protection from bacterial invasion and infection, reduction in fluid, electrolyte, and protein losses from the wound [3]. This can be successfully treated by using skin donated by, and recovered from, persons after death.

Preference
In a patient with a major burn injury or significant skin loss from other causes with paucity of available autologous skin graft donor sites, skin replacement and physiological wound closure can be achieved using deceased donor allograft skin as it has many of the properties of an ideal biological dressing.

Skin allograft is donated from selected donors who are carefully screened and tested. The tissue is procured, processed, stored and distributed through a system of tissue banks, the details of which are discussed elsewhere in companion books to this volume [6, 7].

Human deceased donor skin grafts are generally used for treatment of burns as a split-thickness skin graft and can contain viable cells, supplied as fresh (refrigerated) or cryopreserved (frozen). Alternatively, grafts with nonviable cells can be supplied as irradiated, glycerolized, or freeze dried. The specific type of allograft skin used varies around the world, with viable allograft being popular in North America (fresh or cryopreserved) and non-viable in Europe (glycerolized). In the UK both viable (cryopreserved) and non-viable (irradiated) types are available.

It is thought that fresh human deceased donor skin allograft represents the best alternative when autologous skin is not available for temporary wound closure. Fresh allograft is believed to have the following benefits. It adheres well to the wound stimulating neo-vascularization with inherent growth factors, is rapidly re-vascularized, and prepares the wound bed for autologous skin grafting. Fresh allograft is thought to have inherent anti-microbial properties owing to its competent immune cells and tolerates wound contamination with bacteria more robustly than other forms of allograft [8].

Cryopreserved allograft is an excellent alternative to fresh allograft. In particular it is difficult to maintain stocks of fresh allograft. Cryopreservation allows prolonged storage, increasing the useful lifespan of allograft skin from 14 days to over one year. The cell viability of cryopreserved allograft is less than fresh allograft and continues to decrease over time. However, this decrease in viability is offset by the prolonged availability of a precious resource [8].

Adherence and take

There is continued debate about the superiority or necessity of using viable human deceased donor skin allograft. There have been no studies comparing the use of viable to non-viable allograft in burn wound closure. The choice usually depends on availability and the surgeon's personal preference. However, it is generally felt that fresh skin allograft is the next best skin replacement after skin autograft and is currently considered the "gold standard" for all biological dressings.

After application of any skin substitute there is initial adherence by formation of a film of fibrin, which then coalesces into a matrix. This fibrin matrix is thought to impart many of the benefits of physiological wound closure including reduced evaporative loss, reduced pain, and barrier protection against microorganisms. In the short term, viable allograft provides an advantage because it adheres more readily and lasts longer than other substances. After initial adherence, a phase of fibroblast proliferation and collagen synthesis begins which can encase foreign substances mimicking "take". Revascularization occurs at about 48 hours and capillaries will grow from the host wound bed into the graft, supplying oxygen and nutrients; this can be defined as true "take". This can only occur if the graft is alive and structurally intact.

Subsequently, over days and weeks if vascularization is poor, the epidermal cells die, slough off, and epidermolysis occurs.

The dermis is less antigenic with fewer cells and can withstand initial grafting while provoking relatively little rejection. It is possible for allograft

> **Box 11.3 Uses of human deceased donor skin allograft**
> There are a number of clinical indications for the use of human deceased donor skin allograft where it has a benefit, including:
>
> - Coverage of extensive burn wounds or other wounds where donor sites are not available
> - Coverage of widely meshed autologous skin grafts
> - Extensive partial thickness burns
> - Extensive desquamative skin conditions (Stevens–Johnson syndrome, toxic epidermal necrolysis, staphylococcal scalded skin syndrome)
> - To prepare and test a wound bed for autografting
> - To provide a vascularized dermal bed in a staged procedure for application of cultured epithelial autograft

dermis to survive for prolonged periods, although over months the collagen is eventually replaced with autologous collagen through the process of remodelling. During this time the dermis can serve as a scaffold for autologous epidermal ingrowths.

Once skin allografts have become vascularized, they function as living skin, providing an effective vapor barrier, reducing inflammation, and allowing the active and ongoing elimination of infection by circulating white blood cells. This stable coverage lasts until rejection occurs. Human deceased donor skin allograft will survive longer on patients with large burn wounds as rejection is a function of immune competence and the metabolic state of the patient. The superiority of viable allograft over all other alternatives is widely acknowledged and viable allograft remains the reference to which all other substances are compared.

The indications listed in Box 11.3 will be discussed in a little more detail.

Physiological wound closure in extensive full-thickness wounds

In major burn wounds where donor sites are lacking, physiological closure of the burn wound can be achieved with human deceased donor skin. The allograft must be readily and copiously available to allow immediate cover and closure of an extensive wound. The allograft is usually applied either unmeshed or minimally expanded with a maximum mesh expansion ratio of 2:1. This optimizes physiological wound closure and prevents desiccation of the underlying wound bed beneath the mesh interstices, which can lead to subsequent wound infection and graft loss.

The allograft is usually removed or replaced when autologous donor sites become available after healing. Further skin allograft application may be repeatedly required with a massive burn during the process of resurfacing the wound.

Intermingling skin allograft/autograft techniques

There have been several techniques developed that describe intermingling use of autograft and allograft skin.

The original technique described by Mowlem called "tiger striping" used alternating sheets of autograft and allograft skin placed onto a granulating or excised wound. Both autograft and allograft skin adhere to the wound bed. This is followed by autologous epithelial cell migration across the wound surface between sheets of autograft and underneath the allograft sheet. The allograft sheet slowly separates, leaving a healed epithelialized wound beneath. This process is termed "creeping substitution".

This intermingling technique was modified and described by Alexander in 1981. In this technique, widely meshed autograft skin (greater than 3:1 expansion ratio) is placed on the wound bed and then is covered by sheet or narrowly meshed allograft (2:1 expansion ratio). If widely meshed skin alone is placed on a wound the interstices or wound between the mesh can desiccate, necrose, and become secondarily infected. Placing the allograft over the autograft using this "sandwich" technique closes the wound bed in the interstices and prevents desiccation, necrosis, and infection, while autologous epithelial cells from the autologous meshed graft migrate across the wound bed to achieve healing. As this happens the allograft spontaneously separates from the wound bed. This overlay technique is now the most commonly used method of resurfacing large burn wounds as significant expansion of autologous skin can be achieved to resurface very large wounds. This technique results in significant scarring and is reserved for major full-thickness burn wounds (greater than 40% body surface area) that cannot be closed with meshed autograft alone (Figure 11.2).

Intermingling of autograft and allograft has also been adapted by Chinese surgeons, who have used very small pieces of autograft or "micro grafts" less than 1 mm in diameter seeded onto the dermis of allograft skin before application to the wound. The autograft epidermal cells proliferate and migrate, and creeping substitution occurs with spontaneous separation of the allograft. This technique can be used to obtain very large expansion ratios; however, scar contracture may be worse using this technique [1].

The use in partial thickness wounds

Human deceased donor skin allograft can be used in partial thickness wounds as a temporary biological dressing. After debridement of any necrotic epidermis and dermis, the allograft skin will adhere to the wound, reducing pain, fluid, electrolyte, and protein losses. Wound care is usually easier with less pain during dressing changes. The partial thickness wound will heal by proliferation and migration of epithelial cells from adnexal structures with re-epithelialization of the wound surface. As this occurs the allograft slowly separates, revealing a healed wound beneath. This technique is especially

CASE STUDY 11.1   (FIGURE 11.2)

Autograft/allograft "sandwich" grafting after full-thickness wound excision of back in patient with 75% full-thickness burn

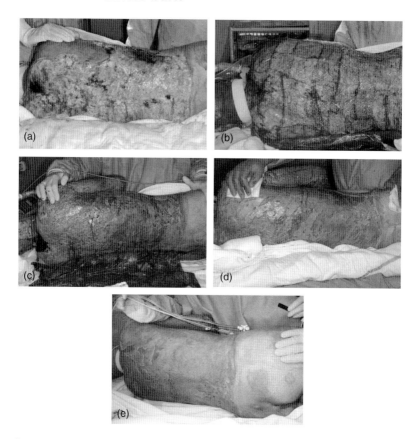

Figure 11.2 (a) Appearance at excision; (b) one week after autograft/allograft "sandwich" grafting; (c) three weeks post grafting – autograft re-epithelializing, allograft not present on wound; (d) five weeks after grafting: continued epithelialization; (e) eight weeks after grafting: approaching complete healing.

useful for large superficial cutaneous wounds where pain, fluid, and electrolyte losses can lead to difficult management problems.

Such large superficial cutaneous wounds include superficial partial thickness burns, drug-induced epithelial loss such as Stevens–Johnson syndrome and toxic epidermal necrolysis, and bacterial toxin-mediated desquamation like staphylococcal scalded skin syndrome [1] (Figure 11.3).

CASE STUDY 11.2   (FIGURE 11.3)

Use of allograft in toxic epidermal necrolysis

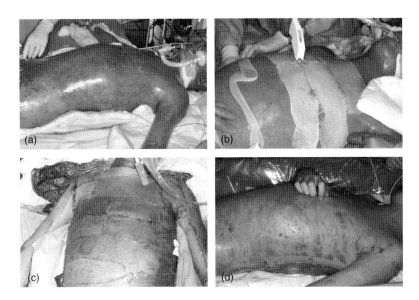

Figure 11.3 (a) 18-year-old male with 90% epidermal loss from TENS; (b) application of allograft after wound cleansing and debridement; (c) appearance of adherent allograft at one week; (d) appearance of re-epithelialized wound at two weeks.

Complications
Transmission of infection
During procurement, processing, dispatch, and clinical use, tissue banks and clinical users screen for pathogenic bacteria, fungi, and viruses. Application of skin allograft has been reported to cause bacterial infection. Although there are data to suggest the safety of low levels of colonization, tissue banks involved in the procurement and processing of human deceased donor skin allograft will not issue skin that has been colonized with pathogenic flora. This is fully discussed elsewhere [6].

Similarly it is mandated by regulations that all tissue donors are now screened for viral transmissible diseases.

A 1992 report of human immunodeficiency virus (HIV) transmission to a few recipients of fresh tissues from a single contaminated donor highlighted the risks associated with allograft usage. There has been one case of HIV-1 transmission to a burn patient from an HIV-1-positive donor, although donor testing results were not known at the time of allograft application and the recipient, who had risk factors for HIV, was not tested before allograft placement [9].

There have been several reports of cytomegalovirus (CMV) transmission from human deceased donor skin with one series reporting over 20% seroconversion in previously CMV seronegative patients. In a review of human deceased donor skin allograft donors, over 60% were CMV positive. However, although CMV transmission is a risk associated with the use of skin allograft, there is little or no evidence about the significance or effect on outcome. At present the decision to use allograft skin from CMV-positive donors rests with the treating clinician.

Rejection

The epidermis of human deceased donor skin allograft contains Langerhans cells, which express type II histocompatibility antigens and serve as the major stimulus to rejection. In immune-competent recipients, allograft epidermis will begin to reject in 1–2 weeks; however, in critically ill burn patients who are immunosuppressed, the allograft can survive for much longer. The rejection process leads to acute inflammation and is often followed by wound infection. Human deceased donor skin when vascularized usually survives for 2–3 weeks. There have been reports of prolonged survival of over 60 days in some patients; however, this would now be unusual with recent improvements in surgery, immune support, and critical care of the burned patient.

There have been numerous attempts made to increase human deceased donor skin survival by reducing its antigenicity. These have included ultraviolet light irradiation and incubation with steroids, with limited success.

Other researchers have used systemic immunosuppressive agents in burn patients including azothioprine and cyclosporine A, reporting prolonged allograft survival. However, rejection occurred soon after stopping the immunosuppression medication except for a few instances of persistent engraftment. Immunosuppression of a burn patient who is already immunosuppressed with the resultant increased risk of infection should not be undertaken lightly.

Allografting from living donors has been used on occasions when suitable donors are available. These donors are usually parents who offer their skin to circumvent cultural issues and assuage guilt. This is a potentially high-risk procedure in terms of pain and morbidity and is only used as a last resort if human deceased donor skin is not available. Skin allograft has also been transplanted in identical twins where one sibling served as a donor for another with an attendant immunological privilege and permanent survival of the allograft [1, 4].

Clinical use

The clinical use and effectiveness of human deceased donor skin allograft is evidenced by its increasing demand. There have been few studies specifically demonstrating the benefit of allograft per se or comparing it with other skin substitutes. The use of allograft has gone hand in hand with a more aggressive excisional approach in burn surgery removing larger amounts of necrotic tissue followed by wound closure with autograft and/or allograft. Studies have repeatedly demonstrated the benefits of this approach [2, 10, 11].

Evidence from direct comparisons between different types of allograft and other skin substitutes is also scarce. One such randomized multicentered trial compared Integra™, a dermal template, with other skin grafting materials. There was no reported difference in "take" between Integra and skin allograft although "take" was not defined [12].

In a cost-constrained environment the use of alternative skin coverings will be limited. This is particularly true in the developing world. There are few or no data evaluating the economics of skin substitute use, particularly when long-term measures of outcome are studied. Without the evidence of long-term benefit the use of skin substitutes in a cost-constrained environment will continue to be limited.

Alternative skin substitutes
Classification of skin substitutes

Skin substitutes can be classified as being either temporary or permanent. They can be used to replace the epidermal portion of the skin, the dermal portion, or both. Their use and effectiveness should be analyzed for how they perform when replacing the specific part of the skin as well as the skin as a whole [13]. Another useful classification is based on the immunogenicity of cells the skin substitute contains. This can also be used for tissue engineered products [8]. These types of human and non-human derived graft options are detailed in Chapter 12. Human-derived grafts that can be considered "alternatives" to conventional fresh, frozen, or lyophilized skin grafts are those that are decellularized, such as Alloderm® and others [14]. Amnion is described next because it is similar to conventional skin allograft.

Amnion

The amnion is the inner layer of tissue that surrounds the fetus in utero, and contains amniotic fluid. Both the inner amnion and the outer chorion layers have been used for many years, but amnion is preferred because it is immunologically privileged and less antigenic. Amnion is commonly used by ophthalmic surgeons to cover damaged corneas as it is immunologically privileged tissue and does not stimulate rejection. Amnion can control evaporative fluid loss and is effective in reducing bacterial counts. It also contains many growth factors that stimulate epithelial proliferation and has antiangiogenic properties.

In view of these specific factors, its main use in burn care has been in partial thickness wounds such as donor sites and partial thickness burns. It has not been extensively used after wound excision. Like any allogeneic material, the risk of disease transmission must be recognized and managed. Restricted availability, small size, and fragility limit its usefulness in burn care. Most reports on its use in burn care have come from the developing world [15].

Cultured skin substitutes

Although a detailed discussion of these options is beyond the scope of this chapter and is covered elsewhere in this book (Chapter 12), this description of skin substitutes would not be complete without a brief mention of tissue-cultured products.

Using tissue culture techniques, epidermal cells (keratinocytes) can be grown in a laboratory and then used to assist wound closure. From a $1\,cm^2$ autologous biopsy, enough cells can be cultured in approximately three to four weeks to cover $1\,m^2$ body surface area. Sheets of these cultured epithelial autografts (CEAs) have been used by burn surgeons for over 20 years.

These cells can be cultured commercially for patients with large burn injuries; however, the cost is significant. This technique only produces the epidermal layer for wound closure and, although there have been many reports of successful use of CEA to close burn wounds, several problems limit their use [16]. The lag time of three weeks from biopsy to production of adequate quantities allows wound colonization and granulation tissue to develop, leading to low take rates compared with split skin grafts. Once applied, the grafts are very fragile and often prolonged immobilization of the patient is required. Even after successful take, the grafted areas remain fragile and blister easily because of poor and delayed basement membrane formation. Attempts to overcome some of these problems have been to graft the CEA onto an allograft dermal bed, as described by Cuono in 1986 [17]. Initially after wound excision, allograft is used for temporary wound closure while CEAs are produced. When ready, the epidermal portion of the engrafted allograft is removed using a dermatome or dermabrasion, leaving a viable dermal allograft bed behind onto which the CEAs are applied. This technique has been reported as having better CEA take with improved basement membrane formation and less fragility and blistering.

More recently the use of subconfluent, autologous keratinocyte suspensions sprayed onto excised wounds has been described. This promising technique has been used directly to treat partial thickness wounds and excised wounds after excision. It has also been used to augment epithelialization by treating interstices of widely meshed skin grafts and skin graft donor sites. Initial results have been promising and many burn surgeons have moved from using sheets of CEA to this subconfluent suspension technique. However, confirmation of the superiority of this technique has yet to be confirmed by a multi-centered trial [16].

In general the use of CEA should be reserved for patients with massive burns (more than 90%) with extremely limited donor sites or major burns where donor sites are limited, difficult to harvest, and cosmetically and functionally important (face, hands, feet, genitalia). A review of patients surviving massive burn injury showed that those treated with CEA had a longer hospital stay, required more operations, and had higher treatment costs than a comparative group treated with conventional techniques [18].

The future

Planning allograft use

It is clear from this discussion that human deceased donor skin graft has an important role in the management of burn patients. As an aggressive surgical approach becomes the standard of care, the subsequent need for allograft will continue to increase. Few published data exist on the amounts of allograft currently being processed, distributed, and used worldwide. However, data from the American Association of Tissue Banks clearly demonstrate an increased demand and usage. This trend is probably replicated across Western Europe. The Eurocet platform (http://www.eurocet.org/) has begun to carry data on European member state tissue donation, including skin, which may give a pattern in donation and use over coming years.

These data are important to enable planning for routine procurement and processing to support use. In addition, they are also important to inform planning for disasters where large numbers of burn victims might be expected.

To give some evidence about allograft use within a burn service, a review of allograft use at St Andrews Centre for Plastic Surgery and Burns, Chelmsford, Essex, UK, was recently undertaken [19]. The aim of the study was to assess allograft use in the past to guide planning for the future. A retrospective observational study looked at a five-year period (January 2004 to January 2009). During this time approximately 3500 burn patients required in-patient admission. Of these, 143 received deceased donor allograft supplied by the National Health Service Blood and Transplant Tissue Services' Skin Bank based in Liverpool, UK. Analysis of data revealed that for patients with burns with a total burn surface area (TBSA) less than 40%, $0.5\,cm^2$ allograft per square centimeter burn excised and grafted was required. This allograft usage index increased exponentially to $1.5\,cm^2$ of allograft per

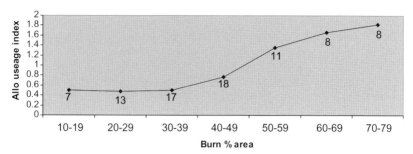

Figure 11.4 Allograft use index square centimeter allograft required per square centimeter burn for increasing percentage TBSA.

square centimeter burn in patients with burns of 60% TBSA, and 1.9 cm^2 of allograft per square centimeter burn in patients with burns over 80% TBSA (Figure 11.4).

Using these data, combined with those on the admission profile of patients being admitted to an individual service, could help the service to estimate the amount of allograft required on a weekly, monthly, and yearly basis and can allow supplying tissue banks to plan their donation, retrieval, processing, and storage requirements.

Disaster planning and skin allograft stocks

We currently live in an unstable environment with an ever-present risk of mass-casualty disasters. Major incidents in the UK are fortunately uncommon owing to increased compliance with health and safety regulations. However, with involvement of United Nations' armed forces in many conflicts across the world within recent years, there is an increased risk of terrorist attacks on home soil of supporting countries.

In major incidents when casualties included burns, studying casualty profiles is a useful starting point for planning resources, including inventory requirements for deceased donor skin allografts. A review examined the casualty profiles of patients involved in major burn incidents in the UK since 1980. The study examined major incidents with 10 or more casualties. Thirty-six major incidents have occurred in the UK since 1980.

An average of 1.29 incidents have occurred per year in the past 28 years. The numbers of incidents have decreased over the past three decades, with 16 major incidents in the 1980s, 13 in the 1990s, and only seven, so far, in this decade. Of the 36 incidents, only two produced more than 100 fatalities. The total fatalities per decade are as follows: 1980s, 710 fatalities; 1990s, 78 fatalities; 2000s, 84 fatalities.

Of the 36 incidents, only 19 were reported to result in burn casualties. In the 19 incidents with burn casualties, the average number of minor injuries was 104.4, the average number of serious injuries was 48, and the average number of fatalities was 38.3. In the incidents of burns, there were many walking wounded but also significant numbers of seriously injured and fatalities. This contradicts findings in previous analyses of casualty profiles which report that people either escape rapidly, sustaining relatively minor injuries, or they become engulfed in the conflagration and sustain lethal injuries. In most burn incidents the traditional pattern is followed of all major incidents where walking wounded numbers are high, then there is a significant number of seriously injured, and then fewer individuals are killed. Our analysis showed that very few casualties reach the hospital with severe burns of greater than 30%.

After the terrorist attacks of September 11, 2001, in the USA, plans to manage thousands of burn casualties have been developed. In addition, historical experiences of previous civilian burn or fire disasters occurring in the USA have been analyzed. A review of these between 1900 and 2000 revealed 73 such disasters, with the number of fatalities per incident steadily decreasing [20]. Examination of the data revealed significant casualty counts with fatalities occurring at the scene or within 24 hours. A second large group comprised the walking wounded who required minimal outpatient care. Most disasters produced fewer than 25–50 patients requiring inpatient burn care. Patients with more severe injury requiring inpatient burn care comprised a small percentage of the total casualty numbers figure but consumed significant resources during treatment.

These figures can be used to predict human deceased donor skin graft storage needs for emergency preparedness. If $1 \, cm^2$ allograft per $1 \, cm^2$ of burn is used as a guide, the following situations can be planned. The body surface area of an adult male is approximately $20,000 \, cm^2$ ($2 \, m^2$). An adult with a 60% burn will require $12,000 \, cm^2$ of allograft, and one with a 40% burn will require $8000 \, cm^2$.

Escalating these figures to a mass casualty incident would have significant implication for emergency preparedness and the need for deceased donor skin stock held within tissue banks.

Fifty patients with an average of 60% burn would require $700,000 \, cm^2$ of allograft. Fifty patients with 40% burns would require $200,000 \, cm^{2.}$ This would have considerable logistic and financial implications; however, the development of a skin allograft index potentially allows efficient use of this limited resource [19]. In the event of a disaster where significant numbers of patients sustain major burn injuries, international cooperation between skin banks could be required to provide sufficient quantities of deceased donor skin.

Cost constraints

After early aggressive surgery and wound excision, it is clear from this discussion that wound closure is vital to survival. The choice of wound closure depends on availability, performance and cost. The "gold standard" is autologous skin, which has the advantage of being usually readily available. All substitutes for autologous skin vary in terms of performance and cost but most surgeons will chose viable allograft as their first choice after autograft. Few comparative studies have been published comparing costs of different skin substitutes.

We reviewed a series of patients with burns greater than 40% TBSA who underwent total or near-total wound excision followed by wound resurfacing with Integra or with our standard approach of allograft/ autograft sandwich technique over a two-year period [21]. All patients survived.

There were seven patients treated with allograft/autograft "sandwich" with a mean age 32 years (range 5–52), a mean total burn size of 60% TBSA (range 43–8) with 49% TBSA (range 40–50) or 8285 cm^2 (range 5000– 14,000) of full-thickness burn.

Another seven patients were treated with Integra™ with a mean age of 15 years (range 2–32), a mean total burn size of 62%TBSA (range 40–85) with 60% TBSA (range 40–85) or 8050 cm^2 (range 4000–1300) being full thickness.

Time to healing in the "sandwich" allograft group was 51.1 ± 8.9 days and in the Integra group 63.9 ± 3.6 days. The "sandwich" allograft group had 5 ± 1 operations while the Integra group had 8 ± 2 operations. Looking at skin replacement requirements, the "sandwich" allograft group required 440 cm^2 per 1% full-thickness burn, with the Integra group requiring 80 cm^2 per 1% full-thickness burn. The difference was attributed to repeated applications and exchanges of allograft. Length of inpatient stay was 62 days (range 52–109) for the "sandwich" allograft group and 88 days (range 43– 164) for the Integra group.

The average Integra cost was calculated as £14,464 per patient or £234 per 1% burn or £1.7 per cm^2 full-thickness burn. This compared with the average allograft "sandwich" cost of £16,671 per patient or £279 per 1% burn or £2.14 per cm^2 full-thickness burn. These costs were based on a price per square centimeter of £4.00 for Integra and £1.50 for allograft skin.

Statistical analysis of all the above data revealed no significant differences in burn demographics, time to healing, length of stay, or cost of skin replacement.

This study highlighted that treatment of major burns is expensive, and that the cost of skin replacement using either method only accounted for about 10% of the total cost of the treatment episode, which was mainly dependent on length of stay [21] (Figure 11.5).

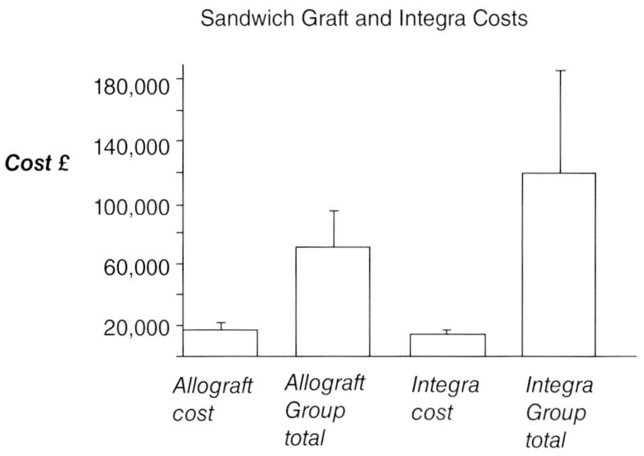

Sandwich Graft and Integra Costs

Figure 11.5 Comparison of skin substitute costs with total treatment cost.

Future of skin substitutes

The current "gold standard" in terms of permanent wound closure remains the split-thickness skin autograft, with viable deceased donor skin being the first choice as a temporary replacement. This hierarchy is likely to be challenged in the future as artificial skin substitutes become cheaper, more reliable, and increasingly sophisticated.

Our concept of skin replacement and wound cover is currently simplistic. We aim to replace dermis and epidermis. Our current technology does not address replacement of adnexal structures such as hair follicles, sebaceous and sweat glands, neurosensory endings, and melanocytes.

Improvements in cost are awaited but, in a cost-constrained environment, the benefits of skin substitutes need to be evaluated and compared in formal, controlled trials. Skin substitutes also need to be produced at lower cost. A combination of improved, proven efficacy with reduced cost and increased availability would increase the use and potential benefit for patients worldwide.

Improvements in reliability could relate to grafts that include epithelial cells engineered to express a variety of growth factors such as platelet-derived growth factor, human growth hormone, and insulin-like growth factor 1, to speed up vascularization and take. In addition, combinations of autologous keratinocytes, fibroblasts, endothelial cells, and melanocytes are likely to be successfully grown in a durable dermal analog.

Further work on reducing the antigenic stimulus of human deceased donor skin grafts may also bring benefits. If allograft can be manipulated to prevent rejection without the need for systemic immunosuppression of the recipient patient, then safe permanent skin replacement with deceased donor skin may yet become possible.

Future advances may initially come from mixing allogeneic and autologous cells and tissues to produce chimeric grafts. This type of mixed skin substitute will have the advantages of autologous tissue culture mixed with readily available allograft tissues, hopefully allowing rapid and reliable production.

Conclusion

The search for the ideal skin replacement remains one of the holy grails of burn care. Despite many advances, one cannot help but acknowledge that, fundamentally, the questions stay the same but the answers may change.

KEY LEARNING POINTS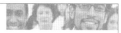

- After burn injury, removal of dead or devitalized tissue saves lives, improves form, and optimizes function.

- Wound closure must be achieved either with autologous skin or a temporary or permanent skin substitute.

- The current "gold standard" in skin replacement after burn injury remains autologous split thickness skin graft.

- Human deceased donor skin allograft represents the best alternative when autologous skin is not available for temporary wound closure.

- This hierarchy is likely to be challenged in the future as artificial skin substitutes become cheaper, more reliable, and increasingly sophisticated.

References

1. Kagan R, Robb E, Plessinger R. The skin bank. In: Herndon D, editor. Total burn care. 3rd edition. Philadelphia: Elsevier; 2007; p. 229–38.
2. Herndon DN, Parks DH. Comparison of serial debridement and autografting and early massive excision with cadaver skin overlay in the treatment of large burns in children. J Trauma 1986;26:149–52.
3. Garner JP, Heppell PS. Cerium nitrate in the management of burns. Burns 2005;31:539–47.
4. Sheridan RL, Tompkins RG. Skin substitutes in burns. Burns 1999;25:97–103.
5. Gilpin DA, Barrow RE, Rutan RL, Broemeling L, Herndon DN. Recombinant human growth hormone accelerates wound healing in children with large cutaneous burns. Ann Surg 1994;220:19–24.
6. Warwick RM, Fehily D, Brubaker SA, Eastlund T (eds). Tissue and Cell Donaton: An Essential Guide. Wiley-Blackwell, 2009.
7. Fehily D, Brubaker SA, Kearney JN, Wolfinbarger L (eds). Tissue and Cell Processing: An Essential Guide. Oxford: Blackwell Publishing Ltd; 2012.

8. Greenleaf G, Hansbrough JF. Current trends in the use of allograft skin for patients with burns and reflections on the future of skin banking in the United States. J Burn Care Rehabil 1994;15:428–31.

9. Pirnay JP, Vandenvelde C, Duinslaeger L, et al. HIV transmission by transplantation of allograft skin:a review of the literature. Burns 1997;23:1–5.

10. Ong YS, Samuel M, Song C. Meta-analysis of early excision of burns. Burns 2006;32:145–50.

11. Mosier MJ, Gibran NS. Surgical excision of the burn wound. Clin Plast Surg 2009;36:617–25.

12. Heimbach DM, Warden GD, Luterman A, et al. Multicenter postapproval clinical trial of Integra dermal regeneration template for burn treatment. J Burn Care Rehabil 2003;24:42–8.

13. Saffle JR. Closure of the excised burn wound: temporary skin substitutes. Clin Plast Surg 2009;36:627–41.

14. Sheridan R. Closure of the excised burn wound: autografts, semipermanent skin substitutes,and permanent skin substitutes. Clin Plast Surg 2009;36:643–51.

15. Kesting MR, Wolff KD, Hohlweg-Majert B, et al. The role of allogeinic amniotic membrane in burn treatment. J Burn Care Res 2008;29:907–16.

16. Wood FM, Kolybaba ML, Allen P. The use of cultured epithelial autograft in the treatment of major burn injuries: a critical review of the literature. Burns 2006;32:395–401.

17. Cuono C, Langdon R, McGuire J. Use of cultured epidermal autografts and dermal allografts as skin replacement after burn injury. Lancet 1986;i:1123–4.

18. Barret JP, Wolf SE, Desai MH, Herndon DN Cost-efficacy of cultured epidermal autografts in massive pediatric burns. Ann Surg 2000;231:869–76.

19. Horner CWM, Atkins J, Simpson L, Philp B, Shelley O, and Dziewulski P. Estimating the usage of allograft in the treatment of major burns. Burns 2011;37:590–3.

20. Barillo DJ, Wolf S. Planning for burn disasters: lessons learned from one hundred years of history. J Burn Care Res 2006;27:622–34.

21. James S, Ghosh S, Simpson L and Dziewulski PA. Comparison Between Integra® and Sandwich grafting for the Treatment of Large Burns. International Society for Burn Injuries Quadrennial Congress, Seattle, USA, August 2002.

12 Skin Substitutes: Burn Treatment and Beyond

Hans-Oliver Rennekampff[1],
Christopher R. Chapple[2], and Glenn Greenleaf[3]
[1]Medical School Hannover, Hannover, Germany
[2]Royal Hallamshire Hospital, Sheffield, UK
[3]LifeCell Corp., Branchburg, NJ, USA

Introduction

Many, if not all, organisms are driven by a strong, innate sense of self preservation. This includes the evolution of mechanisms to deal with injury and disease. The human body and its organ systems are no exception; bleeding stops, broken bones mend, and injured skin heals.

In response to integumental compromise, the body mounts an immediate and concerted effort of containment and repair. When the skin is injured, an elaborate cascade of biochemical and biomechanical reactions is initiated and modulated by a host of cytokines and other cell-mediated factors. The result is an orchestrated release of endogenous proteins and proteinases as well as other chemical signals and targets which trigger cell migration and proliferation, collagen deposition, wound contraction and, ultimately, wound repair.

In some situations, however, the extent of the insult is far too great for effective and timely repair or the healing process has been inhibited or compromised. In other instances, the healing process itself, being predominantly the replacement of differentiated tissue with scar, may result in significant compromise of normal function or appearance. In these cases, the ability to assist the body's natural repair process with biological or synthetic materials has greatly reduced the morbidity and mortality associated with these devastating injuries.

Tissue and Cell Clinical Use: An Essential Guide, First Edition. Edited by Ruth M. Warwick and Scott A. Brubaker.
© 2012 Blackwell Publishing Ltd. Published 2012 by Blackwell Publishing Ltd.

Cutaneous compromise

Each year, hundreds of thousands of people throughout the world suffer severe cutaneous injuries. In the USA alone, the American Burn Association reports that serious burn injuries accounted for over 25,000 admissions to burn centers in 2007 [1]. Although many superficial injuries can be treated with topical dressings, full-thickness injuries must be addressed much more aggressively. Early tangential excision of burn eschar followed by wound closure has increased survival rates and decreased the mortality associated with extensive burns. In full-thickness injuries, use of split thickness autologous skin grafts can provide wound closure and improve the chances of survival. These skin transplants restore the barrier function of the epidermis and deliver a dermal component to the wound that would otherwise heal by intensive scarring and contracture. Although the use of the patient's own non-burned skin effects ultimate wound closure, there can be significant morbidity associated with the resultant skin graft donor sites. The undesirable consequences of autograft donor sites and the fundamental problems associated with the limited availability of non-burned tissue in extensive injuries presents a significant clinical challenge in the treatment of these wounds. Although various methods have been described and used to maximize the use of the patient's own skin including meshing and expansion, Meek (or postage stamp) grafting, and in vitro cell proliferation, clinicians are often challenged to achieve adequate wound closure. Also, in addition to the obvious assault of burn and traumatic injury, other medical conditions resulting in the loss or compromise of integumental integrity or adequate connective tissue present a significant clinical challenge. Every year, tens of thousands of patients suffer ulceration of the skin owing to vascular insufficiency or compromise as the result of diabetes or other metabolic disease processes. In these cases, the normal healing process is challenged resulting in slow or non-healing wounds. The use of autografts in these patients is not generally a viable option. Other conditions such as the loss of abdominal domain, soft tissue defects, urinary incontinence and repair of the pelvic floor require the ability to replace lost connective tissue.

   In all of these cases, the availability of an alternative to autologous tissue has greatly enhanced the clinician's ability to achieve both temporary and permanent wound closure or to ultimately restore form and function.

Temporary dressings

Allograft skin
The use of allograft skin as a temporary biological dressing in the treatment of burn injuries has been extensively described in the previous chapter. As outlined, donated human skin provides an effective bridge between wound

excision and permanent closure; however, there remain some recognized limitations to the use of this tissue.

Limitations of allograft skin

Until fairly recently, the ultimate fate for the majority of all allograft skin grafts was rejection. Under normal conditions, a healthy adult will reject an allograft skin transplant in 7–10 days. Under extremely traumatic conditions, the body's ability to mount an effective immune response may become compromised. In these situations, the length of time to rejection may be significantly increased. Historically, this has been the case in patients with severe burn injury. "Burn induced" immunosuppression has enabled transplanted allografts to survive much longer than would be anticipated, often for several weeks at a time. Aggressive intervention to meet the metabolic needs and to maintain the physiological status of the burn patient has effectively helped to restore the immune status of these patients. As the immune system is returned to a more normal operating level, so follows the body's ability to reject transplanted tissue. This presents a particular dilemma in patients with extensive burn injuries. In these patients requiring large areas of coverage with allograft, the return to immune competence requires that allogeneic skin must be replaced with increasing frequency. This problem is further exacerbated by the development of increased antigenic sensitivity to the skin grafts with each new graft placement.

In efforts to address the historical limitations of allograft skin as well as the limited availability, or contraindication to the use of autologous tissue, clinicians and researchers have pursued the development of synthetic skin substitutes

Skin substitutes

Recognizing that the basic components of the integumental system are the dermis for strength and elasticity and the epithelium for barrier functions, it seems logical that other materials possessing these same properties might have the potential to be used to mimic and ultimately replace these functions. In the early 1980s a plethora of activity surrounded the efforts to produce an artificial skin substitute. A host of synthetic and biosynthetic dressings have been developed and added to the surgical armamentarium.

Strategies in the development of skin substitutes

As with approaches to the engineering of other tissue grafts, strategies for the fabrication of skin substitutes can be allocated to different categories outlined in Table 12.1. The categories include temporary and permanent skin substitutes, epidermal and dermal substitutes, synthetic and biological skin substitutes and cell free and cell-seeded materials. Applications may be

Table 12.1 Skin substitutes grouped according to manufacturing process and materials involved

	Epidermal	Dermal	Epidermal/dermal
Cultured or biological	BioSeed-S, CellSpray, EpiCel, ReCell	AlloDerm, DemaMatrix, FlexHD, Integra, Matriderm, NeoForm	HF/HK in collagen/GAG, Apligraf, OrCel
Synthetic	Biobrane, Suprathel		
Combination of above	Transcyte	Dermagraft	

GAG, glycosaminoglycans; HF/HK, human fibroblasts/human keratinocytes.

Table 12.2 Applications and function

	Function	Product
Temporary	Barrier function/enhanced epithelialization	Biobrane Suprathel Transcyte
Temporary	Enhanced cutaneous healing	Apligraf Dermagraft
Permanent	Epidermal regeneration	CellSpray EpiCel ReCell
Permanent	Dermal reconstruction	AlloDerm Dermamatrix FlexHD Integra Matriderm NeoForm
Permanent	Epidermal and dermal reconstruction	HF/HK in collagen GAG

GAG, glycosaminoglycans; HF/HK, human fibroblasts/human keratinocytes.

targeted to provide a particular function (i.e., barrier versus dermal substrate) and some may overlap. The spectrum of possibilities is outlined in Table 12.2.

Temporary biosynthetic dressings
Biobrane®

As one of the first biosynthetic dressings to offer promise as a replacement to allograft skin for the temporary coverage of burn wounds, Biobrane (UDL Laboratories, Rockford, IL, USA) is a bilaminate membrane composed of nylon-mesh sheet coated with porcine type I collagen peptides. This "dermal" component is bonded to a thin layer of silicone rubber which

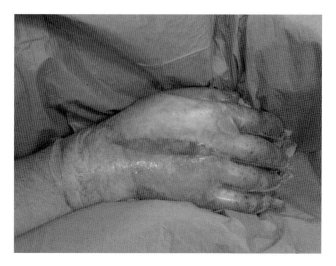

Figure 12.1 Application of a Biobrane glove on a circumferential partial thickens burn of the hand; no secondary dressing is needed.

provides the epidermal, barrier function. Early clinical experience demonstrated that Biobrane was an acceptable dressing when used on partial thickness, clean wounds. After debridement or cleansing of the wound Biobrane is stretched and affixed to the wounds. Wounds must be non-infected and free of eschar with demonstrated capillary blanching. A variety of reports have demonstrated that re-epithelialization is enhanced during Biobrane application on partial thickness burns as well as on donor sites. In two controlled comparative studies on partial thickness burns [2, 3], decreased healing time (9.7 days versus 16.1 days, 13.7 days versus 21.3 days) over silver sulfadiazine cream was reported. In addition, fewer dressing changes are necessary and reduced pain was reported. Owing to the occlusive nature of Biobrane, fluid collections and hematomas often prevent adherence to the wound bed. Fluid accumulation under Biobrane requires prompt aspiration and non adherent material should be removed. Modifications to the original product configuration included addition of fenestrations to allow some fluid release. Provided in a "glove" configuration, Biobrane can be used as an excellent temporary skin substitute to treat partial thickness burns of the hand allowing unrestricted physiotherapy (Figure 12.1). When used as a temporary dressing it tends to slowly separate from the wound bed as the wound re-epithelializes.

Transcyte™ (Dermagraft-TC®)

Transcyte (Advanced BioHealing, Westport, CT, USA), which was originally termed Dermagraft-TC (Advance Tissue Sciences, La Jolla, CA, USA), is essentially human neonatal fibroblasts cultured on a sheet of Biobrane. The fibroblasts attach and grow on the three-dimensional matrix eventually secreting a variety of matrix proteins including growth factors, collagens and several proteoglycans. Factors known to stimulate re-epithelialization, such as keratinocyte growth factor (KGF) and transforming growth factor (TGF-α), have been isolated in high concentrations. This results in a "bioactive" extracellular dermal matrix which mimics the dermal component of the native skin. The silicone rubber component of the mesh provides the barrier function of the epidermis. Transcyte has effectively been used as a temporary dressing in the treatment of all grades of burn injuries from severe to superficial. The efficacy of Transcyte for temporary closure of excised wounds has been demonstrated in controlled clinical trials [4]. Excised wounds were randomized to receive either Transcyte or allograft. Compared with allograft Transcyte, was easier to remove and less bleeding occurred. Subsequent autograft take was equivalent or superior in the Transcyte group. In addition, a controlled prospective randomized study [5] has demonstrated that Transcyte is effective for treating partial thickness wounds leading to rapid re-epithelialization and reduced scarring. Under Transcyte, partial thickness wounds closed up to 7 days faster than under conventional therapy. Long-term results at 3, 6, and 12 months post-burn showed reduced hypertrophic scarring as measured by the Vancouver scar scale.

Transcyte has also been used to treat severe exfoliating disorders such as toxic epidermal necrolysis syndrome and Stevens–Johnson syndrome, conditions in which patients experience critical loss of the epidermis.

Suprathel®

Suprathel (Polymedics Innovation, Denkendorf, Germany) is a copolymer composed of D,L-lactic trimethylene carbonate and ε-capronolacton. The porous material has a water vapor permeability of $40–70\,ml/m^2/hour$ and is biodegradable. The material is intended to be placed on clean, non-infected partial thickness burns. In a randomized, bi-centered clinical study it was shown that Suprathel significantly reduced pain on donor sites as well as on superficial partial thickness burns in comparison to standard petrolatum gauze [6]. The study was not designed to demonstrate a significant improvement in re-epithelialization over controls. Investigators also noted that although Suprathel is more expensive than petrolatum gauze, an overall reduction in total treatment costs was recognized owing to decreased dressing changes.

Dermal substitutes

Although great advances have been made in the acute treatment of burn and other significant integumental injuries, current efforts are now focusing on the restoration of form and function. Although the cellular elements of the epidermis can quickly and effectively replicate and regenerate restoring the barrier function of the skin, the highly organized matrix of the dermis is largely incapable of structured regeneration. The body repairs lost or damaged dermis by a haphazard deposition of granulation tissue. Myofibroblasts located within the granulation bed contribute to wound contraction. Although this combination may present an evolutionary advantage by expediting wound closure, the resultant scarring and contracture can be quite devastating and debilitating. Contractures over joint spaces can lead to loss of function. Similarly, hypertrophic scar and keloid formation remain significant morbidities associated with cutaneous injuries. All are the result of a damaged or inadequate dermal component of the skin. Several recent products have become available to help clinicians address this problem.

Dermagraft®

Dermagraft (Advanced BioHealing, Westport, CT, USA) is a bioabsorbable polyglactin mesh which has been seeded with human neonatal fibroblasts. These fibroblasts populate the three-dimensional architecture of the mesh and deposit several components of an extracellular matrix including growth factors, collagens, and glycosaminoglycans. As originally described by the company that developed this graft (Advanced Tissue Sciences, La Jolla, CA, USA) the intent is to deliver a "dermal-like" substrate to facilitate wound healing. The polyglactin mesh provides the initial structural integrity of the graft and serves as a scaffold for cell migration. The polyglactin mesh is eventually absorbed by hydrolysis, leaving the dermal component behind. Dermagraft has been used to treat cutaneous ulcers successfully. In a randomized, controlled, multi-centered study to evaluate the healing of chronic diabetic foot ulcers in over 300 patients, Marston and colleagues [7] cite complete wound healing in 30% of wounds treated with Dermagraft compared with 18.3% with conventional methods after 12 weeks. Additionally, complications related to diabetic ulcers such as cellulitis, osteomyelitis, and other local wound infections were significantly lower in the Dermagraft group (19% versus 32.5%).

Acellular dermal matrices

The transplantation of a dermal graft has been shown to inhibit contraction and provide a more acceptable cosmetic outcome. AlloDerm® (LifeCell, Branchburg, NJ, USA) represents the first commercially available acellular dermal matrix. In the AlloDerm process, deceased donors' skin grafts are subjected to a process of de-epidermization and decellularization followed by matrix preservation to ultimately provide an acellular dermal matrix complete with a competent basement membrane and essential extracellular matrix proteins. Animal experiments have demonstrated superior results in full-thickness wounds grafted with AlloDerm and cultured keratinocytes in comparison to control wounds without it. A variety of case studies demonstrated good handling characteristics and the ability to simultaneously graft AlloDerm with either split thickness skin grafts or cultured keratinocytes. In a multi-center, non-randomized trial investigators reported similar take rates comparing AlloDerm and simultaneous split thickness autograft application with the standard split thickness skin graft transplantation [8]. Early postoperative evaluation demonstrated normal collagen bundles and retained elastin fibers.

Other acellular dermal products derived from human allograft skin have recently been introduced. NeoForm™ (Mentor, Santa Barbara, CA, USA) is solvent extracted, dehydrated then gamma irradiated resulting in an acellular, cross-linked matrix. DermaMatrix™ and Flex HD™ (Musculoskeletal Transplant Foundation, Edison, NJ, USA) are processed by a series of detergent and acid washes.

Although initially applied to the treatment of full-thickness burn injuries, acellular dermal grafts have been successfully used in a variety of procedures including scar revision, contracture release, soft tissue repair or replacement, duraplasty, pelvic floor reconstruction, periodontal procedures, breast reconstruction, and hernia repair (Figures 12.2, 12.3, 12.4 and Plate 12.1).

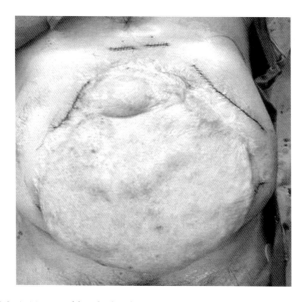

Figure 12.2 A 44-year-old male developed a severe pancreatitis secondary to a motor vehicle accident. This resulted in an extensive loss of abdominal domain. This was closed with autologous skin grafts.

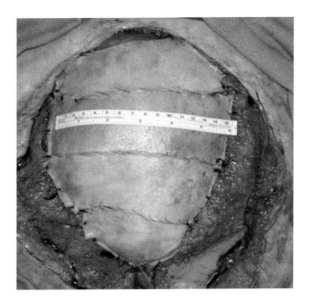

Figure 12.3 Restoration of abdominal integrity with acellular dermal allograft (AlloDerm).

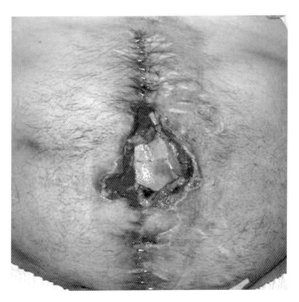

Figure 12.4 Primary skin closure failure with exposure of acellular dermal allograft.

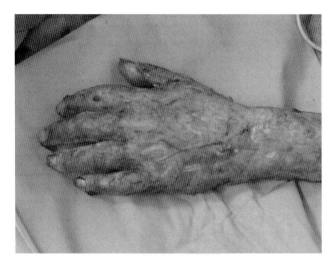

Figure 12.5 Debridment of a full-thickness burn wound down to fat and tendon sheets.

Matriderm®

Matriderm, a bovine non-cross linked collagen /elastin matrix (Dr. Suwelack Skin and Health Care AG, Billerbeck, Germany), has been used as a dermal substitute in experimental animal studies as well as controlled human studies. Matriderm is provided as a lyophilized, sterilized sheet and is reconstituted with saline or Ringer's lactate before application. A split thickness autograft can simultaneously be applied onto this dermal matrix (Figures 12.5, 12.6, 12.7). Experimental studies on full-thickness wounds in animals reported good dermal regeneration and a reduction in wound contraction with fibroblast seeded as well as non-seeded Matriderm. In a controlled clinical trial, an intra-individual comparison was made between Matriderm simultaneously grafted with an autograft and conventional split-thickness autografting. The survival of split-thickness autograft was only minimally affected. Statistical analysis revealed a significant improvement in objective pliability measurements of the dermal substitute-treated site after three months. Long-term evaluation showed an improvement of elasticity of approximately 20% over control wounds [9].

Integra®

In the early 1980s, Yannas and Burke described the use of an artificial skin to treat extensive burns. Integra Dermal Regeneration Template (Integra Life Sciences Corp, Plainsboro, NJ, USA) is a bilaminate membrane consisting of a "dermal" layer of crosslinked bovine type-I collagen and chondroitin-6-sulfate covered with a silastic "epidermis." This material is placed on excised

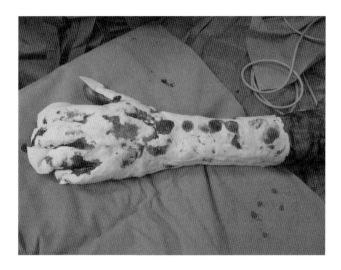

Figure 12.6 Matriderm dermal substitute is applied after debridement.

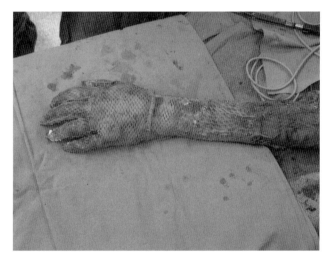

Figure 12.7 Simultaneous transplantation of a 1:1.5 meshed split thickness skin graft.

wounds, where it forms a layer of granulating "neodermis". After two to four weeks, the silicone layer can be peeled away and a thin epidermal allograft or cultured cells can be transplanted onto the wound. In a multi center randomized trial Integra was compared with immediate autografting, temporary placement of allograft and subsequent autografting in a second operation [10]. Integra take was lower than autograft take but there was no

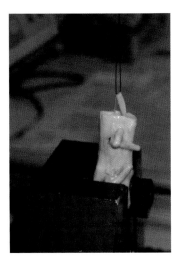

Plate 5.1 Suture-pullout tensile strength testing of a cryopreserved femoral artery allograft.

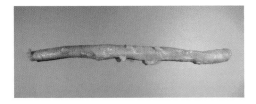

Plate 5.2 Superficial femoral artery specimen prepared for cryopreservation.

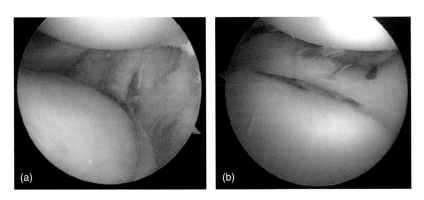

Plate 9.1 The same 15-year-old female as in Figure 9.1. (a) Arthroscopic view showing absence of the lateral meniscus. (b) Arthroscopic view after lateral meniscus allograft transplantation.

Tissue and Cell Clinical Use: An Essential Guide, First Edition. Edited by Ruth M. Warwick and Scott A. Brubaker.
© 2012 Blackwell Publishing Ltd. Published 2012 by Blackwell Publishing Ltd.

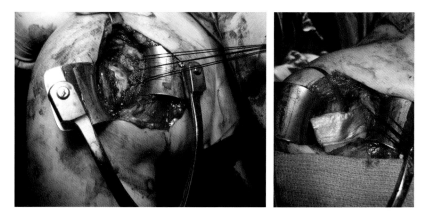

Plate 9.2 Intra-operative photographs (from 30-year-old female in Figure 9.3) showing the Achilles tendon allograft after connection to the glenoid and humeral head.

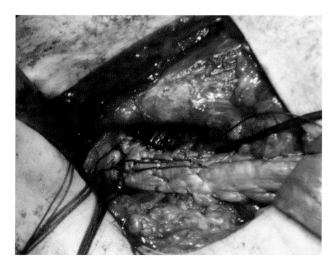

Plate 9.3 Intra-operative photograph (from 40-year-old patient in Figure 9.4) showing the pectoralis major tendon repair augmented with an Achilles tendon allograft sutured to the native pectoralis tendon and then secured to the humerus using suture anchors.

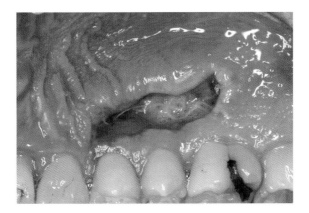

Plate 10.1 Healing palatal donor site one week after procurement of connective tissue graft.

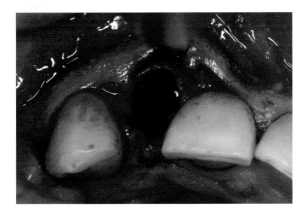

Plate 10.2 Socket immediately after extraction of maxillary lateral incisor. Note preservation of buccal plate of bone.

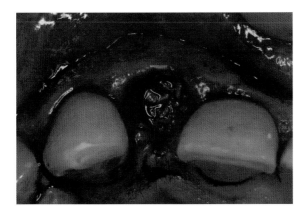

Plate 10.3 Site preservation of the socket from Plate 10.2 grafted with bone allograft.

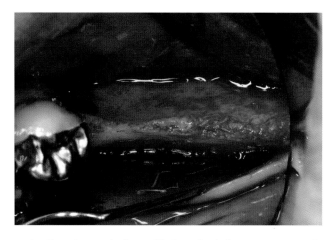

Plate 10.4 Significantly resorbed mandibular ridge before treatment with GBR.

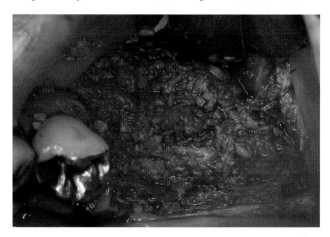

Plate 10.5 Resorbed ridge from Plate 10.4 treated with bone allograft.

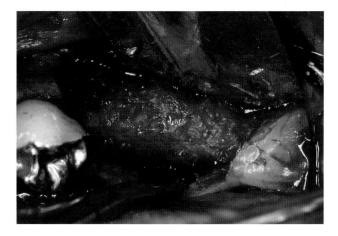

Plate 10.6 Mandibular ridge from Plates 10.4 and 10.5 after four months of healing from GBR treatment. Note the significant improvement in ridge width.

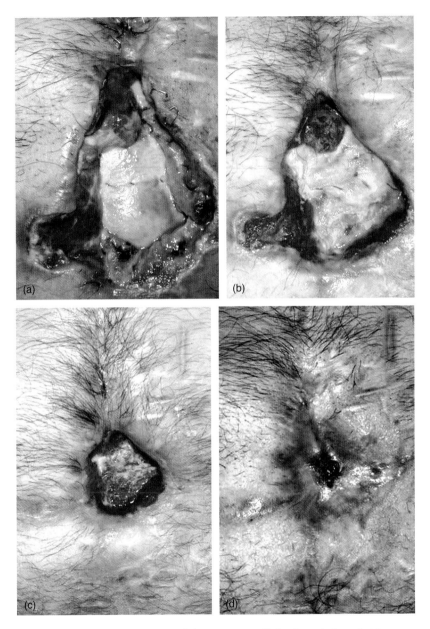

Plate 12.1 (a–d) Progressive wound closure over acellular dermal allograft. (Courtesy of Dr Ronald Silverman, University of Maryland, College Park, MD, USA.)

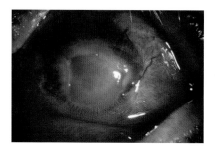

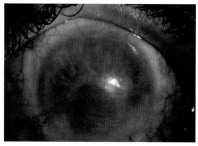

Plate 13.1 Picture of a patient with an alkali chemical injury in the preoperative phase. (Edward J. Holland, M.D.)

Plate 13.2 Same patient as Plate 13.1. Patient has undergone a keratolimbal allograft and has a stable ocular surface. (Edward J. Holland, M.D.)

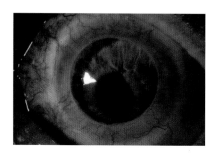

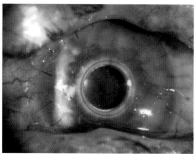

Plate 13.3 Same patient as Plates 13.1 and 13.2. Patient has undergone successful penetrating keratoplasty three months after limbal allograft. (Edward J. Holland, M.D.)

Plate 13.4 Boston type 1 keratoprosthesis. (Edward J. Holland, M.D.)

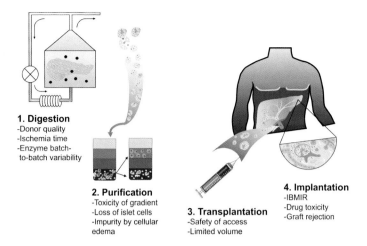

1. Digestion
-Donor quality
-Ischemia time
-Enzyme batch-
 to-batch variability

2. Purification
-Toxicity of gradient
-Loss of islet cells
-Impurity by cellular
 edema

3. Transplantation
-Safety of access
-Limited volume

4. Implantation
-IBMIR
-Drug toxicity
-Graft rejection

Plate 18.1 Current limitations associated with the multiple steps of islet transplantation.

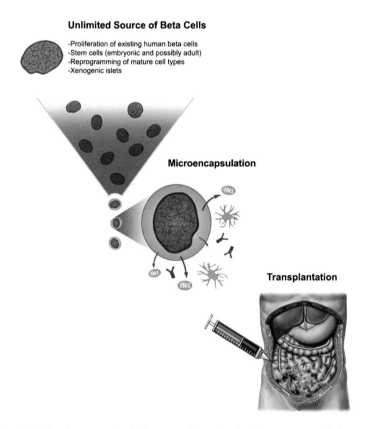

Unlimited Source of Beta Cells
-Proliferation of existing human beta cells
-Stem cells (embryonic and possibly adult)
-Reprogramming of mature cell types
-Xenogenic islets

Microencapsulation

Transplantation

Plate 18.2 The future goal of islet transplantation in the treatment of the type 1 diabetic population from an unlimited donor source without the need for chronic immunosuppressive therapy.

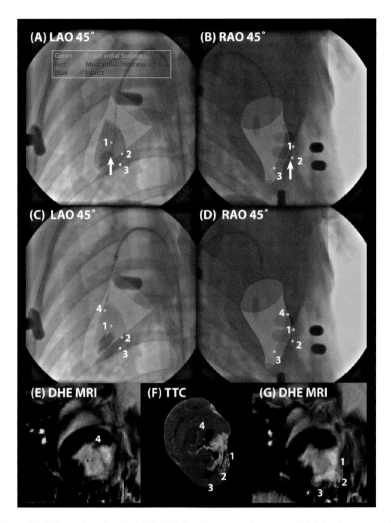

Plate 19.1 X-ray fused with MRI (XFM) to target endomyocardial injections according to infarct location (blue surface) and regional myocardial wall thickness (colored green for wall thickness greater than 6 mm, and red for wall thickness not more than 6 mm) in an animal with a 4-week-old left circumflex artery infarct. These surfaces were displayed on non-contrast enhanced X-Ray acquisitions in orthogonal projections (panels A and B). The position of the endomyocardial injection catheter can clearly be seen to lie in an area of wall thickness not more than 6 mm (arrow); this injection location was therefore rejected before deployment of the injection needle. Panels C and D demonstrate relocation of the injection catheter to a "safe" peri-infarct location with wall thickness greater than 6 mm. After deployment of the needle, X-ray acquisitions in orthogonal views allow reconstruction of the injection location in three dimensions (yellow spot, numbered 4). Previous injection locations (yellow spots, numbered 1–3) are also displayed in these views to help the operator avoid overlapping injections. The three-dimensional injection locations are also displayed superimposed on the prior DHE MRI (panels E and G). A post-mortem TTC-stained heart slice (panel F), located between the MRI slices displayed in Panels E and G, shows tissue-dye staining patterns that correlate well with the XFM-derived injection locations. (Reproduced from de Silva R, Gutierrez LF, Raval AN, McVeigh ER, Ozturk C, Lederman RJ. Circulation 2006;114(22):2342–2350.).

significant difference in take compared with allograft. Autograft take on Integra was reported to be 90%. The use of Integra was associated with a reduced length of stay in severely burned patients with two or more mortality risk factors. Application of Integra showed good results with respect to scarring. As a drawback, poor resistance to infection was noticed and meticulous dressing changes, and local antimicrobial controls are necessary to obtain good take rates of the material. Infected material has to be removed and replaced by new grafts. In a subsequent multicenter controlled clinical trial of Integra for burn treatment, Heimbach et al. reported on 216 patients with life-threatening full-thickness and deep partial thickness thermal injuries [11]. The study demonstrated a 3.1% incidence of invasive infection with a 13.2% rate of superficial infections. The mean take rate of the Integra on the excised burn wound was 76%, whereas the mean take rate of epidermal autografts placed over the Integra prepared wound bed was 87.7%. Integra has also been successfully used to treat other cutaneous injuries such as chronic ulcers, excision of hairy nevi, and revision of scar contractures.

Cultured epithelial substitutes

Keratinocyte sheet grafts

In the early 1980s, in vitro culture techniques were used in efforts to augment the availability of limited amounts of autologous skin. The Rheinwald and Green method for in vitro passaging of single-cell suspensions of keratinocytes is well described [12] and represents a standard for permanent epidermal replacement. Cultured epithelial sheets (Epicel®, Genzyme Tissue Repair, Boston, MA, USA) are now commercially available. One limitation to the use of cultured epithelial sheets is the amount of time required to prepare grafts of a suitable size for clinical use. Starting with a biopsy size of 1–5 cm^2, it takes about three weeks to cultivate a sufficient number of autologous epithelial sheets to cover an adult (17,000 cm^2) with a 70% total body surface area burn. Historically, these autologous cells have been seeded onto animal sourced feeder layers (i.e., irradiated mouse cells) which may present consideration of the transmission of zoonotic diseases such as retroviruses. Furthermore, cultured epithelial grafts are very expensive and are difficult to handle. Confluent and stratified sheets (four to six cell layers thick) are transferred to a backing material before grafting. Numerous reports on the clinical use of cultured epidermal sheets have appeared with variable results. Early and late graft losses and friability of healed skin are reported. Early take rates of cultured epithelium are reported from as low as 40–80% depending on the individual technique [13]. Actual take rates at discharge were reported even lower. Non-adherence and the long-term tendency to form blisters following mechanical stress may be caused by disturbed adhesion properties of the keratinocytes and abnormal structure of anchoring fibrils.

Despite many drawbacks of cultured epithelial sheets, cultured grafts are used in the treatment of extensive skin loss in the absence of sufficient autologous donor skin. Cultured epithelial sheet grafts have also been reported for the treatment of superficial partial thickness wounds of the face and rapid healing with reduced scarring has been noted. Advances in generation and release of cultured epithelial sheets could significantly enhance the use of these products. These advances include the elimination of non-human cell feeder layers by using transplantable substrates (autologous or allogeneic cells or tissues, biocompatible synthetics) which can also negate the need for enzymatic release of the cells.

Alternative delivery systems for keratinocytes

Delivery and durability of the extremely fragile keratinocytes sheets are one limitation to their use. Additional challenges include the enzymatic removal of the cultured cells from the flask with resultant graft shrinkage as well as the requirement to culture the cells on a fibroblast feeder layer. Efforts to address these limitations have met with varying success. The culture of cells directly on a carrier system such as Laserskin® (FIDIA, Advance Biopolymers, Italy), a membrane composed of a semi-synthetic derivative of hyaluronic acid or Hydroderm®, a synthetic hydrophilic polyurethane membrane dressing, has been explored. Use of these grafts has met with some clinical success but they are not readily available and therefore, not currently a viable clinical option.

Keratinocytes in suspension

Single-cell transplantation of keratinocytes can also be achieved via aerosolized or spray delivery of suspended autologous cultures. Two suspended autologous keratinocyte delivery systems have been commercialized. These include cultured keratinocytes suspended in fibrin glue (BioSeed-S™, BioTissues Technology AG, Germany) and cultured keratinocytes suspended in liquid media (CellSpray, Avita Medical Limited, Australia), both of which can be sprayed onto the wound.

Fibrin glue has wide spread applications in various surgical fields and has been shown to be effective for the fixation of meshed skin grafts and the subsequent healing of these grafts. The application of suspended autologous keratinocytes in a fibrin glue was first reported by Hundyadi [14]. Now various clinical reports document the success of cultured keratinocyte suspensions in fibrin glue for re-epithelialization of deep partial and full-thickness wounds [15]. Most clinical reports lack information on seeding densities per treated area and on objective quality of subsequent epithelial coverage. Therefore it remains to be seen how keratinocytes in fibrin glue suspension will perform compared with cultured epithelial sheets and other

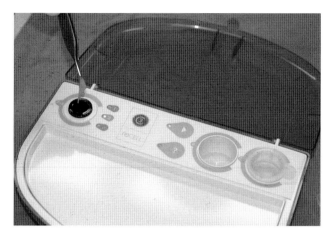

Figure 12.8 ReCell® kit allows on-site preparation of an autologous keratinocyte suspension from a small split thickness skin biopsy in the operating theater. Skin biopsy is placed in preheated trypsin for enzymatic disassociation of the cells.

described methods, in terms of time, costs, and quality of wound coverage. One of the advantages is that the fibrin glue suspension method is technically easy to perform, particularly because fibrin glue is commercially available in most European countries.

Fiona Wood and her group from Australia have demonstrated good re-epithelialization of debrided wounds using cultured as well as non cultured autologous keratinocytes suspended in media (ReCell®, Avita Medical Limited, Australia; Figure 12.8). A spray nozzle was used to deliver keratinocytes to the wound bed which was then covered by a dressing. Minimal cell loss was demonstrated and an even distribution of cells noticed. This method has also achieved success in reseeding melanocytes to the epidermis which has a clinical application such as restoration of skin color after burn wound coverage.

There have been some reports of treatment of wounds with non-confluent sheets or cell suspensions of cultured allogeneic keratinocytes. There is continued discussion as to whether these cells actually persist on the wounds or if they are stimulating the recruitment of host cells which in turn provide ultimate wound healing.

Composite grafts

Clinical results in transplanted epithelium have led to a consensus among most clinicians that a dermal substitute is needed to enhance the function of epithelial grafts. Therefore efforts were taken to combine dermal substitutes and cultured keratinocytes in vitro before grafting. Handling properties of the "composite" grafts were dramatically improved and the composite nature of the grafts eliminates the need to enzymatically remove sheets of cells from culture vessels. The delivery of either a single layer of keratinocytes or a differentiated epithelium on a dermal substrate as a composite graft has been subject to extensive work that is still ongoing. It seems obvious that applying a functional skin replacement rather than an "epidermal only" component most closely resembles the eventual need for tissue. Several variants on this technique have been described. In general these include dermis-derived lattices, collagen-derived matrices, and cultured substrates.

A promising technique was developed by Steven Boyce and colleagues from the University of Cincinnati, USA. A dermal lattice composed of collagen and glycosaminoglycans (collagen-GAG) was inoculated with autologous fibroblasts and seeded with autologous keratinocytes in vitro. Inoculation with fibroblasts was necessary to promote epithelial growth on the upper surface. The autologous composite graft can then transplanted onto the debrided burn wounds. Long-term follow-up studies showed good results [16]. A major problem with dermal substrates for the delivery of keratinocytes as a composite graft is the limited availability for grafting of extensive wounds. Currently a complete epidermal–dermal autologous product is not commercially available.

Apligraf® (GraftSkin)

Apligraf (Organogenesis) is a living bilayered graft composed of human fibroblasts seeded in a bovine collagen matrix covered with an epidermal layer of human keratinocytes. Apligraf is approved for application to carefully selected, slow-healing venous leg ulcers and diabetic foot ulcers.

OrCel®

OrCel (Forticell Bioscience, New York, NY, USA) is another bi-layered composite graft in which neonatal fibroblasts and allogeneic keratinocytes are seeded onto a coated type I bovine collagen sponge. The allogeneic fibroblasts secrete extracellular matrix proteins including growth factors and cytokines. OrCel has been approved by the US Food and Drug Administration for use in the reconstruction or treatment of recessive dystrophic epidermolysis bullosa of the hands.

Beyond burns

Although the use of allograft skin has historically been limited to that of a temporary topical biological dressing, the development of acellular matrices and biosynthetic skin substitutes has greatly expanded the clinical applications of these grafts. Moving beyond the realm of cutaneous injuries, these grafts are now being used to treat a variety of conditions requiring the repair or replacement of other connective tissues and organ systems. In fact in the USA today, more allograft skin transplants are being performed for non-burn applications than for temporary burn dressings.

Similarly, the use of biosynthetic skin or dermal substitutes has not been limited to applications historically associated with these tissues. The use of these artificial substitutes in urological applications stands as a case in point.

Substitution urethroplasty for urethral stricture disease has been performed using autologous penile or scrotal skin, bladder mucosa or, more recently, buccal mucosa. Various factors have contributed to the recognition of buccal mucosa grafts as an ideal substitute for the urethra. These include easy accessibility and handling, resistance to infection, compatibility with a wet environment, a thick epithelium, and a thin lamina propria which allows for early inosculation. The versatility of buccal mucosa grafts has been well documented, whether used dorsally or ventrally or when used in one or two stage repairs. Use of these grafts has resulted in good medium-term results which are at least comparable to full-thickness skin grafts.

Although buccal mucosa grafts can be recovered from either the inner cheek or lower lip, lengthy strictures require the recovery of extensive tissue grafts. In these instances, the availability of a robust, biocompatible tissue-engineered product could facilitate a successful substitution urethroplasty while eliminating or minimizing donor site morbidity.

Tissue engineering in urological reconstruction has come a long way from the first report of in vitro culture of transitional cell epithelium by Bunge in 1955 to the recently described use of tissue-engineered autologous bladder for cystoplasty by Atala et al. [17]. Organic and synthetic materials have been used both in clinical and experimental settings to provide a urethral substitute. These have included acellular bladder matrices, acellular porcine intestinal submucosa, woven meshes of dexon, collagen matrices, and poly-tetrafluoroethylene (Gore-Tex). Unfortunately, these grafts have usually met with limited success owing to mechanical, structural, or biocompatibility problems.

A major limitation in developing tissue-engineered materials for urethral reconstruction is to find a suitable biomaterial; an ideal biomaterial should be biocompatible, promote cellular interaction and possess appropriate mechanical and functional properties. Biocompatibility of biomaterials is essential so as to minimize the inflammatory or foreign body response once implanted. The ideal biomaterial should also encourage appropriate regulation of cell behavior, such as adhesion, proliferation, migration and differentiation, to promote and facilitate the development of the best quality new tissue. It is also important that biomaterials possess appropriate mechanical properties for the regeneration of tissues of predefined sizes and shapes.

Vascularization of these biomaterials can pose a significant challenge, as an adequate blood supply is required for supporting both the growth and proliferation of seeded cells. In efforts to produce an "off-the-shelf" replacement graft for lengthy urethral strictures, autologous buccal keratinocytes and fibroblasts have been isolated, cultured, and expanded in vitro, then seeded on a de-epidermized dermal matrix to produce a full-thickness tissue-engineered buccal mucosa (TEBM) matrix [18].

It has been demonstrated that an adequate number of good quality cells can be obtained from a small oral biopsy and that this is adequate to prepare TEBM to substitute a full length of the urethra without any paucity of tissue. If all the cultured cells were used for preparation of TEBM it would be possible to culture 10 strips of $3 \, cm \times 5 \, cm$ of TEBM for each patient.

The use of a de-epidermized dermis allows for easy surgical handling of tissue and provides an excellent scaffold for cellular proliferation which is biocompatible with the native urethra. Studies have shown early vascularization of these constructed implants. This could be attributed to the rich vascular supply of the urethra and the porosity of de-epidermized dermis. Also, the presence of cells (in particular keratinocytes) may allow for early inosculation by secretion of several cytokines which are vital for neo-angiogenesis.

Although TEBM may in the future offer a clinically useful autologous replacement tissue for the urethra, there has been a significant inflammatory reaction to the dermal substrate used. Chapple and colleagues (Royal Hallamshire Hospital, Sheffield, UK) are currently researching these issues before further clinical evaluation is undertaken.

Future perspectives

The use of allograft skin has become the standard of care in the treatment of extensive burn injuries. Fresh or cryopreserved allograft skin can provide effective barrier functions and restore the physiological environment of the wound bed; however, allograft tissue is ultimately rejected and therefore can only function as a temporary biological dressing. The development of techniques to isolate and preserve the native structure of the dermis while removing the antigenic properties of allograft skin effectively converts this tissue to a universal matrix graft with multiple applications.

Biosynthetic skin substitutes can effectively address some of the functional characteristics of native tissues. Although over three decades of research and clinical applications have yielded great strides in the development of tissue substitutes, we have yet to deliver the perfect skin replacement.

Exciting new developments in the field of gene manipulation may pave the way for selective seeding of the appropriate dermal scaffold. Specific cell types might be targeted to produce angiogenic factors, growth hormones, and other modulators of wound healing or, perhaps, inhibitors of scarring and contracture. Recent publications from the University of Alberta Burn

Center on adenovirus-infected indoleamine 2,3-dioxygenase expressing fibroblasts have focused on immuno-protection of allogeneic and xenogeneic grafts [19]. The generation of a gene-manipulated non- immunogenic keratinocyte combined with other manipulated cell types (melanocytes, Langerhans cells) seeded on a dermal matrix may allow the transplantation of an off-the-shelf product. Concurrently, mesenchymal stem cell research has given insight into new possibilities in dermal and other tissue regeneration. Some effort has been taken to expand mesenchymal stem cells which could then be used to accelerate re-epithelialization [20]. Legal and regulatory restrictions in most countries have required research strategies to focus on autologous adult derived stem cell therapies.

Although patient survivability is the acute goal of the treatment of cutaneous injuries or connective tissue compromise, short-term repair of these deficits is suboptimal if the ultimate results are scarring, contracture, and loss of function. The ideal tissue-engineered graft will ultimately provide a bioactive scaffold that will facilitate and/or direct the body's natural tendency of tissue regeneration. Although great advances have been made in the design and development of skin and connective tissue substitutes, the elegant simplicity yet ultimate complexity of human tissues continues to present significant challenges.

KEY LEARNING POINTS

- Over the past 30 years, clinicians and researchers have mounted a focused attempt toward development of a skin/connective tissue substitute, but efforts have experienced a mixed degree of success, and the search for the ideal autologous skin/connective tissue replacement continues.

- The ability to assist the body's natural repair process with biological or synthetic materials has greatly reduced the morbidity and mortality associated with devastating burn injuries by greatly enhancing the clinician's ability to achieve both temporary and permanent wound closure or ultimately to restore form and function.

- Donated human skin provides an effective bridge between wound excision and permanent closure; however, there remain some recognized limitations to its use, which have led clinicians and researchers to pursue development of synthetic skin substitutes.

- A host of synthetic and biosynthetic dressings have been developed and can be categorized to include temporary and permanent skin substitutes, epidermal and dermal substitutes, synthetic and biological skin substitutes, and cell-free and cell-seeded materials.

(Continued)

- The development of acellular matrices and biosynthetic skin substitutes (tissue-engineered materials) has greatly expanded possibilities for clinical applications beyond the realm of cutaneous injuries, and these grafts are now being used to treat a variety of conditions requiring the repair or replacement of other connective tissues and organ systems.

- The ideal tissue-engineered graft will ultimately provide a bioactive scaffold that will facilitate and/or direct the body's natural tendency of tissue regeneration.

References

1. Burn incidence and treatment in the US: 2007 fact sheet. American Burn Association Web site. http://www.ameriburn.org/resources_factsheet.php (accessed July 26, 2010).
2. Gerding RL, Imbembo AL, Fratianne RB. Biosynthetic skin subsitute versus 1% silver sulfadiazine for treatment of inpatient partial-thickness thermal burns. J Trauma 1988;28:1265–69.
3. Barret JP, Dziewulski P, Ramzy PI, et al. Biobrane versus 1% silver sulfadiazine in second-degree pediatric burns. Plast Recon Surg 2000;105:62–5.
4. Hansbrough JF, Mozingo DW, Kealey GP, et al. Clinical trial of a biosynthetic temporary skin replacement, Dermagraft Transitional Covering, compared with cryopreserved human cadaver skin for temporary coverage of excised burn wounds. J Burn Care Rehab 1997;18:43–51.
5. Noordenbos J, Dore C, Hansbrough JF. Safety and efficacy of Transcyte for the treatment of partial-thickness burns. J Burn Care Rehab 1999;20:275–81.
6. Schwarze H, Kuntscher M, Uhlig C, et al. Suprathel, a new skin substitute in the management of partial thickness wounds: results of a clinical study. Ann Plast Surg 2008;60:181–5.
7. Marston WA, Hanft J, Norwood P, Pollak R. The efficacy and safety of Dermagraft in improving the healing of chronic diabetic foot ulcers. Diabetes Care 2003;26: 1701–5.
8. Wainright D, Madden M, Luterman A, et al. Clinical evaluation of an acellular allograft dermal matrix in full-thickness burns. J Burn Care Rehab 1996;17: 124–36.
9. Van Zuijlen PPM, Vloemans JPM, Van Trier AJM, et al. Dermal substitution in acute burns and reconstructive surgery: A subjective and objective long-term follow up. Plast Recon Surg 2001;108:1938–46.
10. Heimbach D, Luterman A, Burke J, et al. Artificial dermis for major burns. A multicenter randomized trial. Ann Surg 1988;208:313–20.
11. Heimbach DM, Warden GD, Luterman A, et al. Multicenter post-approval clinical trial of Integra dermal regeneration template for burn treatment. J Burn Care Rehab 2003;24:42–8.

12. Rheinwald JG, Green H. Serial cultivation of strains of human keratinocytes – the formation of keratinizing colonies from single cells. Cell 1975;6:331–43.
13. Rue LW III, Cioffi WG, McManus WF, Pruitt BA Jr. Wound closure and outcome in extensively burned patients treated with cultured autologous keratinocytes. J Trauma 1993;34:662–7.
14. Hundyadi J, Farkas B, Bertenyi C, et al. Keratinocyte grafting: A new means of transplantation for full thickness wounds. J Dermatol Surg Oncol. 1989;14:75–8.
15. Kopp J, Jeschke MG, Bach AD, et al. Applied tissue engineering in the closure of severe burns and chronic wounds using cultured autologous keratinocytes in a natural fibrin matrix. Cell Tissue Bank 2004;5:89–96.
16. Boyce ST, Supp AP, Wickett RR, et al. Assessment with the dermal torque meter of skin pliability after treatment of burns with cultured skin substitutes. J Burn Care Rehab 2000;21:55–63.
17. Atala A, Bauer SB, Soker S, et al. Tissue-engineered autologous bladders for patients needing cystoplasty. Lancet 2006;367:1241–6.
18. Bhargava S, Chapple CR, Bullock AJ, et al. Tissue-engineered buccal mucosa for substitution urethroplasty. BJU Int 2004;93:807–11.
19. Li Y, Tredget EE, Kilani RT, et al. Expression of indoleamine 2,3-dioxygenase in dermal fibroblasts functions as a local immunosuppressive factor. J Invest Dermatol 2004;122:953–64.
20. Fu X, Li H. Mesenchymal stem cells and skin wound repair and regeneration: possibilities and questions. Cell Tissue Res 2009;335:317–21.

13 The Use of Allograft Corneas and Cells in Ophthalmic Surgery

Diego Ponzin[1], Stefano Ferrari[1], Edward J. Holland[2], and Joseph M. Biber[2]
[1]The Veneto Eye Bank Foundation, Venice, Italy
[2]Cincinnati Eye Institute, Cincinnati, OH, USA

The past

According to the World Health Organization, diseases affecting the cornea are a major cause of blindness worldwide, together with cataract, glaucoma, and age-related macular degeneration (www.who.int/blindness). Severe ocular surface diseases such as chemical or thermal injuries, Stevens–Johnson syndrome, ocular cicatricial pemphigoid, neurotrophic keratopathy, chronic limbitis, and severe microbial keratitis cause significant morbidity and even corneal blindness. Over recent decades, tremendous clinical and scientific advancements have been developed, leading to new treatments for the management of severe ocular surface diseases.

More than 100 years ago, on December 7, 1905, Edward K. Zirm performed the world's first successful full-thickness human corneal transplant. This milestone did not lead to relatively "routine" keratoplasty success for several more decades. A measure of this success is that in more developed countries corneal transplant surgery is now scheduled as an elective procedure. However, penetrating keratoplasty (PK) is not devoid of problems and, importantly, is not a definitive solution for all ocular surface disorders.

First, a stable ocular surface and adequate stem cell function are required for PK success.

Secondly, long-term PK studies have demonstrated poor long-term graft survival rates in some corneal diseases, primarily because of the continuous loss of donor endothelial cells, eventually leading to graft failure. In the USA, the Cornea Donor Study Investigator Group has recently reported a 70%

Tissue and Cell Clinical Use: An Essential Guide, First Edition. Edited by Ruth M. Warwick and Scott A. Brubaker.
© 2012 Blackwell Publishing Ltd. Published 2012 by Blackwell Publishing Ltd.

endothelial cell loss in the five years after PK, with a slight association between cell loss and donor age (69% cell loss in subjects who received a cornea from a donor 12–65 years old, 75% when received from a donor 66–75 years old). The Australian Corneal Graft Registry has shown that the one-year graft survival rate after PK was 90% and dropped to 59% at 10 years. In India, the survival rates at one, two, and five years were 79.6%, 68.7%, and 46.5%, respectively. In Italy, the CORTES study was the most extensive survey on corneal transplantation performed. Graft survival after PK in patients with keratoconus was 98% for the whole period of observation, whereas patients with other indications reported survival rates (after PK) ranging from 92% after one year to 52% after three years.

In addition, conventional PK is not a solution in pathologies or injuries leading to partial or total limbal stem cell deficiency (LSCD). To be successful, conventional PK is, in fact, dependent on the gradual replacement of the donor's corneal epithelium with the recipient's. LSCD, instead, allows for, or may even stimulate, conjunctival cell ingrowth with accompanying neovascularization and inflammation, resulting in cornea graft failure. Patients with total LSCD are therefore poor candidates for conventional PK.

To find potential treatments for the management of severe ocular surface diseases that could not be cured with just conventional PK, several new therapeutic strategies were developed. In 1940, De Rotth reported the first therapeutic use of amniotic membrane (AM) in ocular surgery by describing the use of fetal membranes in the repair of conjunctival defects. In 1946, Sorsby and Symons reported the successful use of AM overlay patch grafts in the treatment of acute ocular chemical injury. In 1984, Fox and colleagues described the beneficial effects of artificial tears made with autologous serum in patients with keratoconjunctivitis sicca. However, the single most important breakthrough in managing ocular surface failure was probably related to the identification of the location and function of limbal stem cells. In 1989, Kenyon and Tseng pioneered the clinical application of the limbal stem cell theory by transplanting grafts of bulbar conjunctiva and limbus (called conjunctival limbal autografts, CLAU) (Figure 13.1) harvested from the normal fellow eye to manage a series of 26 consecutive cases with unilateral LSCD [1]. In cases of bilateral LSCD, limbal allografts were performed using tissue from a living relative donor with healthy eyes (a procedure known as living-related conjunctival limbal allograft (LR-CLAL)). Or, a deceased donor can be the source where tissue is obtained either from a corneo-scleral disc or whole eye (keratolimbal allograft transplantation, KLAL) (Figure 13.2). Whether autograft or allograft, outgrowth of epithelial cells from transplanted sectors of limbal tissue onto the affected eye resulted in repopulation of the corneal surface with corneal epithelial cells.

Despite being successful when first described, all these pioneering treatments have been further refined in the past 10–20 years. New insights into

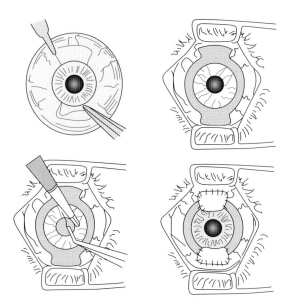

Figure 13.1 Schematic diagram illustrating surgical technique of conjunctival limbal autograft (CLAU). Top left: Donor tissue harvesting. Gentian violet marking pen marks areas of conjunctiva to be used. Dissection is then performed starting with the bulbar conjunctival portion and extending anteriorly onto the peripheral cornea to ensure supply of limbal stem cells. Top right: Preparation of recipient eye. A 360 degree limbal peritomy removing at least 2–3 mm of bulbar conjunctiva. Tenons is often resected as well. Bottom right: Superficial keratectomy is performed removing abnormal epithelium and scar tissue. Bottom left: The two conjunctival limbal grafts are sutured with 10 nylon or glued with tissue adhesives into proper position at the 6 and 12 o'clock meridians. (Reproduced with kind permission from Springer Science+Business Media: Croasdale CR, Holland EJ, and Mannis MJ: Conjunctival Limbal Autograft. In Holland EJ, Mannis MJ, editors: Ocular Surface Disease. New York, 2002.)

the use of autologous serum eye drops, AM graft, anterior and posterior lamellar keratoplasty, and limbal stem cell transplantation have provided ophthalmologists with new and powerful tools in the armamentarium of therapies available for patients with severe ocular surface diseases. These are reviewed next.

The present

Anterior/posterior lamellar keratoplasty as alternative to penetrating keratoplasty: the impact of new surgical techniques

Although PK remains the most common procedure for cornea transplantation with at least one million transplants performed since 1961

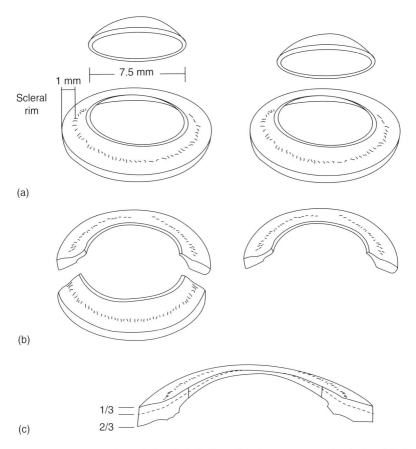

Figure 13.2 Preparation of the limbal allograft using a corneoscleral rim. (a) A 7.5 mm donor corneal button is trephined. (b) The corneoscleral rim is divided in half. (c) A crescent blade is used to dissect the tissue. The authors advocate using two rims and three segments of allografts for transplantation. (Reproduced from Schwartz GS, Tsubota K, Tseng S, et al: Keratolimbal allograft. In Holland EJ, Mannis MJ, editors: Ocular Surface Disease. New York, 2002, Springer-Verlag. Used with kind permission.)

(www.restoresight.org), improvements in microsurgical techniques and introduction of new devices have led to increasing numbers of lamellar keratoplasty (LK) procedures being performed. This appears to be true both for the anterior lamellar keratoplasty (ALK) replacing the anterior stroma [2], and for the posterior lamellar keratoplasty (PLK) also known as endothelial keratoplasty (EK), which involves the replacement of deep stromal and endothelial layers [3].

ALK involves the exchanging of corneal stroma and epithelial layers only and therefore avoids the replacement of the deepest layer of the cornea, the

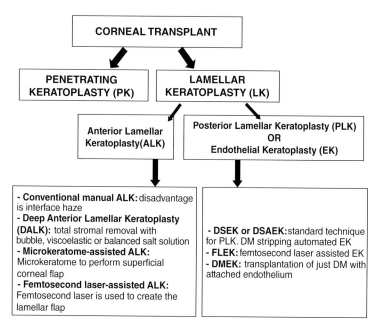

Figure 13.3 Schematic diagram illustrating the different types of keratoplasty procedures available. DM: Descemet membrane.

endothelium, thus diminishing potential risks of endothelial immunological graft rejection. A variety of ALK procedures have been described (Figure 13.3) and include the following: (1) conventional manual ALK surgery; (2) deep anterior lamellar keratoplasty (DALK) with total corneal stromal replacement; (3) microkeratome-assisted ALK; and, (4) femtosecond laser-assisted ALK.

The major advantage of ALK is the avoidance of unnecessary replacement of healthy endothelium, thus obviating the problems of endothelial rejection and hence subsequent endothelial graft failure. In addition, being a non-penetrating extraocular procedure, complications such as expulsive hemorrhage, glaucoma, cataract, and endophthalmitis are greatly reduced. A few reports have recently shown that clinical outcomes after DALK using the big-bubble technique in patients with keratoconus are comparable to standard PK. The major disadvantages of ALK include a steep learning curve and the possibility of suboptimal visual outcomes owing to interface related problems.

In up to 50% of all PK procedures, the clinical indication for surgery is endothelial decompensation and, provided there are no stromal opacities or high-degree astigmatism, new endothelial cells are all that is needed for the cornea to become clear. For this reason EK, also known as Descemet

Stripping Automated Endothelial Keratoplasty (DSAEK) (Figure 13.3), was developed and in recent years has gained widespread popularity. In the USA, statistics show that in 2008 the numbers of corneas provided for EK procedures increased by 23% to 17,468 from 14,159 in 2007. With this procedure the recipient's ocular surface and stroma are maintained, with the exception of the complex Descemet membrane and endothelium, which are removed from the central part of the posterior corneal surface. The donor graft consists of a thin lamella (usually 9.0 mm in diameter, between 100 and 200 μm in thickness) of deep stroma carrying the donor Descemet membrane and endothelium and is attached to the recipient cornea by means of an air bubble in the immediate postoperative period. Although cornea clarity is re-established by DSAEK in a relatively short period of time, the resulting stromal interface is sometimes considered as a limiting factor for final visual acuity.

A major advantage of EK over PK is that it is a closed eye procedure, thus minimizing the risks of severe complications. EK is performed though a small incision (typically 4 or 5 mm), which may require only a couple of sutures. The refractive changes are more predictable hence there is less likelihood of an astigmatic shift, even if hyperopic shift has been reported. EK has been shown to be successful in previously failed grafts and is less invasive than repeat PK.

EK is, however, not devoid of complications. Donor graft dislocation may occur in up to 50% of cases and attempts at re-attaching the donor tissue with a repeat air injection further exacerbate endothelial cell loss. Another disadvantage of DSAEK is that endothelial loss determined one to two years postoperatively is substantially higher than that observed for conventional PK. Folding of the donor button in a "taco" configuration (60:40 fold), squeezing of the graft between forceps for insertion, crushing of the tissue while passing through the surgical wound, and further manipulation often necessary to unfold the graft inside the anterior chamber are the primary causes of endothelial damage, resulting in reduced postoperative endothelial cell density. In 2008, Busin and colleagues described the prototype of a glide specially designed to facilitate graft delivery and minimize surgical trauma. The graft passing through the opening of the glide is shaped like a flat cylinder, with the endothelium protected against traumatic contact. The tissue roll can be easily pulled into the anterior chamber while its sides freely slide on each other to conform to the characteristics of the clear cornea tunnel. The tissue is therefore not crushed as in the "taco" technique and trauma is minimized. Most importantly, the donor endothelium remains protected during the entire procedure, thus limiting endothelial cell loss to levels recorded after conventional PK. A recent study showed that Busin guide-assisted DSAEK results in a lower percentage of endothelial cell loss compared with forceps insertion, six months after surgery. Several new delivery mechanisms are being investigated.

In the near future we might expect increasing numbers of more tailored surgical procedures being performed with the aim of changing only the endothelium when the pathology is owing to endothelial failure (through EK), or just the anterior part when the corneal disease involves the stroma, thus leaving a healthy and intact endothelium (with ALK). Eye banks can have a major role in this field as: (1) precut corneal tissue preparation and distribution could help reduce the manipulation of the donor tissue at the time of surgery, (2) routine graft preparation by skilled eye bank technicians could overcome the variability and poor quality of grafts likely to occur when LK procedures are not performed routinely by surgeons, and (3) potential drawbacks occurring during graft preparation (misshapen cuts, damages, etc.) could be easily solved by using additional corneas stored in the incubators. The last is an opportunity that surgeons might not have when grafts are prepared before surgery, thus inevitably leading to delays in the scheduled intervention. In addition, these procedures might broaden the donor cornea pool by enabling tissues that cannot be used for PK to be used for anterior or endothelial transplantation. As our understanding of these new procedures evolves, our techniques and outcomes will continue to improve.

A further important issue worth discussing is how cornea processing and storage might influence the postgrafting course. There are currently two main methods for cornea preservation: hypothermic storage (HS) at 2–6°C and organ culture (OC) held at 31–37°C. Prolonged storage time in OC may allow better outcomes in patients at high risk for immune rejection. In fact, storage of corneas for longer than 7 days results in the complete migration of donor dendritic cells from the cornea into the culture media. On the other hand, OC up to 12 days allows delivery of corneas with higher endothelial cell density. Despite these speculations, prospective studies analyzing short (one to two years) or long-term (up to 14 years) follow-ups of PKs did not find any statistically significant difference in corneal thickness, endothelial cell density or clinical outcome between corneas stored in HS or OC. Newly developed grafts for ALK or PLK might have different needs, thus challenging the storage methods with regard to postoperative results and adequacy of the method itself.

Corneal transplantation in the setting of ocular surface disease

Reconstruction of the ocular surface is often a stepwise approach that ultimately culminates in optical keratoplasty. The goals of the surface reconstruction procedures that precede the corneal transplant are to maximize conditions for optical function by ensuring a normal interface between the lids and the globe, normal tear function, and, finally, cellular replacement or reconstruction. The important steps to ensure successful integration of this new tissue into the host include acceptance of the transplant by the host immunologic system, successful epithelialization of the donor tissue, and an adequate shape and clarity of the tissue for refractive success. Although all are necessary components of successful LK or PK, the ingrowth of a normal ocular surface is the most crucial aspect in treating patients with ocular surface disorders. In the context of ocular surface failure, approximately 50% of patients will need corneal transplantation to clear the resultant corneal opacity. As mentioned above, there are multiple sources of cells (CLAU, LR-CLAL, KLAL, and ex vivo cultured and engineered cells) that can be used to stabilize the ocular surface before transplantation.

Once the decision to proceed with corneal transplantation has been made, two key questions must be answered. (1) When to perform the keratoplasty? Either simultaneously with ocular surface reconstruction or staged in a two-step procedure with keratoplasty after ocular surface reconstruction by 3 months (or once stabilized). (2) What type of keratoplasty to perform? Either lamellar, penetrating, or keratoprosthesis.

For the timing of keratoplasty, Croasdale et al. [4] presented a series of 36 cases using staged stem cell transplantation followed by penetrating keratoplasty approximately three months later. They used two eyes from the same donor for the keratolimbal tissue and a third donor for the corneal transplant (Plates 13.1 and 13.2). In a subsequent expansion of this series to 54 patients with keratolimbal allograft (personal communication), 35 patients underwent lamellar or penetrating keratoplasty three to four months after stem cell graft and were followed for at least one year. Forty of these patients (74%) were stable and 60% (21 of 35) had successful corneal grafts (Plate 13.3). Of the 14 failed grafts, three succumbed to endothelial graft rejection and 11 to recurrent ocular surface disease. In 2004, Shimazaki et al. [5] presented a case series of 32 eyes of 32 patients with chemical or thermal corneal burns who underwent amniotic membrane transplantation with either conjunctivolimbal autograft transplantation or keratolimbal allograft transplantation. Of these 32 patients, 21 underwent penetrating keratoplasty with 15 performed simultaneously and six in a two-step process. The incidence of endothelial rejection was significantly higher in eyes with simultaneous penetrating keratoplasty than those with a staged procedure (53.3% versus 0%, $p = 0.019$). Although not statistically different, the eyes with a staged procedure had higher rates of corneal epithelialization and clearer grafts than those with simultaneous keratoplasty. Based on the largest series with the longest follow-up, as well as on their clinical impressions, the authors favor a staged approach, which is more protracted but allows for surface stabilization and resolution of ocular surface inflammation before keratoplasty.

As for type of keratoplasty, we commonly advocate three types of transplant. The health of the endothelial layer is vital to deciding between penetrating and lamellar keratoplasty. In cases of abnormal endothelium, we use PK. Due to advantages of LK discussed earlier, we offer deep anterior lamellar keratoplasty to our patients with a healthy endothelium. The

Boston Keratoprosthesis is a viable option in patients without a stable ocular surface, or for those unable to tolerate surface reconstruction and immuno-suppression (Plate 13.4).

Systemic immunosuppression in ocular surface transplantation

Owing to the vascularity of the limbus, limbal allografts are at higher risk of rejection than conventional corneal transplantation. In addition, the antigenic challenge to the host is higher in limbal transplanted tissues because of their higher number of Langerhans cells. Several studies have confirmed the importance of systemic immunosuppression in patients undergoing limbal stem cell transplantation. One study found 87% of patients that were treated with systemic immunosuppression had a stable ocular surface compared with 62% that were not treated with immunosuppression [6]. Systemic side effects of immunosuppression include severe adverse events such as death, myocardial infarction, cerebrovascular event, and secondary tumors; and minor adverse events of immunosuppression include alterations in biochemisty, increased cardiovascular risk factors, and infections requiring hospitalizations. In a large retrospective series [7] of 136 patients undergoing limbal stem cell transplantation and systemic immuno-suppression with a mean follow-up of 4.5 years, only 1.5% had a severe adverse event and 15.4% had minor adverse events. Therefore, we strongly advocate systemic immunosuppression in all patients undergoing donated limbal stem cell transplantation (either from a living related donor or deceased donor), even in those with HLA-matched tissues (LR-CLAL). In cases of perfect HLA-match, the duration of the treatment may be reduced.

Close monitoring by a transplant immunologist is advised in patients on immunosuppression. Our current regimen includes tacrolimus and myco-phenolate mofetil for one to two years, and a short course (three months) of oral prednisone.

The multiple uses of the amniotic membrane

The AM derives from the innermost layer of the placental membranes and is composed of a single epithelial layer, a thick basement membrane and an avascular stroma. Both fresh and preserved AM function equally well when transplanted onto the ocular surface. However, preserved (either cryopre-served or lyophilized) AM allows more flexibility in scheduling surgery. Importantly, the epithelial cells in fresh or preserved AM graft are poorly viable or non-viable, an important feature since the viability of amniotic epithelial cells may be associated with low-grade inflammatory response. Besides the lack of immunogenicity, AM has a unique combination of prop-erties [reviewed in reference 8]. First, it is known to promote epithelial cell migration thus supporting the growth of epithelial progenitor cells. This effect explains why AM transplantation facilitates epithelialization for persistent corneal epithelial defects with stromal ulceration. Secondly, it is known to suppress the expression of certain inflammatory cytokines, to attract and sequester inflammatory cells, and to contain various forms of protease inhibitors. This might explain some of its anti-inflammatory properties. Finally, the AM stromal matrix is known to suppress transforming growth factor (TGF)-β signaling, proliferation and myofibroblastic differentiation of normal corneal and limbal fibroblasts as well as normal conjunctival and pterygium fibroblasts. This action may explain why AM transplantation helps reduce scars during conjunctival surface reconstruction, prevents recurrent scarring after pterygium removal or glaucoma surgery, and reduces corneal haze after photorefractive keratectomy. Three different surgical techniques for AM transplantation have been described: (1) inlay or graft technique (the AM is tailored to the size of the defect and acts as a scaffold to allow migration of the surrounding epithelial cells); (2) overlay or patch technique (the AM use is akin to a biological contact lens to protect the healing surface defect and to reduce inflammation); and (3) filling-in or layered technique (the entire depth of an ulcer crater is filled with small pieces of AM trimmed to the size of the defect). After the first therapeutic applications reported by De Rotth in 1940 and Sorsby and Symons in 1946, AM transplantation has been used widely in ocular surgery as an epithelial surrogate after excision of large ocular surface neoplasias, reconstruction of conjunctival fornix, pterygium, severe or refractory neurotrophic corneal ulcers, conjunctival surface reconstruction, and to improve comfort after acute ocular burns. In a prospective noncomparative interventional case series study, Gunduz et al. reported that nonpreserved human AM appears useful for ocular surface reconstruction after excision of extensive ocular surface neoplasia. In another study, sterilized, freeze-dried AM resulted in complete epithelialization, early resolution of ocular inflammation, and no recurrence of pterygium over a follow-up period of 13.9 ± 6.0 months. However, Joseph et al. reported that AM did not improve the overall success rate of ocular surface restoration nor preserve the integrity of the eye in patients with severe acute chemical and thermal burns, whether used alone or in conjunction with other surgical procedures. An interesting perspective is that shown by a recent study demonstrating the use of AM in an animal model to assist in the healing of bacterial keratitis. One of the newer applications of AM has been its use as a scaffold for propagation and transplantation of limbal stem cells onto the eyes of patients with LSCD [9]. AM was also used to cultivate and expand conjunctival cells for the regeneration of the conjunctival epithelium. Future progress in this field might include availability of low-heat dehydrated AM, sutureless applications with fibrin glue, topical applications of AM extracts, and AM attached to a soft contact-lens-sized conformer for easier insertion.

Table 13.1 Comparison of the biochemical properties of normal, unstimulated human tears and serum. (Reproduced from Geerling G et al. Br J Ophthalmol 2004;88:1467–74 with permission from BMJ Publishing Group Ltd.)

Parameter	Tears	Serum
pH	7.4	7.4
Osmolality	298	296
EGF (ng/ml)	0.2–3.0	0.5
TGF-β (ng/ml)	2–10	6–33
NGF (pg/ml)	468.3	54.0
IGF (ng/ml)	0.31	105
PDGF (ng/ml)	1.33	15.4
Albumin (mg/ml)	0.023	53
Substance P (pg/ml)	157	70.9
Vitamin A (mg/ml)	0.02	46
Lysozyme (mg/ml)	1.4	6
Surface immunoglobulin A (µg/ml)	1190	2
Fibronectin (µg/ml)	21	205
Lactoferrin (ng/ml)	1650	266

Autologous serum eye drops as alternative to tear supplements

Eye drops made from autologous serum (AS) are a new therapeutic approach for ocular surface disorders. Serum is the fluid component of full blood that remains after clotting. Although artificial tears commercially available offer little to no nutrition, eye drops made from AS have tear-like biochemical characteristics with regard to pH and osmolarity and contain a large variety of growth factors, fibronectin, vitamins, and immunoglobulins (Table 13.1). The use of AS was first described by Fox and colleagues in 1984 in their search for a preservative-free tear substitute. The recent renaissance of this therapy began in 1999 when Tsubota and colleagues described its successful use in eyes with persistent epithelial defects (PED) and dry eye. It was found that in 16 eyes with PED treated with AS drops, 62.6% were healed within 1 month while their mean duration of PED before serum drops was 7.2 months. A comprehensive review of the clinical studies published from 1984 to 2004 has shown that serum eye drops have been used to treat 255 patients with diseases including PED, severe dry eye and superior limbal keratoconjunctivitis, recurrent erosion syndrome as well as a supportive measure in ocular surface reconstruction. Protocols to prepare and use AS eye drops vary considerably between the studies and range from concentrations of 20–100%. However, there is no universal consensus on how AS eye drops should be prepared. For example, in the UK, anemia is a contraindication and patients are screened for blood-borne viruses including hepatitis and HIV. The number of complications reported was small, with most authors reporting no complications at all. A few isolated cases of microbial keratitis, bacterial conjunctivitis, increased discomfort, or epitheliopathy and eyelid eczema have been described. However, these complications may easily be attributed to the natural course of the disease being treated. Because of all these variables, the rate of success was difficult to establish with objective/ subjective scores ranging from 21 to 100%.

In vitro toxicity studies suggest that serum eye drops might be more appropriate than pharmaceutical tear substitutes in maintaining intracellular ATP levels and cell membrane integrity of cultured human corneal epithelial cells. A few randomized studies were performed to compare the effectiveness of serum eye drops against artificial tears. In all cases AS drops were found to be superior to conventional treatments as evidenced by improvement in ocular surface health and subjective comfort [10], higher tear stability, faster closure of corneal epithelial wounds and prolongation of the tear break-up time.

In 2003, the University Hospital of Lubeck estimated the costs associated with the production of serum eye drops and reported that the total costs of a day dosage was 2.27 euros for 20% and 4.61 euros for 100% serum eye drops. This was reported to be approximately equivalent to the costs of one bottle of preserved pharmaceutical lubricant.

Potential disadvantages of serum eye drops are limited stability (especially when stored at 4°C) and risk of infection both for patients and personnel handling serum. In addition, there has been no report so far on the effects and risks of prolonged application of autologous serum to the human ocular surface. There remains the possibility that serum contains active components that may adversely affect the ocular surface when applied in the wrong concentrations for prolonged periods.

Clinical application of ex vivo cultured limbal stem cells

As previously outlined, in pathologies or injuries leading to partial or total LSCD, conventional PK is not very successful. In 1989, recognition of the need to replenish the stem cell population in LSCD led to the development of limbal autograft and allograft as means of restoring corneal epithelial stem cells in the eyes of patients affected by unilateral or bilateral LSCD, respectively. It became evident that these strategies were not devoid of risks. In case of autologous limbal transplantation, one serious limitation is the requirement for a sizeable limbal donation, as up to 30–40% must be harvested from the contralateral donor eye. This may harm the structural integrity of the remaining healthy eye, and prevent repetition of the procedure in case of failure. Similar risks are also present in allogeneic limbal transplantation. In LR-CLAL, there is concern regarding damage to the healthy donor eye by removal of limbal tissue. KLAL carry higher risks of rejection caused by the abundance of HLA antigens in the graft material, requiring the recipient to receive long-term systemic immunosuppression (prednisone, cyclosporine, etc.) together with topical steroids to prolong graft survival.

For all these reasons, in the past 10–15 years, ex vivo expansion of autologous limbal stem cells and proper cultivation techniques have been actively investigated. Stem cells of the corneal epithelium are located in the basal layers of the limbus. In 1997, in a landmark report, Pellegrini et al. described the successful reconstruction of the ocular surface in two patients with severe LSCD using transplantation of corneal epithelial stem cells previously expanded in vitro onto a feeder-layer of lethally irradiated murine 3T3-J2 cells [11]. They demonstrated that (1) keratinocyte stem cells can be isolated from $1\,mm^2$ limbal biopsies thus reducing the likelihood of the aforementioned complications; (2) grafting of autologous cultured corneal epithelial cells with/without keratoplasty leads to disappearance of clinical symptoms and restoration of visual acuity; and, (3) long-term follow-up showed the stability of regenerated corneal epithelium. Many other studies describing the clinical application of limbal stem cells expanded in vitro have since been reported, with a range of follow-up times (Table 13.2). The protocols used to cultivate cells vary widely. Some studies used the "explant culture system," in which harvested limbal tissue (autologous or allogeneic) is placed directly onto amniotic membrane (used as a surrogate environmental stem cell niche) and the limbal epithelial cells migrate out of the biopsy and proliferate to form an epithelial sheet. Alternatively, limbal stem cells are isolated from the biopsy using an enzymatic treatment (dispase followed by trypsin) and seeded onto an amniotic membrane or a feeder-layer of lethally irradiated murine 3T3-J2 fibroblasts [12]. Scaffolds used to transfer the cells to the eye include fibrin glue, amniotic membrane and poly(N-isopropylacrylamide) polymers. Very recently, a promising new technique was developed to achieve ocular surface rehabilitation. In three patients with LSCD, contact lenses approved by the US Food and Drug Administration were used both as substrate for limbal stem cell expansion and as carrier/bandage for transfer and protection of cells. A stable transparent corneal epithelium was restored and best-corrected visual acuity increased in each patient. However, to our knowledge, only limbal stem cells cultured onto 3T3-J2 feeder-layers and transferred to the diseased eye using fibrin as carrier were shown to maintain undifferentiated phenotypes and the ability to generate holoclones.

Recent evidence suggests that transplantation of limbal stem cells cultured onto human AM may be an alternative to limbal allografting. In a recent case report of 1 patient with severe Stevens–Johnson syndrome and bilateral total LSCD, more effective minimization of corneal scarring and better vision improvement were demonstrated using cultured limbal stem cells in the right eye compared with transplantation of four quadrants of limbal allografts onto the recipient limbal region of the left eye. Observation period lasted for four years after surgery. Complete corneal epithelialization was achieved in two days using cultivated limbal stem cells, whereas it took three weeks to achieve the same results with limbal allografts. In addition,

Table 13.2 Summary of clinical studies for the reconstruction of the corneal epithelium with *ex vivo* cultured stem cells

Study	Technique	Patients (eyes)	Follow-up: mean and range (months)	Success rate
Pellegrini (Lancet 1997)	Autologous limbal stem cells cultured onto lethally irradiated murine feeder-layers	2 (2)	24	2/2
Schwab (Trans Am Ophthalmol Soc 1999)	Autologous (17 cases) and allogeneic (two cases; living related donors) limbal stem cells cultured onto murine feeder-layers using different carriers (corneal stroma, type 1 collagen, soft contact lenses, collagen shields, and AM)	19	10 (2–24)	63%
Tsai (N Engl J Med 2000)	Autologous limbal epithelial explants cultured on human AM	6 (6)	15 (12–18)	6/6
Schwab (Cornea 2000)	Autologous (10 cases) and allogeneic (four cases) cultured limbal stem cells seeded onto a matrix derived from AM	14 (14)	13 (6–19)	60%
Koizumi (Ophthalmology 2001)	Allogeneic limbal epithelial cells cultured onto murine feeder-layers for four weeks and denuded AM with air-lifting.	11 (13)	11.2 (12–27)	92%
Rama (Transplantation 2001)	Autologous limbal stem cells cultured onto murine feeder-layers. Fibrin-glue was used as scaffold.	18 (18)	17.5 (12–27)	78%
Shimazaki (Ophthalmology 2002)	Allogeneic (seven deceased donor and six living related donors) limbal epithelial explants cultured on human amniotic membrane	13 (13)	Not available	46%

(Continued)

Table 13.2 (Continued)

Study	Technique	Patients (eyes)	Follow-up: mean and range (months)	Success rate
Sangwan (Biosci Rep 2003)	Autologous limbal or conjunctival or mixed epithelial explants cultured on human amniotic membrane	125	Not available	100%
Nakamura (Br J Ophthalmol 2004)	Autologous oral mucosal epithelial cells cultured onto murine feeder-layers and air lifting on human amniotic membrane	4 (6)	14 (11–17)	6/6
Nishida (N Engl J Med 2004)	Autologous oral mucosal epithelial cell sheets	4	14	4/4
Daya (Ophthalmology 2005)	Allogeneic (nine deceased donors and one living related donor) limbal epithelial cells cultured on plastic	10	28 (12–50)	70%
Inatomi (Am J Ophthalmol 2006)	Autologous oral mucosal epithelial cell sheets	12 (15)	20	67%
Sangwan (Indian J Ophthalmol 2006)	Autologous limbal epithelial explants cultured on human amniotic membrane	86 (88)	18.3 (3–40.5)	73%
Nakamura (Ophthalmology 2006)	Allogeneic (seven cases) and autologous (two cases) corneal cells cultivated with autologous serum on amniotic membrane	9 (9)	14.6 (12–20)	100%
Ang (Arch Ophthalmol 2006)	Autologous serum-derived cultivated oral epithelial transplants	10 (10)	12.6 [6-19]	100%
Shortt (Ophthalmology 2008)	Allogeneic (seven cases) and autologous (three cases) limbal epithelial cells cultured on human amniotic membrane.	10	13	60%

the intensity of ocular inflammation and lacrimal levels of IL8 declined more rapidly in the eye with cultivated limbal stem cells, likely owing to the anti-inflammatory activity of the AM. The eye receiving limbal allograft demonstrated more severe corneal scarring and opacification after four years [13].

Although success rates after limbal stem cell transplantation are relatively high (ranging from 46 to 100%, Table 13.2), the mechanism of how grafts of limbal stem cells regenerate a stable transparent corneal epithelium remains a debated issue. Several DNA genotyping studies indicate that the transplanted donor cells persist for only seven to nine months and are then replaced by host cells. Rather than transplanting a new source of limbal stem cells, many investigators hypothesize that donor transplanted cells may stimulate the niche where stem cells are localized (limbal epithelial crypts between the palisades of Vogt), thus regenerating the host limbal stem cell population and their progeny. Conversely, however, there is some evidence generated using polymerase chain reaction (PCR) amplification of DNA satellites, indicating persistence of donor epithelial cells for up to 3.5 years after transplantation.

The future

Many challenges lay ahead in the field of ophthalmic allograft/autograft usage and regenerative medicine that could further change ophthalmic care. It is important to highlight that many of the studies reported below and describing innovative products or applications are just preliminary. Results will therefore have to be confirmed and validated before any of these new advances are used in a clinical setting.

Future advances in corneal transplantation

Although DSAEK surgery is still the main surgical technique of EK surgery, in 2006, G. Melles reported the development of a new procedure known as Descemet membrane endothelial keratoplasty (DMEK). Surgical challenges with DMEK are considerable, as the Descemet membrane with attached intact endothelium has to be carefully stripped off the donor cornea and attached to the recipient cornea. Currently, the technique has a high endothelial cell loss and dislocation rate, thus suggesting that further refinements are needed before it can replace DSAEK. A further innovation in ALK and EK surgical procedures is the use of femtosecond lasers to perform the surgery. Several platforms are currently available including IntraLase™ FS Laser FEMTEC™ Laser Microkeratome and VisuMax. However, although superficial lamellar flap dissection with these lasers has been well-refined, deep lamellar dissection poses new challenges and current results with femtosecond laser-assisted ALK and EK (FLEK) do not match non-laser surgical results.

New challenges for cell therapy

Stem cell-based therapies have recently been classified as medicinal products by the European Union (EU) and are therefore regulated according to the manufacture of biological medicinal products for human use [14]. Groups providing cellular therapies within the EU will have to comply with EU laws, which require that grafts are only produced by accredited tissue banks under the defined conditions of good manufacturing practice. Recently, the results of the first study describing the use of ex vivo limbal stem cells cultured in compliance with good manufacturing practice standards and the EU Tissues and Cells Directive were reported. It is also likely that regulations will become more stringent in the next few years and will limit the current use of murine feeder-layers and growth media containing serum of bovine origin. The discovery that human embryonic stem cells cultured on such feeder-layers begin to express animal glycoproteins on their surfaces has raised concerns about the use of these cells in clinical cultures [15]. Similarly, serum of bovine origin has the potential for transmission of prions and animal viruses. In the near future, many efforts will have to be made toward the development of animal serum-free and murine feeder-free culture systems.

New cell sources for LSCD

Patients with bilateral total LSCD require transplantation of allogeneic donor-derived limbal stem cells, with the prospect of lifelong immunosuppressive treatments and the associated risks. An interesting new approach would be to transplant stem cells from alternative sources. Four studies have reported the transplantation of ex vivo cultured autologous oral mucosal epithelial cells to treat patients with bilateral LSCD. The rationale behind these studies is that transplantation of oral mucosa to the eye is a well-documented surgical procedure. Inatomi et al. showed that corneal clarity, improved visual acuity and stable corneal surface persisted in 67% of the patients after a mean follow-up period of 20 months. Conjunctival epithelial cells have also been considered for the treatment of patients with LSCD. Among all stratified epithelial tissues, in fact, the conjunctival cells are the ones that more resemble the biological characteristics of corneal epithelial cells, thus suggesting that they may serve some of the functions of corneal epithelial cells when transplanted onto the corneal surface. A recent study has clearly demonstrated the potential of human conjunctival epithelial cells cultivated onto amniotic membrane to be an alternative tissue source for replacement of the corneal epithelium in rabbit animal models. If results were confirmed, this might be a potential new therapeutic treatment for patients with total bilateral LSCD.

Other investigators have proposed the use of embryonic stem cells or bone marrow-derived mesenchymal stem cells, but results have so far been obtained only in animal models of cornea damage. It is also exciting to speculate whether other autologous stem cell sources such as hair follicles and bone marrow have the potential to open novel therapeutic opportunities for patients with bilateral LSCD. These studies are indeed interesting as they would reduce the need for immunosuppressive therapy and minimize risks associated with allograft immunologic rejection. However, because these cells are not of "cornea" or "limbus" origin, it will be important to perform long-term studies aimed at assessing the restoration of corneal avascularity and clarity, the tear film function and objective visual functions.

Engineering the conjunctiva

The conjunctival epithelium may be damaged by a variety of ocular disorders, such as chemical burns, Stevens–Johnson syndrome, ocular cicatricial pemphigoid, or after wide-field excision of tumors. In addition, loss of goblet cells and changes in keratin or mucin/glycocalix expression are usually found in squamous metaplasia, a hallmark of different forms of dry eye and ocular surface disorders. The use of bioengineered conjunctival equivalents would therefore be an important alternative for disorders involving the conjunctiva and it would avoid harvesting conjunctival autografts and causing iatrogenic injury to the remaining ocular surface. Autologous cultured conjunctival epithelial cells have recently been transplanted for the treatment of primary pterygium [16], recurrent viral papillomata and other disorders of the conjunctiva. However, long-term results need to be examined. Gradual corneal neovascularization has been reported after transplantation of oral mucosa epithelium. Because the conjunctival epithelium is known to have pro-angiogenic characteristics, corneal neovascularization might be seen after transplantation of cultured conjunctival epithelium. Secondly, better protocols to isolate, characterize and expand human conjunctival goblet cells should be identified. The ability to obtain enriched goblet cell cultures might open up new perspectives for the treatment of disorders caused by conjunctival goblet cell deficiency.

Engineering the endothelium

Eye diseases causing dysfunction or a low density of human corneal endothelial cells (HCECs) require transplantation of full- or partial-thickness corneas containing a healthy endothelium. A desirable alternative would be to cultivate HCECs in vitro, thus regenerating a sheet that could be grafted onto patients affected by a diseased corneal endothelium. The main hurdle is that HCECs do not normally replicate in vivo and are arrested in the G1 phase of the cell cycle. Despite this, several studies have evaluated protocols to isolate and expand HCECs in vitro starting from donor corneas. Studies in primates have also shown that monkey corneal endothelial cells can be cultured in vitro, transplanted and maintain a clear cornea for approximately two years postoperatively. In the future, it might be possible to expand HCECs into autologous human endothelium monolayers from surgical biopsy samples. Potential future perspectives might involve strategies based on the long-term genetic modification of HCECs for endothelial disorders such as Fuchs endothelial corneal dystrophy, pseudophakic bullous keratopathy and graft failure. A few in vivo and ex vivo studies have already been reported, with results showing that recombinant lentiviruses are very efficient in transducing corneal endothelial cells. Data are, however, limited to evaluation of reporter gene expression.

Gene therapy approaches

The cornea is a particularly suitable tissue for gene-therapy based approaches, as it can be preserved for several days/weeks allowing time for ex vivo gene alteration before surgery. In addition, corneal cells are easily accessible (as in direct contact with the storage medium) and therefore amenable to gene transfer. Gene therapy strategies to improve graft survival have so far focused on inhibiting neovascularization (by expression of soluble vascular endothelial growth factor (VEGF) receptors or short interfering RNAs (siRNAs) against VEGF before PK), reducing inflammation (by endothelial expression of interleukin-10), promoting tolerance or preventing endothelial cell death (through anti-apoptotic gene expression). Alternatively, gene therapy treatments might be administered in vivo, with anti-inflammatory and anti-angiogenic transgenes helping "to quiet" the eye before surgery, thus improving graft survival.

Gene therapy might also be used to treat hereditary disorders of the ocular surface. These comprise a heterogeneous group of diseases including ectrodactyly–ectodermal dysplasia–clefting (EEC) syndrome (mutations in *p63* gene), aniridia (mutations in *pax6* gene), Meesman corneal dystrophy (mutations in keratin 3/12 genes), keratoconus, macular corneal dystrophy I and II (mutations in CHST6 gene), several stromal dystrophies, Fuchs endothelial corneal dystrophy, and many others. No definitive cures are available to treat these diseases, which eventually lead to visual impairment. The only effective management for these patients would be to transplant *ex vivo* cultured genetically engineered cells of the ocular surface back onto the patient's eye. Some gene transfer vectors, including retroviral, lentiviral, and adenoviral vectors, have already shown promising in vitro results. Although these approaches might be challenging for genetic disorders affecting the conjunctiva/endothelium (cell culture techniques have not been fully validated) or the corneal stroma (stem cells have not yet been characterized), transplantation of genetically corrected autologous limbal stem cells could represent a valid and alternative treatment for genetic disorders of the corneal epithelium. Protocols to culture and amplify limbal stem cells are, in fact, fully established and already used for cell therapy applications in patients with LSCD.

New sources of eye drops

As outlined earlier, autologous serum eye drops are effective in treating conditions such as primary and secondary causes of dry eye, persistent epithelial defects, neurotrophic ulcers, and after ocular surface reconstructive surgery. In the future, allogeneic serum preparations (for example from blood donors) might be prepared and used for patients not able to donate their own blood for various reasons (i.e., anemia). In addition, ophthalmologists might be able to use umbilical-cord serum eye drops. Some studies have already reported higher effectiveness in decreasing symptoms and keratoepitheliopathy in severe dry eye syndrome and increasing goblet cell density in Sjogren syndrome when umbilical-cord serum was compared with autologous serum eye drops. Recent studies also reported that topical applications of amniotic membrane extracts might be equally promising.

CASE STUDY 13.1

Immunosuppression after KLAL

A 31-year-old man presented to our clinic six months after a chemical injury with anhydrous ammonia. The patient had been followed closely by his local ophthalmologist and managed with conservative therapy. At presentation in our clinic, the patient had a central epithelial defect and a stromal melt with 50% loss of stromal tissue (Plate 13.1). His visual acuity was Hand Motion at face. Patient also had a significant amount of conjunctival inflammation. Although it is our preference to wait about 12 months after a chemical injury to let the conjunctival inflammation resolve, we proceeded with an emergent KLAL because of our concerns with his ongoing melt and impending perforation. It should also be noted that the patient's intraocular pressure was stable on a single medicine. For these patients, we advise glaucoma management and oculoplastics consultation before performing ocular surface reconstruction. Three donor segments from two deceased donor eyes from one donor were placed 360 degrees at the patient's limbus. The patient was begun on systemic immunosuppression with tacrolimus, mycophenolate mofetil, and a short course of oral prednisone. The patient was followed closely in the postoperative period and the epithelial layer was healed 100% at day 10. Plate 13.2 shows the patient at three months postoperatively. At three months, we performed a penetrating keratoplasty. The patient has been followed in the postoperative period and has done very well. His visual acuity improved to 20/40 at one year after his corneal transplant (Plate 13.3). As for his immunosupression the patient was tapered off the oral prednisone at four months and was tapered off the tacrolimus by two years. He remained on monotherapy mycophenolate mofetil for over four years and has done very well without any adverse events from the immunosuppression and without an episode of rejection of either the corneal or limbal stem transplants. His care was closely monitored by a transplant immunologist from our local hospital.

CASE STUDY 13.2

Autologous serum eye drops for neurotrophic keratitis

In January 2006, a 54-year-old male patient diagnosed with "a corneal ulcer in the left eye" was referred to our center. Despite being treated with conventional lubricants, topical steroids and antibiotics for the previous four months, his ocular conditions had progressively worsened. He had undergone head surgery because of left trigeminal neuralgia due to a neurinoma, with ocular symptoms in the ipsilateral eye starting six months after surgery. His former ocular history was unremarkable.

Upon examination, his visual acuity was 20/20 in the right eye and 20/200 in the left eye. The right eye was normal. The left eye presented a central cornea epithelial defect, with initial involvement of the anterior stroma. The epithelium surrounding the ulcer was hazy and loosely attached to a clear stroma while a punctuate keratopathy was present in the inferior sector. The ocular surface was mildly inflamed, with normal lids and a low blinking rate. The anterior segment was normal. The symptoms observed were severe photophobia, recurrent foreign body and burning sensation, that the patient described as "severe ocular discomfort." The corneal mechanical sensitivity was severely impaired.

A "neurotrophic keratitis" was diagnosed and the cornea covered with a soft contact lens as a permanent, therapeutic bandage. He started topical therapy with 40% autologous serum eye drops administered hourly in the daytime, and preservative-free topical antibiotics, four times a day. Seven days later, the contact lens was gently removed. Both the epithelial defect and the punctuate keratopathy were reduced, and the patient symptoms were already improved. We discontinued the contact lens and antibiotics, and maintained the patient under treatment with autologous serum eye drops every two hours. After two months, the epithelial ulcer had disappeared, the epithelium was stable, and the ocular symptoms greatly reduced. The central anterior stroma showed some mild opacity, but visual acuity had improved to 20/50. The patient has since maintained the treatment with autologous serum eye drops, five times a day. When discontinued, an immediate worsening of the symptoms was observed. The visual acuity in the affected eye is stable, and the ocular surface has remained stable since.

Neurotrophic keratitis is a degenerative condition caused by dysfunctional corneal innervation and can be considered as the worst form of dry eye. The use of autologous serum eye drops successfully limited a worsening of the patient's conditions and restored the patient's quality of life to acceptable levels.

CASE STUDY 13.3

Donor-to-host transmission of *Acanthamoeba* from an asymptomatic cornea donor

A 30-year-old man underwent uneventful PK for keratoconus. A week later, at the follow-up visit, he presented ocular pain, ciliary injection, and keratic precipitates in an edematous corneal graft. He was treated with antibiotics and steroids with no significant improvement. A month later, the surgeon re-grafted the patient and the excised corneal button revealed the presence of cysts deeply embedded within the corneal stroma. These were later recognized as *Acanthamoeba* cysts. The patient was treated with topical desomedin and 0.02% polyhexamethylene biguadine. Keratitis occurred also in the second graft. Pharmacological treatments were strengthened and, after one month, a third PK was performed because of melting of the second graft. The patient is currently being treated for epithelization defects, with no signs of *Acanthamoeba* infection. Visual acuity is limited to counting fingers.

The fellow cornea from the same donor was transplanted onto a 73-year-old German woman with ocular trauma. As in the first case, a worsening postgrafting course led to treatments with oral and topical antibiotics. A second PK was therefore performed. As with the mate tissue, the explanted graft revealed stromal *Acanthamoeba* cysts. The patient was treated with aminoglycoside, 0.02% polyhexamethylene biguadine and 0,1% propamidinisoethionate eyedrops. She is currently being treated for secondary glaucoma and has no light perception.

The corneas were from a 45-year-old male donor who died after a motorbike accident. He never wore contact lenses and never complained about ocular discomfort or redness and nor did his relatives. The donor was still wearing his helmet when pronounced dead and the eyes were not exposed to any known source of contamination until the corneas were retrieved, 26 hours later. Slit lamp and light microscopy confirmed that both corneas were suitable for transplantation. No stromal abnormalities were observed and microbiological tests were negative. PCR analysis of 18S ribosomal subunit was performed on DNAs extracted from both explanted grafts using forward *JDP1* and reverse *JDP2* primers. PCR bands of 440 base pairs were sequenced and BLASTed (basic local alignment search tool), revealing 98% homology to GenBank-deposited *Acanthamoeba* sp. and *Acanthamoeba castellani* 18S sequences. Sequences of the PCR amplified bands from the two explanted corneas were identical, suggesting a common and unique origin of the *Acanthamoeba* infection source. We therefore suspect that a donor-to-host transmission of *Acanthamoeba* from an asymptomatic subject might have occurred, with the cysts residing in the donor corneas being in a dormant state without evidence of active infection or morbidity [17].

KEY LEARNING POINTS

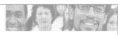

• Although penetrating keratoplasty (PK) remains the most common procedure for cornea transplantation, improvements in microsurgical techniques and introduction of new devices have led to increasing numbers of lamellar keratoplasty procedures being performed. This appears to be true both for the anterior lamellar keratoplasty replacing the anterior stroma, and for the posterior lamellar keratoplasty also known as endothelial keratoplasty, which involves the replacement of deep stromal and endothelial layers.

• Autologous serum eye drops have beneficial effects in patients with ocular surface disorders refractory to conventional treatments. A few randomized studies comparing the effectiveness of serum eye drops against tear supplements found that autologous serum drops were superior to conventional treatments as evidenced by improvement in ocular surface health and subjective comfort, higher tear film stability, faster closure of corneal epithelial wounds and prolongation of the tear break-up time. Umbilical-cord serum eye drops and amniotic membrane extracts are also being evaluated.

• Amniotic membrane (AM) is routinely used for ocular surface reconstruction, as epithelial surrogate after excision of large ocular surface neoplasias, for reconstruction of conjunctival fornix, pterygium (a fibrovascular subepithelial ingrowth of degenerative bulbar conjunctival tissue with a typical triangular shape growing over the limbus and onto the cornea), severe or refractory neurotrophic corneal ulcers, bacterial keratitis, conjunctival surface reconstruction, and to improve comfort after acute ocular burns. AM has also been used as a carrier for limbal stem cells expansion, transport, and transplantation in patients with limbal stem cell deficiency (LSCD).

• Many studies have described the clinical application of limbal stem cells in patients with total LSCD. Four sources of limbal stem cells have been routinely used: (1) deceased donor tissue (keratolimbal allograft, KLAL); (2) living-related conjunctival limbal allografts (LR-CLAL); (3) limbal stem cells harvested from the fellow eye (conjunctival limbal autograft, CLAU) in unilateral injuries; and (4) ex vivo cultured limbal stem cells. Studies evaluating the efficacy of mesenchymal and embryonic stem cells are under scrutiny.

• Autologous cultured conjunctival epithelial cells have been transplanted for the treatment of primary pterygium, recurrent viral papillomata, and other disorders of the conjunctiva. Human corneal endothelial cell culture techniques are also being developed. Gene therapy protocols might be used to improve graft survival and correct hereditary diseases of the ocular surface.

References

1. Kenyon KR, Tseng SC. Limbal autograft transplantation for ocular surface disorders. Ophthalmology 1989;96:709–22.
2. Shimmura S, Tsubota K. Deep anterior lamellar keratoplasty. Curr Opin Ophthalmol 2006;17:349–55.
3. Melles GRJ. Posterior lamellar keratoplasty. DLEK to DSEK to DMEK. Cornea 2006;25:879–81.
4. Croasdale CR, Schwartz GS, Malling JV, et al. Keratolimbal allograft: recommendations for tissue procurement and preparation by eye banks, and standard surgical technique. Cornea 1999;18:52–8.
5. Shimazaki J, Shimmura S, Tsubota K. Donor source affects the outcome of ocular surface reconstruction in chemical or thermal burns of the cornea. Ophthalmology 2004;111:38–44.
6. Djalian AR, Bagheri MM, Swanson PJ, Schwartz GS, Holland EJ. Keratolimbal allograft for the treatment of limbal stem cell deficiency. Oral presentation, Castroviejo Cornea Society Annual Meeting, October 1999, Orlando, FL.
7. Holland EJ, Mogilishetty G, Alloway R, Biber JM. (2009) A decade of immunosuppression in patients undergoing ocular surface transplants. Oral Presentation, Symposium on Eye Banking and Cornea, October 2009, San Francisco, CA.
8. Sangwan VS, Burman S, Tejwani S, Mahesh SP, Murthy R. Amniotic membrane transplantation: a review of current indications in the management of ophthalmic disorders. Indian J Ophthalmol 2007;55:251–60.
9. Tsai RJ, Li LM, Chen JK. Reconstruction of damaged corneas by transplantation of autologous limbal epithelial cells. N Engl J Med 2000;343:86–93.
10. Noble BA, Loh RSK, MacLennan S et al. Comparison of autologous serum eye drops with conventional therapy in a randomized controlled crossover trial for ocular surface disease. Br J Ophthalmol 2004;88:647–52.
11. Pellegrini G, Traverso CE, Franzi AT, Zingirian M, Cancedda R, De Luca M. Long-term restoration of damaged corneal surfaces with autologous cultivated corneal epithelium. Lancet 1997;349:990–3.
12. Shortt AJ, Secker GA, Notara MD, et al. Transplantation of ex vivo cultured limbal epithelial stem cells: a review of techniques and clinical results. Surv Ophthalmol 2007;52:483–502.
13. Ang LPK, Sotozono C, Koizumi N, Suzuki T, Inatomi T, Kinoshita S. A comparison between cultivated and conventional limbal stem cell transplantation for Stevens-Johnson syndrome. Am J Ophthalmol 2007;143:178–80.
14. European Commission. EUDRALEX, Vol. 4, Medicinal Products for Human and Veterinary Use: Good Manufacturing Practice. Annex 13, Revision 1. Brussels. 2003 July. Manufacture of investigational medicinal products, Available from: pharmacos. eudra.org/F2/eudralex/vol-4/pdfs-en/anx13en030303Rev1.pdf.
15. Martin MJ, Muotri A, Gage F, Varki A. Human embryonic stem cells express an immunogenic nonhuman sialic acid. Nat Med 2005;11:228–32.
16. Ang LP, Tan DT, Cajucom-Uy H, Beuerman RW. Autologous cultivated conjunctival transplantation for pterygium surgery. Am J Ophthalmol 2005;139:611–9.
17. Camposampiero D, Caramello G, Indemini P, et al. Two red eyes and one asymptomatic donor. The Lancet 2009;374:1792.
18. Geerling G, MacLennan S, Hartwig D. Autologous serum eye drops for ocular surface disorders. Br J Ophthalmol 2004;88:1467–74.

14 Vascularized Composite Allotransplantation

David Otterburn and Linda C. Cendales

Emory University, Atlanta, GA, USA

The past

The development of vascularized composite allotransplantation (VCA), also known as composite tissue allotransplantation, is the result of advances in organ transplantation and microsurgical techniques, which have followed exquisitely scripted, stepwise evolutions. An initial idea experienced failed attempts but was followed with focused research that showed promising results followed by their application and clinical use in recipients. VCA refers to the non-autologous transplantation of peripheral tissues including skin, muscle, nerve, and bone as a functional unit (e.g., hand) to replace tissue defects that cannot be reconstructed.

The first recorded attempt at a VCA was performed in the third century. Although it was most likely that vascular connections were not made, Saints Cosmas and Damian replaced the gangrenous leg of a Roman nobleman with the leg of a recently deceased slave [1]. This has been depicted in iconography throughout the ages, however, no follow up to the procedure was documented. The images demonstrate our natural inclination to replace damaged tissue with healthy, like tissue.

It would take many years and the dawn of modern medicine to understand why this ancient methodology would not have worked. As our understanding evolved from the four bodily humors (fluids) to tissue oxygenation, we understood the need for revascularization, and immunosuppression.

There have been innumerable contributors to medicine and science over the past 150 years who not only have their place in history but our

Tissue and Cell Clinical Use: An Essential Guide, First Edition. Edited by Ruth M. Warwick and Scott A. Brubaker.
© 2012 Blackwell Publishing Ltd. Published 2012 by Blackwell Publishing Ltd.

Table 14.1 Relevant contributors to medicine and science in regard to VCAs

1902	Alexis Carrel describes the modern vascular anastamosis which made reattaching large vessels possible, which was recognized for its significance by receiving the Nobel prize in medicine and physiology (1912).
1944	Peter Brian Medawar described the immunological basis for graft failure (Nobel prize in medicine and physiology, shared with Sir Frank Macfarlane Burnet, 1960).
1949	Sir Frank Macfarlane Burnet and Fenner hypothesize that the immune system differentiates between self and nonself.
1957	Sir Frank Macfarlane Burnet describes the process of self tolerance (Nobel prize in medicine and physiology, shared with Peter Brian Medawar, 1960).
1954	Joseph Murray performs the first solid organ transplant (Nobel prize in medicine and physiology, shared with Donnall Thomas, 1990).
1962	Ronald Malt performs first upper extremity replant.
1964	Harold Kleinert and Kasdan perform the first thumb revascularization.
1964	Roberto Gilbert Elizalde performed the first hand transplant in 1964, in Guayaquil, Ecuador. Although it required amputation 2 weeks later owing to acute rejection, it provided the impetus to a new area in VCA.
1968	Komatsu and Tamai reported the first successful replantation of an amputated thumb.
1998	Jean Michel Dubernard performs the first successful hand transplant in Lyon, France.
2005	Jean Michel Dubernard and Devauchelle perform the first partial face transplant in France.

appreciation for allowing us to stand on their shoulders. As it would be impossible to list all of them, we attempt to list a few (see Table 14.1).

The multidisciplinary team

Selection of appropriate patients for VCA cannot be overemphasized. As a visible transplant, recipients undergo extensive psychological evaluation. Usually, a hand or face transplant recipient has suffered a traumatic loss that is also associated with significant psychological injury.

Similar to organ transplants, VCA uses a multidisciplinary team, composed of several surgeons and health professionals, to ensure a safe and successful outcome for patients. Patient preoperative care includes an extensive preoperative evaluation including psychosocial assessment to ensure proper patient selection, which is continued in the postoperative period. The postoperative care is directed by the surgical team and the medical transplant team including immunologists, pharmacists, and pathologists. Once the perioperative period is complete, therapists play a crucial role in the patient's recovery. All members of the VCA team are essential to the success of the patient's outcome and the program: transplant and reconstructive surgeons;

medical transplant physicians; nurse coordinators; clinical pathologists; clinical pharmacologists; mental health providers; rehabilitation medicine; tissue typing specialists; data entry personnel; an infectious disease specialist; social worker; dietitian; and clinical laboratory personnel.

An invaluable and required constituent for the success of VCA is participation of the organ procurement organization community. Simulation sessions leading up to procurement procedures must be integrated into the multi-organ donor process to avoid jeopardizing other organs being procured for transplant.

Alternatives to allografts and their limitations

VCA is a procedure for a select group of patients. Many patients are functional with a prosthesis after amputation, however, no option is free from complications. Even though amputees receive great benefit from these devices, many use more than one prosthesis for their functional needs so may be fitted with more than one type of prosthesis [2]. Two common types of prostheses are myoelectric and body powered. The myoelectric type uses small electrical motors to provide function. It relies on the concept that whenever a muscle in the body is contracted or flexed there is a small electrical signal created by the chemical interaction in the body. Once recorded, the signal is amplified and then processed by a controller that switches the motors on or off in the hand, wrist, or elbow to produce movement and function. A body-powered prosthesis is powered and controlled by gross body movements. These movements, usually of the shoulder, upper arm, or chest are captured by a harness system attached to a cable connected to a terminal device (hook or hand). For a patient to be able to control this type of prosthesis, he/she must possess at least one or more of certain gross body movements (i.e., glenohumeral flexion, scapular abduction or adduction, shoulder depression and elevation, and chest expansion). Even advanced prostheses have problems. Skin problems, caused by ill-fitting devices, are commonly seen on amputation stumps. These include edema often accompanied by eczema, contact dermatitis, infections (both bacterial and fungal), friction blisters, chronic ulcers, verrucous hyperplasia, epidermoid cysts, squamous cell carcinoma, traumatic neuroma, and sarcoma. Dermatologic problems resulting from friction, pressure, occlusion, and allergic dermatitis also restrict the normal use of a prosthetic limb [3, 4]. Newer prostheses, such as smart prosthesis with integrated biofeedback and neurosensitization, are being developed and used experimentally.

The functionality brought by hand transplant has shown to exceed that of prosthesis in several aspects: it is a human hand; it provides protective sensation due to nerve regeneration; and, it restores body image. The international registry on hand and composite tissue transplantation reported the results of 30 patients after hand transplantation [5]. All patients developed protective sensibility with 90% of them developing tactile sensibility, and 72% developed discriminative sensibility. Complications included rejection in 85% (most of them reversed with treatment similar to other transplants), infections, hyperglycemia, and avascular necrosis of the hip, a well-described complication of steroid use. Using the Carroll test, which grades objectively how functional the limb is, hand transplant recipients have outscored prosthesis patients [6]. Others have claimed that the immunosuppression for an otherwise healthy individual decreases the life expectancy of the patients, and performing a VCA is not effective. Decision analysis studies show that the quality of life after face transplantation with the immunosuppression and its side effects is far superior to life without transplantation and no immunosupression [7].

The present

Currently, over 80 patients worldwide have received a vascularized composite allograft including hands, digits, face (Figure 14.1), larynx, knee, diaphyseal bone, uterus, and abdominal wall [8]. VCA is currently a field under experimentation and not regulated. Nonetheless, most VCA investigators worldwide define the VCA graft as an "organ." Discussions are taking place both in Europe and the USA about the definition of VCA from the biologic and regulatory standpoint. On May 1, 2008, the US Health Resources and Services Administration put forward a Request for Information about VCA and held a meeting [9]. Professional societies from the reconstructive, transplantation [10], and procurement community in the USA, supported the

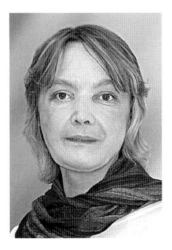

Figure 14.1 Recipient of the first partial face transplant. (Reprinted from First human face allograft: early report. Devauchelle B, Badet L, Lengelé B, Morelon E, Testelin S, Michallet M, D'Hauthuille C, Dubernard JM. Lancet. 2006 Jul 15;368(9531):203–9, with permission from Elsevier.)

inclusion of the VCA graft within the definition of an organ recovered for transplantation described in the National Organ Transplant Act, and that the process should be managed by the Organ Procurement and Transplantation Network. Arguments in support of such a designation are based on similarities of VCA with organ transplantation such as (1) vascularized allografts, like organs, also require matching and a short warm ischemia time, (2) VCAs are susceptible to ischemia after procurement and are not banked, nor are they stored, for more than 36 hours, and (3) they are susceptible to allograft rejection and thus require the recipient to take immunosuppressive drugs [10]. The major function of the Organ Procurement and Transplantation Network is to provide controls for allocation of every organ. However, allocation of grafts used for VCA is not yet established but would need to be defined. We believe that, like other transplant fields, VCA transplants should be performed at centers capable of responding to complications of surgery, infection, immunosuppression, social and financial stresses, and other complexities well described in solid organ transplantation. In addition, defining the VCA graft as an organ provides assurance that all centers performing VCA will follow similar reporting rules.

Matching and selection of the donor

The VCA donor is normally a multi-organ donor and as such, undergoes thorough screening. As we move forward, it is a focus of the VCA scientific community to delineate the specificities of VCA as they pertain to infectious agents and extended criteria. Currently, HLA matching is determined and studied retrospectively.

Up to now, donor selection has been based on matching size, gender, skin pigmentation, and ABO type. For face transplantation, age is given more credence. Owing to the developmental stages of the field, currently, children are excluded as donors and recipients. Thus, donors are generally included between 18 and 65 years of age. Nonetheless, as we move forward, it is anticipated that pediatric patients will be included as VCA donors and recipients and that matching will be patient centered for gender and skin pigmentation. In the case of face transplantation, cadaveric studies have shown that recognition of the recipient's face as that of the donor should not occur unless extensive bony reconstruction is performed [11].

Recipient selection

The selection of a recipient of a vascularized allograft is complex and its importance cannot be overemphasized. The risk–benefit analysis between immunosuppression (see below) and improving quality of life has been a point of interest and controversy for years.

Owing to the limited number of clinical cases performed worldwide, so far, VCA is experimental and thus, in the USA, it requires approval by institutional review boards. Age limits are arbitrary, but generally the upper limit is placed at 65. However, as experience with VCA grows along with life expectancy, the age limit will most likely change.

The patient must be motivated and must understand the research nature of the procedure. They must understand the need for continual follow-up with surveillance for rejection, infection, and other transplant-related complications. A thorough preoperative evaluation with psychological support (see emotional complications below) will help in this evaluation. Continuous research will allow the development of a validated mechanism to select when and for whom this quality-of-life transplant should be performed.

Immunosuppression

Like all other organ transplants, vascularized composite allografts are susceptible to allograft rejection, thus requiring the recipient to take immunosuppression for as long as they have the transplant. So far, most patients have developed some rejection within the first 12 months. The severity of rejection has varied from mild to severe based on the standardized classification system developed by international consensus at the Ninth Banff Conference on Allograft Pathology in 2007. Briefly, the scoring system includes four grades: grade 0 (no specific changes), grade I (mild rejection), grade II (moderate rejection), grade III (severe rejection), and grade IV (necrotizing rejection) [12].

Other complications have included cytomegalovirus disease and reactivation, *Clostridium difficile* enteritis, herpes simplex blisters, cutaneous mycosis, ulnar osteitis owing to *Staphylococcus aureus*, Cushing's syndrome, diabetes mellitus type 2, serum sickness, and avascular necrosis of the hip. The patient suffering from this last complication underwent unilateral hip replacement [4]. Treatments have varied widely and included systemic and/or topical steroids and tacrolimus, and the use of monoclonal and/or polyclonal antibodies, with one patient receiving all four [13].

Emotional complications

Of all handicaps, perhaps the loss of a hand and/or a face is one of the most socially devastating. Our hands are the direct reflection of our brains and our face is much more than only the home of different functional systems such as visual, olfactory, and ingestion. The human face identifies origin, emotions, health, and personal identity. Thus, face disfigurement interrupts fundamental aspects of appearance and functionality. As such, research reveals that the most common problems experienced by individuals with facial differences are secondary to social interactions with others [14].

Disfigured individuals and amputees may view the prospect of recovering their face or a hand differently than might those who are anatomically complete individuals. They may perceive this quality-of-life transplant as an opportunity and thus they are willing to accept the risks to return to a more normal facial appearance and independence.

At the time of writing this chapter, no emotional complications after the receipt of a VCA have been reported in the literature. Patients have reported "ownership" of the hands at different stages; some at the time of first seeing the hand, and others at the time of sensory recovery to the fingertips. Face transplant recipients have reported adaptation to their visible grafts and improvement of function compared to their condition before the transplant.

Outcomes

So far, over 80 patients have been reported to receive a VCA [8]. The last report from the International Registry on Hand and Composite Tissue Transplantation published the results from 33 hand transplant patients [8]. Eight of these patients received bilateral transplants (both hands). The results revealed three graft losses secondary to rejection and one mortality. Discriminative sensation varied between grade S2 and S4 according to the Higher Scale as modified by Dellon et al. [15]. Grip strength was reported as being between less than 2.5 kg in two patients and greater than 10 kg in four patients. Pinch strength ranged from 0.5 to 2 kg whereas intrinsic muscle activity was shown by electromyographic studies in eight hands. The registry also reported that all patients had returned to work. Nine hands and two digital transplants have been reported from China. All nine hands underwent revision amputation owing to rejection. Graft loss was due, primarily, according to the reports from the Chinese group, to the inability of the patients to get access to chronic immunosuppressive medicine owing to financial limitations. Complications included vessel thrombosis, opportunistic infections, hyperglycemia, increase in creatinine values, hypertension, and necrosis of the hip in one patient who required bilateral hip replacements. Reversible acute rejection was experienced in 85% of the patients within the first year, except in a patient with graft loss owing to subtherapeutic levels of immunosuppression [16]. No graft-versus-host disease has been reported by any group.

At the time of writing this chapter, 13 patients have received a face transplant. The first partial face transplant was reported in France in a female who sustained extensive trauma from animal bites. The 18-month outcome revealed sensitivity to light touch, psychological acceptance, labial contracture allowing complete mouth closure, and a satisfactory esthetic result. Complications included decrease of creatinine clearance at 14 months and reversible acute rejection episodes. Recipients of a face transplantation following the French case include both males and females. Results from a near-total human face transplant performed in a female patient in the USA showed good short-term outcome both physically and psychologically. The patient had good acceptance of her new face, and six months after surgery the recipient was able to breathe through her new nose, smell, taste, and speak intelligibly, eat solid foods, and drink from a cup. Complications included transient leukopenia during the third week after transplant [17].

Additional cases have been performed in the USA, France, Spain, China, and the registry reported a case in Egypt [18–21]. These cases include partial to total face transplants.

At the time this chapter was written, two patients have died after face transplantation. One patient, in China, succumbed owing to inaccessibility to immunosuppressive medication, and another one in France owing to infection after receiving a simultaneous face transplant and bilateral hand transplants [22, 23].

The future

Advances in transplantation, reconstructive surgery, and microsurgery have allowed the emergence of VCA and its inclusion as a partner in transplantation. VCA is in its experimental phase; however, it is at a stage where clinical development is appropriate for patients with no other means of reconstruction with autologous tissue or synthetic possibilities. So far, the successful ability to perform the procedures has clearly been demonstrated and cost-effectiveness studies are ongoing. It is likely that VCA will experience a growth period in the next decade. VCA has the potential to assist with answering scientific questions that can positively impact several fields in medicine.

KEY LEARNING POINTS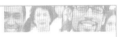

- Vascularized composite allotransplantation (VCA), also known as composite tissue allotransplantation, includes connection of non-autologous peripheral tissues including skin, muscle, nerve, and bone as a functional unit (e.g., hand), and continues to evolve as a new option for limb replacement and reconstruction of major tissue defects.

- Similar to organ transplants, VCA uses a multidisciplinary team, composed of several surgeons and health professionals, to provide a safe and successful outcome for patients.

- The selection of a qualified recipient for VCA is complex and its importance is critical.

- Decision analysis studies show that the quality of life after face transplantation including the need for immunosuppression and its side effects is superior to life without transplantation or immunosupression.

- The functionality brought by hand transplant has been shown to exceed that of prosthesis in several aspects: it is a human hand; it provides protective sensation owing to nerve regeneration; and it restores body image.

- VCA is in its experimental phase; however, it is at a stage where clinical development is appropriate for patients with no other means of reconstruction with autologous tissue.

References

1. http://www.sscosmandamiano.com/history.html (accessed 20 March 2011).
2. Millstein SG, Heger H, Hunter GA. Prosthetic use in adult upper limb amputees: a comparison of the body powered and electrically powered prostheses. Prosthet Orthot Int 1986;10:27–34.
3. Gucluer H, Gurbuz O, Kotiloglu E. Kaposi-like acroangiodermatitis in an amputee. Br J Dermatol 1999;141:380–1.
4. Lyon CC, Kulkarni J, Zimerson E, Van Ross E, Beck MH. Skin disorders in amputees. J Am Acad Dematol 2000;42:501–7.
5. Petruzzo P, Lanzetta M, Dubernard J, et al. The International Registry on Hand and Composite Tissue Transplantation. Transplant 2010;90:1590–4.
6. Petit F, Minns AB, Dubernard JM, Hettiaratchy S, Lee A. Composite tissue Allotransplantation and Reconstructive Surgery: First Clinical Applications. Ann Surg 2003; 237:19–25.
7. Cugno S, Sprague S, Duku E, Thoma A. Composite tissue allotransplantation of the face: Decision analysis model. Can J Plast Surg 2007;15.
8. www.handregistry.com (accessed March 20, 2011).
9. Department of Health and Human Services. Health Resources and Services Administration. Federal Register 2008;73:11420–2.
10. Cendales L, Granger D, Henry M, et al. Implementation of vascularized composite allografts in the United States: recommendations from the ASTS VCA Ad Hoc Committee and the Executive Committee. Am J Transplant 2011;11:13–7.
11. Baccarani A, Follmar K, Das R, et al. A pilot study in sub-SMAS face transplantation: defining donor compatibility and assessing outcomes in a cadaver model. Plast Recon Surg 2007;119:121–9.
12. Cendales L, Kanitakis J, Schneeberger S, et al. The BANFF 2007 working classification of skin containing composite tissue allograft pathology. Am J Transplant 2008; 8:1396–400.
13. Schneeberger S, Kreczy A, Brandacher G, et al. Steroid- and ATG- resistant rejection after double forearm transplantation responds to Campath-1H. Am J Transplant 2004 Aug; 4(8):1372–4.
14. Storey B, Furr A, Banis J, et al. Psychosocial issues in composite tissue allotransplantation. In Transplantation of Composite Tissue Allografts (ed. Hewitt, Lee and Gordon). Springer, pp. 452–9.
15. Dellon A, Curtis R, Edgerton M. Reeducation of sensation in the hand after nerve injury and repair. Plast Reconstr Surg 1974;53:297.
16. Breidenbach W, et al. Update of World Hand Transplant Programs. Presented at the 9th Symposium of the International Hand and Composite Tissue Allotransplantation Society, Spain, 2009.
17. Siemionow M, Papy F, Alam D, et al. Near total human face transplantation for a severely disfigured patient in the USA. Lancet 2009;374:203–9.
18. Lantieri L, Meningaud JP, Grimbert P, et al. Repair of the lower and middle parts of the face by composite tissue allotransplantation in a patient with massive plexiform neurofibroma: a 1-year follow up study. Lancet 2008;372:603–4.
19. Pomahac B, Lengele B, Ridgway EB, et al. Vascular considerations in composite midfacial allotransplantation. Plast Reconstr Surg 2010;125:523–4.

20. Eaton L. First patient to receive complete face transplant can leave hospital. BMJ 2010;341:c4088.

21. Cavadas P, Landin L, et al. Update on Face Transplantation. Presented at the 10th Symposium of the International Hand and Composite Tissue Allotransplantation Society, Atlanta, GA, 2011.

22. Lantieri L. Presented at the 2010 American Transplant Congress.

23. http://www.dailymail.co.uk/health/article-1193131/Face-transplant-patient-30-dies-just-weeks-pioneering-operation.html (accessed March 20, 2011).

24. Devauchelle B, Badet L, Lengelé B, et al. First human face allograft: early report. Lancet 2006;368:203–9.

15 The Role of Bone Marrow, Peripheral Blood Stem Cells, and Cord Blood Hemopoietic Stem Cells in Autologous, Related, and Unrelated Transplants

Rachael Hough[1] and John E. Wagner[2]
[1]University College Hospital, London, UK
[2]University of Minnesota, Minneapolis, MN, USA

Introduction

Over the past five decades, the transplantation of autologous and allogeneic hemopoietic stem cells (HSCs) after the administration of chemotherapy, with or without radiation, has cured or ameliorated underlying life-threatening malignant or nonmalignant disease in thousands of children and adults. The HSCs are derived from the bone marrow, hematopoietic growth factor mobilized peripheral blood, or umbilical-cord blood and are most often obtained from the patient (autologous), sibling or other related donor, closely human leukocyte antigen (HLA)-matched altruistic, unrelated adult volunteer, or banked umbilical-cord blood (allogeneic). HSC transplantation (HSCT), however, is associated with substantial risk; for this reason, it is reserved for those patients who have either failed previous chemoradiotherapy as in the treatment of a malignant disease or have no other therapeutic option (e.g., congenital immunodeficiency disorders or marrow failure). The risks of this treatment modality are due to the high doses of chemotherapy and radiation therapy often used and the immunological reactions frequently observed in allogeneic HSC recipients. This chapter summarizes the expected outcomes with HSCT, key advances in the field of

Tissue and Cell Clinical Use: An Essential Guide, First Edition. Edited by Ruth M. Warwick and Scott A. Brubaker.
© 2012 Blackwell Publishing Ltd. Published 2012 by Blackwell Publishing Ltd.

HSCT, the current use of this procedure, and postulates how this technology might be used in the future.

The past

Initial interest in the therapeutic potential of HSCT was prompted by the growing threats of "radiation poisoning" at the dawn of the atomic age [1]. Studies in murine and canine models demonstrated that the marrow aplasia associated with radiation exposure could be reversed by shielding the spleen or femur or by the infusion of splenocytes or bone marrow cells from a healthy donor. It also became apparent that when the donor cells were not identical to the recipient, an immunological reaction occurred which either resulted in loss of donor cells (graft rejection) or a defined disease in the recipient, later referred to as "graft-versus-host disease" (GVHD). In the following years, with the identification of the HLA system in the early 1960s, development of immunosuppressive agents that would allow engraftment, such as cyclophosphamide and radiation, and increased availability of broad-spectrum antibiotics and transfusion support, the foundations for modern HSCT era were laid.

Autologous HSCT

The first attempt to transplant human autologous HSCs was performed by McGovern et al. in 1959 in a patient with "terminal" acute lymphoblastic leukemia. After total body irradiation and infusion of autologous bone marrow, the patient remarkably achieved a complete remission although they subsequently relapsed [2]. Technological advances in the procurement, cryopreservation, and storage of recipient HSC collected when the patient was in a state of complete marrow remission has allowed wide use of this technique. Autologous HSCT essentially allows higher than conventional doses of chemotherapy and/or radiotherapy, previously restricted by prolonged marrow aplasia and pancytopenia, to be administered to the patient, with bone marrow and immune function being "rescued" by previously harvested bone marrow or peripheral blood stem cells. It was postulated that the higher doses of chemotherapy and radiation, which could not be given previously, would enhance the treatment's anti-tumor effect, leading to a higher chance of cure in those with malignant disease. More recently, the restoration or "re-setting" of the immune system achieved by autologous HSCT has also been exploited in the treatment of autoimmune diseases.

Although the most common reason for treatment failure after autologous HSCT is disease recurrence, nonrelapse causes of death are related to end-organ toxicity from the chemoradiotherapy itself, infections, or hemorrhage that occur during the brief period of pancytopenia. The outcome of autologous HSCT is dependent on the quality of recipient HSCs [3]. In inherited metabolic, immunodeficiency, and bone-marrow failure syndromes, autologous stem cells are generally affected by the genetic disease and cannot therefore be used for transplantation. In malignant diseases with a predilection to bone marrow involvement, harvested recipient cells may also contain occult malignant cells with the potential to repopulate the patient if re-infused [4]. For such patients, the use of allogeneic HSCT is the only suitable option.

Allogeneic HSCT

Allogeneic HSCT offers the potential for curing a variety of high-risk hematological malignancies, especially in patients known to be high risk for relapse after autologous HSCT. Historically and today, a healthy HLA-matched sibling is the "donor of choice". Although preferred, an HLA-matched sibling donor is not available for nearly 70% of all patients. It is for this reason that volunteer marrow donor registries were developed, with the Anthony Nolan Registry being the precursor to Bone Marrow Donors Worldwide and the National Marrow Donor Program. Today, over 14 million people have been HLA typed with an expressed interest in voluntarily serving as a donor of HSC.

Depending upon the patient's racial and ethnic background, the probability of identifying an HLA-matched unrelated adult volunteer donor varies. Furthermore, a significant proportion of patients being considered for unrelated donor transplantation will die, have progressive disease, or otherwise become ineligible before they can get to transplant because of the slow process of identifying and clearing an unrelated adult donor, which may take months.

To expand the donor pool, unrelated umbilical-cord blood has been investigated as an alternate HSC source. As with marrow and mobilized peripheral blood, umbilical-cord blood also provides an unaffected, healthy source of HSC. In addition, umbilical-cord blood appears to be less likely to cause GVHD, allowing a reduction in the "standard" HLA matching required for adult HSC sources [5]. Together, adult volunteer donors and banked cryopreserved umbilical-cord blood have made allogeneic HSCT nearly universally available.

Sibling HSCT

The first allogeneic HSCT was reported by Thomas and colleagues in 1959 [6]. They observed a short-lived remission in a patient with end-stage leukemia after total body irradiation and infusion of bone marrow from her identical twin. Further experience was soon gained in other patients with a range of diseases using HLA-identical sibling bone marrow transplantation (BMT) [7]. By the late 1970s, it was clear that HLA-identical sibling BMT could reverse immunodeficiency states and aplastic anemia as well as achieve long-term remissions in a proportion of patients with end stage, refractory

Table 15.1 Outcomes of sibling HSCT (IBMTR data)

Disease	Transplant-related mortality	Overall survival at 6 years
Acute lymphoblastic leukemia	10%	25–30%
Acute myeloid leukemia	10%	45%
Chronic phase CML	10%	65%
Aplastic anemia	10%	70–85%

IBMTR, International Bone Marrow Transplant Registry.

Table 15.2 Outcomes of unrelated donor HSCT. (Reproduced from Hough R, Cooper N, Veys P. Allogeneic haemopoietic stem cell transplantation in children: what alternative donor should we choose when no matched sibling is available? Br J Haematol. 2009 Aug 25.)

Disease	Engraftment	Transplant-related mortality	Relapse	Overall survival
Acute leukemia	>90%	20%	40%	40%
Aplastic anemia	>90%	0–20%	—	80–100%
Fanconi anemia	>90%	10–50%	—	30–50%
SCID	—	25–30%	—	60–90%
Hurler's syndrome	65%	30%	—	50%

leukemia. It was also observed that the risk of leukemic relapse was reduced in patients who had experienced GVHD, demonstrating that donor-derived immune cells were capable of eliminating malignant cells that had survived conditioning chemoradiotherapy [7].

Based on this early success, sibling BMT has become an increasingly used treatment strategy and an HLA-identical sibling remains the "preferred" donor for allogeneic HSCT (Table 15.1).

Unrelated donor HSCT

Initial attempts of unrelated donor HSCT in patients with aplastic anemia and severe combined immunodeficiency (SCID) were frustrated by nonengraftment [8, 9]. However, in 1979, the Seattle group transplanted a 10-year-old girl with acute lymphoblastic leukemia in second remission using an unrelated donor. Although, she ultimately relapsed and died two years after the transplant, she did engraft donor cells and had no significant GVHD, proving the principle that this approach was feasible [10]. Since then, thousands of children and adults have been cured of a range of diseases by unrelated donor HSCTs (Table 15.2).

Early experience with unrelated donor HSCT was associated with higher rates of graft failure and GVHD, resulting in poorer outcome than that achieved by sibling BMT. However, improvements in HLA typing and modification of conditioning regimens has dramatically reduced the incidence of nonengraftment (graft failure). Attempts to reduce the risk and severity of

GVHD by removing T cells from the graft (T-cell depletion), the cells responsible for the alloreactive response, has been shown to be effective, but has not improved survival in most cases because the lower GVHD advantage has been offset by a higher rate of nonengraftment, opportunistic infection, and relapse in specific diseases. The use of more stringently HLA-matched unrelated donors and further optimization of methods of GVHD prophylaxis are now being explored to reduce the incidence of this complication. However, GVHD continues to present a significant challenge to the use of unrelated donors, particularly when used in the treatment of nonmalignant disorders for which a graft versus malignancy effect is not required.

As previously stated, the likelihood of identifying a "suitably" matched unrelated volunteer donor is determined by the ethnicity of the recipient. Although this may be around 50% for Caucasians, the likelihood falls to 10% or less for those of certain ethnic or mixed race backgrounds who are generally less well represented on the unrelated donor registries. Although the use of more stringent molecular HLA typing methods has optimized donor selection and improved transplant survival outcomes, it has also prolonged the search process and reduced the likelihood of finding any HLA-matched donor. In addition, even if a donor is identified, the individual may be unable to donate for several reasons, including medical disqualification, unavailability, or a change in the desire to donate. The impact of the prolonged search process on transplant outcome is hard to quantify; however, it is clear that some patients will succumb to their disease or develop complications during the search interval that could negatively impact the chance of survival.

However, ongoing improvements in HLA typing, conditioning regimens, graft manipulation, and supportive care have led to overall survival rates after unrelated donor HSCT which are now approaching those expected for sibling allografts. For now, an HLA-matched unrelated adult volunteer donor is the preferred alternative donor when an HLA-matched sibling donor is not available. However, the limitations described above have led to investigation of mismatched (haploidentical) related donor and unrelated umbilical-cord blood transplantation.

Haploidentical family member donor transplantation

Haploidentical family member donor (HFD) HSCT has been increasingly and successfully used over the past 20 years, particularly in children. HFDs are matched to only half of the recipient's HLA alleles, which presents specific challenges to HSCT, consequent on the requirement to cross major histocompatibility barriers.

Early experience of HFD HSCT met with a prohibitive incidence of GVHD and nonengraftment. Over time, the risk of GVHD has been reduced to a level comparable to matched unrelated donor transplants by the vigorous depletion of alloreactive T cells. The barrier to engraftment has been partly overcome by the infusion of very high numbers

Table 15.3 Outcomes of HFD HSCT. (Reproduced from Hough R, Cooper N, Veys P. Allogeneic haemopoietic stem cell transplantation in children: what alternative donor should we choose when no matched sibling is available? Br J Haematol. 2009 Aug 25.)

Disease	Engraftment	Transplant-related mortality	Relapse	Overall survival
Acute leukemia	90%	20%	55%	30%
Aplastic anemia*	—	—	—	—
Fanconi anemia*	—	—	—	—
SCID	—	35–50%	—	70–90%
Hurler's syndrome	85%	40%	—	50%

*Sporadic case reports only. SCID, severe combined immunodeficiency; HFD, haploidentical family member donor.

("megadose") of granulocyte colony-stimulating factor (GCSF) mobilized peripheral blood stem cells. Primary engraftment is now being reproducibly achieved in over 90% of patients, the risk of GVHD is comparable to that observed after unrelated donor transplants, and encouraging disease-free survivals in selected malignant and nonmalignant diseases are being reported (Table 15.3) [11].

The principal limitation of HFD HSCT is the marked delay in immunological recovery (immune reconstitution), which results in an increased and ongoing risk of relapse and life-threatening opportunistic infection. Aggressive infection surveillance and early preemptive treatment are therefore essential elements of post-HFD HSCT care.

Unrelated umbilical-cord blood transplantation

In 1988, the first related umbilical-cord blood transplant was performed for the treatment of bone marrow failure in a boy with Fanconi anemia [12]. This confirmed murine data suggesting that cryopreserved and thawed umbilical-cord blood contained sufficient hemopoietic stem cells to reconstitute hemopoietic and immune function safely in humans. Following the subsequent success of related donor umbilical-cord blood transplantation, umbilical-cord blood banks were quickly established to facilitate unrelated donor cord blood transplants (UCBTs). On the basis of registry data and other publications it is estimated that these banks have grown rapidly across the world with a cumulative repository exceeding 600,000 units and have supported over 20,000 UCBTs so far.

Initial experience in children demonstrated that, compared with unrelated donor HSCT, UCBT was associated with a lower cumulative probability of engraftment, longer duration of neutropenia, lower incidence and severity of acute and chronic GVHD allowing a less stringent donor-recipient HLA-match, equivalent relapse incidence and equivalent overall survival.

The cell dose of the umbilical-cord blood unit infused and HLA match between unit and recipient were shown to be critical determinants of

Table 15.4 Outcomes of umbilical-cord blood transplantation. (Reproduced from Hough R, Cooper N, Veys P. Allogeneic haemopoietic stem cell transplantation in children: what alternative donor should we choose when no matched sibling is available? Br J Haematol. 2009 Aug 25.)

Disease	Engraftment	Transplant-related mortality	Relapse	Overall survival
Acute leukemia	>80%	20%	40%	30%
Aplastic anemia*	75%	20%	—	75%
Fanconi anemia*	60%	50%	—	40%
Severe combined immunodeficiency	—	35–50%	—	70–90%
Hurler's syndrome	85%	10%	—	85%

engraftment, transplant-related mortality and overall survival. A threshold pre-thaw cell dose of around 2×10^7 to 3×10^7 total nucleated cell count per kilogram or 2.0×10^5 CD34$^+$ cells per kilogram (CD34 is a marker of HSC) which needed to be exceeded in order to achieve a satisfactory outcome was identified [13]. Increasing HLA disparity was also shown to be associated with poorer outcome although the deleterious effects of an increase in HLA disparity could be overcome, at least partly, by an increase in cell dose of the unit infused.

As experience has grown and the selection of a suitable graft has been informed by the above findings, clinical outcomes of UCBT have improved significantly such that UCBT is equivalent to matched unrelated donor HSCT in children and mismatched unrelated donor HSCT in adults (Table 15.4). The principal obstacle to the wider use of UCBT has been delayed hematopoietic recovery and inferior engraftment. Several strategies designed to abrogate the duration of neutropenia have been investigated, the most successful of which so far has been the co-infusion of two umbilical-cord blood units [14], which has improved the likelihood and speed of engraftment. Interestingly, only one unit prevails as the long-term contributor to hemopoiesis, although the mechanism for this remains unclear.

Reduced intensity transplants

Another key advance in the field of allogeneic HSCT has been the development of reduced-intensity conditioning regimens. Historically, it was impossible to treat older patients (above 45 years) or patients with other significant medical conditions, because the risks of toxicity or death after myeloablative conditioning regimens were too high. Reduced-intensity conditioning regimens use immunosuppressive rather than ablative agents, which facilitate engraftment of donor cells. Donor-derived immune function subsequently eradicates residual host hemopoiesis and disease. This approach also provides a platform for further modulation and "boosting" of donor immune function, by the infusion of donor lymphocytes in those cases where the donor is not an unrelated cord blood donor. Reduced-intensity conditioning HSCT is effective, irrespective of stem cell source, and is tolerated in those patients previously precluded from allogeneic HSCT. The number of such transplants performed worldwide has increased exponentially in recent years.

The present

Indications for HSCT

Autologous and allogeneic HSCTs are now established therapeutic options for children and adults with selected life-threatening conditions (Table 15.5) [5].

Autologous transplantation can provide curative consolidation therapy in the management of malignant lymphomas and solid tumors, where there is no contamination of the recipient's bone marrow with malignant cells. Remissions of a year or more may also be achieved in multiple myeloma by this approach. More recently, autologous HSCT is being used to induce remission or amelioration of symptoms in severe autoimmune diseases.

Allogeneic HSCT is the strategy of choice where a "healthy" source of stem cells and/or graft versus malignancy effect is required. The indications for

Table 15.5 Predominant indications for autologous and allogeneic HSCT

Autologous HSCT	Allogeneic HSCT
Malignant diseases Hodgkin's lymphoma Non-Hodgkin's lymphoma Multiple myeloma Solid tumors (e.g., Ewing's sarcoma, neuroblastoma, germ cell tumors)	**Malignant diseases** Acute lymphoblastic leukemia Acute myeloid leukemia Hodgkin's lymphoma Non-Hodgkin's lymphoma Multiple myeloma Chronic lymphocytic leukemia Myelodysplastic syndromes Myeloproliferative disorders
Autoimmune disorders Systemic lupus erythematosus	**Bone marrow failure syndromes** Aplastic anemia Fanconi anemia Inherited hemoglobinopathies
	Metabolic diseases Hurler's disease
	Immune deficiency disorders Severe combined immunodeficiency Wiscott–Aldrich syndrome

these procedures include malignant disorders of the bone marrow, bone marrow failure syndromes, and immune deficiency disorders, where aberrant bone marrow and immune cells are replaced by normal donor cells. Metabolic disorders include a range of enzyme deficiencies and transport protein defects that result in progressive and often fatal organ damage as a consequence of accumulation of toxic substrates within tissues. Engrafted donor cells, in this context, provide a continuous source of normal enzymes and can arrest the progression of clinical disease in affected patients.

Complications of HSCT

HSCT is a highly complex procedure, with many potential complications occurring at different periods from the infusion of HSC (summarized in Figure 15.1).

The toxicity of the conditioning regimen is dependent on the intensity used (reduced-intensity conditioning or ablative) and the specific agents incorporated. Most patients will develop aplasia (requiring red-cell and platelet transfusion support), immune suppression, mucositis (sore mouth and diarrhea), nausea, vomiting, and alopecia. Specific side effects, such as hemorrhagic cystitis secondary to cyclophosphamide or veno-occlusive disease secondary to drugs such as busulfan, may also occur. The more intensive regimens used are associated with greater early toxicity.

Infections are the most common cause of death after allogeneic HSCT. During the interval between conditioning and hemopoietic recovery (engraftment), the patient is susceptible to bacterial, fungal, viral, and protozoal infections. With neutrophil recovery, the risk of bacterial and fungal infection diminishes, but the risk, particularly of viral reactivation, continues until normal immune reconstitution is achieved. Antimicrobial prophylactic

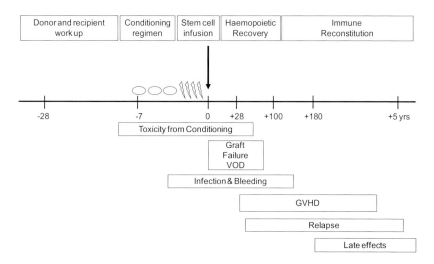

Figure 15.1 Schedule and complications of HSCT. VOD = veno-occlusive disease.

drugs are given to reduce the incidence of this complication but surveillance and early instigation of treatment of infection are critical.

Graft failure is an increasingly uncommon complication of HSCT and may be primary or secondary. The risk factors for primary graft failure include nonmalignant diseases, alloimmunization of the recipient before transplant, minimal previous exposure to chemotherapy, the use of mismatched unrelated HSC or umbilical-cord blood units, low graft cell dose and the use of T-cell depletion. Secondary graft failure may arise as a consequence of drugs or viral infection. Optimization of the conditioning regimen, graft manipulation, and donor selection, for any given patient, reduces the risk of this complication. However, when it does occur, graft failure presents a significant risk of death and requires urgent further infusion of stem cells either from reharvesting of a related or unrelated volunteer donor or from a "backup" unit in the case of umbilical-cord blood transplantation.

Veno-occlusive disease is a recognized complication of the conditioning used before HSCT in which microthrombi form in the hepatic venules and sinusoids as a result of the chemoradiotherapy (particularly busulfan and total body irradiation). The clinical features usually occur before day +30, but may occur later, and include weight gain, hepatic enlargement and pain, jaundice, renal impairment, ascites, and refractoriness to platelet transfusions. The severity ranges from a mild, self-limiting illness to a life-threatening condition, with a mortality of 60% without treatment. Prophylactic treatment with ursodeoxycholic acid, continuous low-dose heparin or defibrotide is generally given to those at highest risk. Treatment for established veno-occlusive disease includes intensive supportive care and defibrotide.

GVHD is a syndrome which results from immunocompetent donor cells reacting against recipient tissues and may occur within the first 100 days after transplant (acute GVHD) or later (chronic GVHD). GVHD is more likely with increasing age (patient and donor), if the donor is female, with increasing donor-recipient HLA disparity, and use of unmanipulated mobilized peripheral blood HSC. Strategies developed to reduce the risk of GVHD include the preemptive use of immune suppressive agents (e.g., methotrexate, ciclosporin) or depletion of alloreactive T cells from the graft. Acute GVHD predominantly affects the gut (diarrhea), liver (jaundice), and skin (rash). First-line therapy with steroids is usually effective, but second-line approaches, including anti-thymocyte globulin or monoclonal antibodies, may be necessary. Chronic GVHD may be restricted to the skin and/or liver (limited) or can be a multisystem disorder, affecting almost any organ (extensive). Treatment can be difficult, but therapeutic options include steroids, immune suppressive agents (e.g., ciclosporin, thalidomide), and photopheresis.

HSCT is also associated with several long-term sequelae, secondary to either the conditioning regimen or GVHD. These include neuroendocrine dysfunction, impairment of growth and development, infertility, cardiac disease, cataracts, musculoskeletal disease, secondary malignancy, autoimmune disorders, and psychosocial effects. The severity and likelihood of specific toxicities are determined by the type of HSCT performed, the age of the patient at transplant, and the nature of any early complications. Modification of the conditioning regimen and GVHD prophylaxis has reduced these complications where possible, but lifelong surveillance and intervention remains necessary for most patients.

Advantages and disadvantages of different HSC sources

The profile of benefits and limitations of HSCT varies with HSC source, as illustrated in Table 15.6.

Autologous peripheral blood stem cells can be harvested in a high proportion of patients. The cells are cryopreserved and available for use when clinically indicated with easy re-arrangement of infusion date if necessary. Autologous HSCT is associated with a very low transplant-related mortality (TRM) of less than 2% in most centers. The principal disadvantages of using autologous cells are the potential for re-infusion of occult malignant cells, capable of causing a relapse, and their inappropriateness for use in metabolic disorders and other acquired or congenital lympho-hematopoietic disorders, at least until the development of improved genetic modification strategies.

HLA identical siblings remain the donors of choice when an allogeneic procedure in indicated. Stem cells are rapidly available with easy scheduling of transplant date. Engraftment is reliably achieved and compared with alternative HSC sources, TRM, risk of severe acute GVHD and time to immune reconstitution are low [13]. The limitations of using an HLA identical sibling are that such a donor is often not available and there is a poorly defined psychosocial impact on the donor should the patient not survive.

The advantages of using unrelated adult volunteer donors for HSCT include the wealth of experience gained by transplant centers over the past four decades, the reproducible quality of HSC product used, the low risk to the donor during the HSC collection and the ability to obtain additional HSC or lymphocytes in the event of graft failure and falling chimerism or relapse, respectively. However, the principal obstacles to the wider use of this approach are lack of HLA-matched donors, the long duration of the search process and higher risks of acute and chronic GVHD, particularly when HLA-mismatched donors are used.

Haploidentical family donors are highly motivated donors, identifiable for nearly all allograft candidates and are available for harvest or re-harvest as clinically indicated. Engraftment is achieved rapidly and reliably. However, long-term outcome is compromised by very slow immune reconstitution, with an ongoing risk of life-threatening infections and relapse. Also, more intensive conditioning, graft manipulation, and viral/fungal monitoring requirements have limited the generalization of this transplant approach.

The overall survival after unrelated donor UCBT is similar to that observed with an HLA-matched sibling or unrelated adult volunteer donor at least for

Table 15.6 Advantages and disadvantages of different stem cell sources

	Autologous HSCT	HLA identical related donor HSCT	Unrelated donor HSCT	Unrelated donor UCBT	Haplo-identical related donor HSCT
Available donor pool	—	—	>14 million	>600,000	—
Estimation of likelihood of suitable donor	>90%	Approx 30%	10/10 = 40% 9/10 = 70% Ethnic minority = 20%	≥5/6 = 40% ≥4/6 = 70%	>90%
Speed of access	Immediate	Immediate	3–4 months	3–4 weeks	Immediate
Cost of graft	Low	Low	High	High	Low
Ability to re-arrange infusion date	Easy	Easy	May be difficult	Easy	Easy
Ability to re-access	Impossible	Yes	Possible	No	Yes
Quality of product	Assured	Assured	Assured	Variable	Assured
Speed of engraftment	Fast	Moderate	Moderate	Slow	Fast
Risk of graft failure	Low	Low	Moderate	High	Moderate
Risk of transplant related mortality	Very low	Low	High	High	High
Risk of GVHD	None	Moderate	High	Moderate	Low
Speed of immune reconstitution	Rapid	Moderate	Moderate	Moderate	Very slow
Risk of viral transmission	None	Yes	Yes	None	Yes
Risk of transmission of congenital disease	Yes	Yes	No	Yes	No

adults and children with acute leukemia. Several important logistical advantages to the use of this HSC source have also emerged, including rapid access to donor cells, easy change in transplantation date, lack of risk to the donor, lack of donor attrition, expansion of the donor pool by targeting collections to ethnic groups poorly represented on volunteer unrelated donor panels and a preserved graft-versus-graft-versus-malignancy effect. The principal disadvantage remains a relatively high early TRM, which is in part due to delayed hemopoietic reconstitution.

In the light of these advantages and disadvantages, donor selection algorithms have been proposed to aid physician choice. As yet, there is no international consensus on such algorithms but Table 15.7 and Figure 15.2 summarize the current UK consensus and University of Minnesota guidelines [14].

Choice of HSCT approach

The remarkable achievements that have been made in the field of HSCT over the past four decades now allow a donor to be identified for almost all patients requiring a transplant. The successful use of reduced intensity conditioning regimens has extended access to older patients or those with pre-existing comorbidities. For any given patient, the physician is now faced with a myriad of potential options: autologous versus allogeneic HSC, non-myeloablative versus reduced dose versus myeloablative conditioning, method of graft manipulation if any (CD34 selection versus other method of T-cell depletion), and choice of HSC source, namely mobilized peripheral blood versus marrow versus umbilical-cord blood. Although treatment consistency may be critical in the implementation of a clinical trial, tailoring the therapy to fit the circumstances of the patient is common (Table 15.8). Factors that potentially influence the final treatment plan include disease, remission status, age, comorbidities, and donor availability for an individual patient. Outcomes of HSCT are superior at "experienced" centers, which have extensive local expertise and an appropriate infrastructure equipped to deal with such complex and costly (medically and financially) procedures.

The future

The field of HSCT is developing at a rapid and exciting rate. It is likely that progress in extending access and speed to acquisition of donor HSC, improving supportive care and optimizing the graft, development of nontransplant therapeutic alternatives, and the use of marrow and umbilical-cord blood "stem cell" populations in the treatment of diseases beyond those involving the lympho-hematopoietic system, will potentially change the face of this field considerably in the next decade.

Table 15.7 UK consensus donor selection algorithm

(a) Malignant disease

Choice	Family donor	Unrelated donor	Unrelated cord
1st	Matched family donor Matched UCB (sibling)		
2nd		10/10 9/10	6/6 5/6 (>3 × 10^7 TNC/kg)
3rd	≤4/6	8/10	5/6 (<3 × 10^7 TNC/kg) 4/6

(b) Primary immunodeficiency/metabolic disorders

Choice	Family donor	Volunteer unrelated donor	Unrelated cord
1st	Matched family donor Matched cord (sibling)		
2nd		10/10	6/6
3rd		9/10	5/6 (>3 × 10^7 TNC/kg)
4th	≤4/6		5/6 (>3 × 10^7 TNC/kg) 4/6

(c) Bone marrow failure syndromes

Choice	Family donor	Volunteer unrelated donor	Unrelated cord
1st	Matched family donor Matched cord (sibling)		
2nd		10/10	
3rd		9/10	6/6 5/6 (>3 × 10^7 TNC/kg)
4th	≤4/6		5/6 (<3 × 10^7 TNC/kg) 4/6

TNC/kg, total nucleated cell count per recipient kilogram body weight.
These algorithms consider only HLA matching and cell dose and may be modified by other important factors (e.g., availability of donor, need for further cell infusions from same donor, CMV status, or donor gender). HLA matching in unrelated donor refers to matching at high/intermediate resolution for HLA-A, -B, -C, -DRB1, -DQB1 (i.e., 10 alleles). HLA matching in UCB refers to matching at low resolution for HLA-A, -B, and intermediate/high resolution for -DRB1 (i.e., six alleles). For each level of "choice", centers should take their individual experience and expertise into consideration.

Single unit selection

Based on the interaction between cell dose and HLA matching, it is clear that a higher cell dose is required in recipients of more mismatched units. With this principle in mind, an adequate unit is defined as 6/6 match with a minimum cell dose of 3.0×10^7 nucleated cells per kilogram or a 5/6 match with a minimum cell dose of 4.0×10^7 nucleated cells per kilogram or a 4/6 match with a minimum cell dose of 5.0×10^7 nucleated cells per kilogram actual recipient body weight. If there is no adequate single unit as defined above, then they may be eligible for a double UCB transplant.

Double unit selection (table below – order of preference of unit selection given 1–15)

The method of selecting two units is detailed in figure 1. The principles are that each unit must contain a minimum cell dose of 1.5×10^7 nucleated cells per kilogram, the total combined cell dose must contain a minimum cell dose of 3.0×10^7 nucleated cells per kilogram and the two units must be partly HLA matched with each other. Although there is no proof of the need for interunit matching, the decade of experience at the University of Minnesota has been with the proposed interunit matching with a maximum of two mismatches between units and the recipient.

If the UCB is to be composed of two 4/6 UCB units

Step 1) Unit 1 is the 'best' single unit that is available
Step 2) Unit 2 is the second 'best' unit that is available
Unit 2 must be partially HLA matched with Unit 1

HLA Match	Cell Dose Levels						
	1.5-2.0	2.1-2.5	2.6-3.0	3.1-3.5	3.6-4.0	4.1-4.5	4.6-5.0
HLA 6/6	3	2	1				
HLA 5/6	8	7	6	5	4		
HLA 4/6	15	14	13	12	11	10	9

New unit selection parameters under consideration

Retrospective analysis of data from the COBLT Study in the USA suggested that high-resolution HLA typing at HLA-A, -B, -C, -DRB1, and -DQB1 might have a place in unit selection in that those patients with a 9–10/10 matched donor have a particularly high survival rate. Therefore, allele-level typing might be requested for patients with a 5–6/6 matched donor as determined by conventional HLA matching for UCB. The 9–10/10 HLA-matched unit with a highest cell dose should be selected.

Unpublished data from the New York Blood Center suggest that unit blanks or homozygosity at an HLA antigen (i.e., GVHD vector) might be associated with improved outcome. Based on these data, units with a blank at a given antigen might be considered matched at that antigen and the level of HLA mismatch downgraded accordingly.

Figure 15.2 University of Minnesota donor selection algorithms.

Table 15.8 Choice of transplant approach

	Indications	Relative contraindications
Transplant type		
Autologous HSC	Acute myeloid leukemia, lymphoma, multiple myeloma	Minimal residual disease, chemoresistant disease
Allogeneic HSC	Acute lymphoblastic leukemia, chronic myeloid leukemia, genetic diseases, marrow failure syndromes	Preexisting comorbidities and infections
Conditioning		
Nonmyeloablative/ reduced intensity	Preexisting comorbidities and infections, older age	Early relapsed malignant disease
Myeloablative	Healthy, younger age, acute lymphoblastic leukemia	Poor end-organ function
Allogeneic HSC source		
PBSC	Adults	Children
Marrow	Poor peripheral blood stem cell mobilization	Previous pelvic irradiation
Umbilical-cord blood	Urgent need; unavailable HLA 8/8 unrelated adult volunteer donor	Low cell dose; preexisting potential requirement for donor lymphocyte infusion
Allogeneic graft manipulation		
T-cell depletion	High risk of GVHD; HLA-mismatched donor	Chronic myeloid leukemia, myelodysplastic syndrome

Extended access and speed to acquisition of unrelated donor cells

International attempts to increase the likelihood of finding an unrelated volunteer donor are focused on expanding targeted racial and ethnic representation within the marrow donor registries, reducing the marked attrition rate by continued education efforts and donor engagement, and improving international collaboration with sophisticated information technology.

In parallel, umbilical-cord blood banking efforts internationally are rapidly increasing in size. With greater standardization and regulation of collection, processing, and storage, the quality of product available for transplantation has markedly improved. As more units with larger cell doses are placed in the international inventory, the greater is the chance of finding a single HLA 5–6/6 matched umbilical-cord blood unit for children and adults. It is already known that the collection of umbilical-cord blood is a means for overcoming some of the ethnic and racial barriers plaguing adult donor registries, improving our chance to serve all populations of patients in need of allogeneic HSC for transplantation.

Improvements in HSCT procedure

Future refinements in conditioning regimens, GVHD prophylaxis strategies, and graft manipulations will likely improve patient outcomes, irrespective of HSC source. Attempts to ameliorate the delayed immune reconstitution commonly observed after allogeneic HSCT in general, in particular haploidentical-related donor HSC, is the next big obstacle to tackle. Efforts are focused on protecting the thymus (radiation shielding, hormonal therapies, use of keratinocyte growth factor), adoptive transfer of viral- or fungal-specific T cells or allodepleted donor lymphocytes (e.g., using anti-CD25 immunotoxin) and infusion of immunomodulatory cells, such as mesenchymal stem cells, regulatory T cells, or other tolerizing agents. Additional work is being done to speed neutrophil recovery, particularly in the area of umbilical-cord blood transplantation; these include interosseous injection, co-infusion of haploidentical family CD34+-selected PBSCs or "off-the-shelf" myeloid progenitors, use of ex vivo expansion culture techniques, and strategies to enhance homing of the HSC to the marrow microenvironment.

Development of nontransplant alternatives

As our understanding of the fundamental biology of many diseases increases, the opportunity for developing targeted, disease-specific treatments becomes a reality. This has already been achieved in chronic myeloid leukemia (CML) and selected metabolic disorders. Leukemogenesis in CML is driven by a reciprocal translocation between chromosomes 9 and 22 (the Philadelphia chromosome), which results in juxtaposition of the *BCR* and *ABL* genes. The resulting *BCR–ABL* fusion gene encodes a protein with tyrosine kinase activity. Identification of this biology enabled the design of tyrosine kinase inhibitors, the first of which was imatinib. This drug has revolutionized the management of CML and has obviated the need for allogeneic HSCT in a high proportion of patients. Similarly, exogenous enzyme replacement therapy may be effective in neuronopathic metabolic disorders, again removing the requirement for an allograft. It is likely that similar progress in other diseases will mandate reappraisal of the role of HSCT over time.

New indications

There is much current scientific interest and exploration of deriving non-HSC stem cells from bone marrow or umbilical-cord blood for use in the treatment of nonhemopoietic conditions. Non-HSC stem-cell-based therapies offer the promise of ameliorating serious diseases for which no disease-modifying treatment is currently available. The scope is potentially enormous and could ultimately be incorporated into the treatment armamentarium of many common diseases, including Parkinson's disease, degenerative musculoskeletal diseases such as osteoarthritis, heart failure, and type I diabetes. In addition to stem cells, umbilical-cord blood and adult peripheral blood may be potent sources of regulatory T cells that could be used to ameliorate autoimmune diseases. Although there is great promise for these new indications based on laboratory investigations, future clinical trials will be required to define the power of these novel cellular approaches to treat these diseases.

Funding

HSCTs are very expensive procedures, with costs increasing with more complex procedures, the use of unrelated donors (cord blood and bone marrow), and if significant complications occur. With improvements in transplant technology (such as the use of reduced-intensity conditioning regimens) and increasing identification of suitable donors, the current trajectory of expansion of HSCT indications is set to continue. This technology represents a significant financial burden to health care systems around the world. Whether state funded or insurance based, individual countries need to develop a financial strategy to ensure that the growing number of potential recipients of stem cell therapy will have access to these treatments.

Conclusions

There have been outstanding advances in the field of HSCT over the past 50 years, such that it is now possible to offer this life-saving treatment to almost all patients who might benefit. The complexity of tailoring the "best" transplant for an individual patient mandates that these procedures are concentrated in specialized transplant centers, with the expertise and infrastructure available to optimize clinical outcome. The future of stem-cell-based therapies is potentially enormous and will require considerable investment from international health care systems.

CASE STUDY 15.1

A 7-year-old girl presents with a high-risk relapse of acute lymphoblastic leukemia and requires an HSCT. Mum mentions that they had stored the girl's umbilical-cord blood when she was born. A fully HLA-matched volunteer donor has also been identified and will be available to donate at the time required for the patient. Would you use the girl's own umbilical-cord blood or the unrelated donor?

The risks associated with autologous umbilical-cord blood transplantation are considerably less than an unrelated donor HSCT and there are likely to be enough HSCs in a single unit to transplant a 7-year-old safely. However, the genetic signatures of leukemias developing in children and teenagers have been shown to be present in their blood (Guthrie spots) at birth. Thus the girl's own umbilical-cord blood may contain pre-leukemic cells capable of causing future relapse. In addition, the patient could benefit from the graft-versus-leukemia effect of allogeneic cells to reduce the risk of relapse after HSCT. Together, our recommendation would be to use the HLA-matched unrelated donor. If this child had acquired severe aplastic anemia, however, we would argue that the autologous umbilical-cord blood be considered.

CASE STUDY 15.2

A 24-year-old man is diagnosed with CML. He has received cytoreductive therapy with hydroxyurea and has a normal white blood count. His brother has been found to be HLA identical. Would you proceed with a sibling allograft or use imatinib?

This has been a controversial area and highlights the challenges of incorporating novel agents into clinical practice. Allogeneic HSCT is the only approach that has been proven to be curative in CML, but it is associated with a significant risk of transplant related mortality and morbidity. The early clinical trials of imatinib have demonstrated its ability to achieve a molecular complete remission. However, it was unknown whether the remission would be sustained or what the long-term toxicity would be. The maturing imatinib trial data are encouraging in both respects and new tyrosine kinase inhibitors are being developed. Thus, first-line therapy in CML has changed from an HLA-matched sibling allograft to imatinib for many transplant centers.

KEY LEARNING POINTS

- Autologous and allogeneic HSCT offers potentially curative therapy for patients with a variety of life-threatening diseases.

- HSC can be harvested from the bone marrow, peripheral blood or cord blood of the patient themselves (autologous) or from another related or unrelated individual (allogeneic).

- There are different risks and benefits associated with transplantation of hemopoietic stem cells from different sources.

- The type of transplant and donor choice must be individualized for each patient, based on the risks of their disease, age and physical fitness.

- Stem-cell-based therapies may be used for a wide range of other diseases in the future.

References

1. Mathe G, Jammet H, Pendic B, et al. [Transfusions and grafts of homologous bone marrow in humans after accidental high dosage irradiation.]. Rev Fr Etud Clin Biol 1959;4:226–38.
2. McGovern J, Russel P, Atkins L, Webster E. Treatment of terminal leukaemic relapse by total body irradiation and intravenous infusion of stored autologous bone marrow obtained during remission. N Engl J Med 1959;260:675–83.
3. Scheding S, Brugger W, Mertelsmann R, Kanz L. Peripheral blood stem cells: in vivo biology and therapeutic potential. Stem Cells 1994;12 (Suppl 1):203–10; discussion 211.

4. Brenner MK, Rill DR, Holladay MS, et al. Gene marking to determine whether autologous marrow infusion restores long-term haemopoiesis in cancer patients. Lancet 1993;342:1134–7.

5. Hough R, Cooper N, Veys P. Allogeneic haemopoietic stem cell transplantation in children: what alternative donor should we choose when no matched sibling is available? Br J Haematol. 2009;147:593–613.

6. Thomas ED, Lochte HL, Jr., Cannon JH, Sahler OD, Ferrebee JW. Supralethal whole body irradiation and isologous marrow transplantation in man. J Clin Invest 1959;38:1709–16.

7. Bortin MM. A compendium of reported human bone marrow transplants. Transplantation 1970;9:571–87.

8. Speck B, Zwaan FE, van Rood JJ, Eernisse JG. Allogeneic bone marrow transplantation in a patient with aplastic anemia using a phenotypically HL-A-identifcal unrelated donor. Transplantation 1973;16:24–8.

9. Horowitz SD, Bach FH, Groshong T, Hong R, Yunis EJ. Treatment of severe combined immunodeficiency with bone-marrow from an unrelated, mixed-leucocyte-culture-non-reactive donor. Lancet 1975;2:431–3.

10. Hansen JA, Clift RA, Thomas ED, Buckner CD, Storb R, Giblett ER. Transplantation of marrow from an unrelated donor to a patient with acute leukemia. N Engl J Med 1980;303:565–7.

11. Lang P, Handgretinger R. Haploidentical SCT in children: an update and future perspectives. Bone Marrow Transplant 2008;42 (Suppl 2):S54–9.

12. Gluckman E, Broxmeyer HA, Auerbach AD, et al. Hematopoietic reconstitution in a patient with Fanconi's anemia by means of umbilical-cord blood from an HLA-identical sibling. N Engl J Med 1989;321:1174–8.

13. Barker JN, Weisdorf DJ, DeFor TE, et al. Transplantation of 2 partially HLA-matched umbilical cord blood units to enhance engraftment in adults with hematologic malignancy. Blood. 2005;105:1343–7.

14. Shaw BE, Veys P, Pagliuca A, et al. Recommendations for a standard UK approach to incorporating umbilical cord blood into clinical transplantation practice: conditioning protocols and donor selection algorithms. Bone Marrow Transplant 2009; 44;7–12.

16 Mesenchymal Stem Cells: Application for Immunomodulation and Tissue Repair

Nicole J. Horwood[1], Francesco Dazzi[2], Walid Zaher[3,4], and Moustapha Kassem[4]

[1]Kennedy Institute of Rheumatology, University of Oxford, London, UK
[2]Imperial College, London, UK
[3]King Saud University, Riyadh, Kingdom of Saudi Arabia
[4]University Hospital of Odense, Odense, Denmark

Introduction

Bone-marrow-derived mesenchymal stem cell (MSC) populations (also known as skeletal stem cells, bone marrow stromal cells, or, as recently suggested by the International Society for Cytotherapy, multipotent mesenchymal stromal cells [1]) are present among the bone marrow stroma and capable of multi-lineage differentiation into mesoderm-type cells such as osteoblasts, adipocytes, and chondrocytes [2] and possibly, but still controversially, other non-mesoderm type cells, for example neuronal cells or hepatocytes [3–4]. Moreover, MSCs provide supportive stroma for growth and differentiation of hematopoietic stem cells (HSCs) and hematopoiesis [5].

The identification and systematic characterization of MSCs was initiated through the pioneering work of Friedenstein and co-workers in Russia [6] and later Owen and co-workers in the UK [7]. Friedenstein's group were studying the effects of radiation on bone marrow cells with special focus on bone marrow stroma. Their clonal analysis and in vivo transplantation studies of bone marrow stromal cells led to the identification of the multipotent MSCs. Recently there has been increased interest in understanding the

Tissue and Cell Clinical Use: An Essential Guide, First Edition. Edited by Ruth M. Warwick and Scott A. Brubaker.

© 2012 Blackwell Publishing Ltd. Published 2012 by Blackwell Publishing Ltd.

biology of MSCs because of their potential therapeutic use in a variety of skeletal and non-skeletal disorders. This chapter focuses on the properties of MSCs that make them suitable for the modulation of immune responses and in the treatment of autoimmune disorders as well as their potential in the arena of tissue repair.

Definition, isolation, and characterization of MSCs

MSCs are fusiform, fibroblast-like cells. During their initial growth in vitro, they form colonies (termed by Friedenstein, in analogy with HSC, colony-forming unit-fibroblasts (CFU-f)) [7–9]. The cells are negative for hematopoietic cell surface markers CD34, CD45, and CD14, and positive for CD29, CD73, CD90, CD105, CD166, and CD44 [1, 10–11]. Unfortunately, these markers are not specific for MSCs as they are expressed on other fibroblast-like cells. Therefore, MSCs are usually defined by their ability to differentiate into osteoblastic, adipocytic, and chondrocytic cells (i.e., multipotentiality) in vitro or by demonstrating their ability to form bone upon transplantation subcutaneously in immune-deficient mice, which is considered to be "the gold standard" for MSC phenotype [12]. Traditionally, MSCs have been isolated based on their selective adherence to plastic surfaces [9, 13, 14]. One disadvantage of this approach is unavoidable hematopoietic cell contamination and the phenotypic heterogeneity of cultures. Clonal analysis of plastic-adhered bone marrow-derived MSCs has demonstrated that around 30% of the clones are multipotent and thus by definition MSCs [15]. The remaining cells are considered to be more committed progeny. We have recently reported the presence of clonal heterogeneity amongst MSC with respect to their bone-forming capacity [16] and that committed populations of pre-osteoblastic or pre-adipocytic cells exist among MSC populations [17]. Thus, one of the active areas of investigations is the identification of specific surface markers that can distinguish multipotent MSCs from more committed progeny. One approach that has been used is the development of monoclonal antibodies. Haynesworth et al. generated three monoclonal antibodies, SH2, SH3, and SH4 that were non-reactive with hematopoietic cells and mature osteoblasts, suggesting specificity for early stage cells of the osteoblastic lineage [18]. SH2 is known now to recognize endoglin (CD105) whereas both SH3 and SH4 react with CD73 (ecto-5'nucleotidase). Similarly, the monoclonal antibody SB-10 was generated, and its epitope ALCAM [19] and HOP-26 identifies CD63 [20]. STRO-3 is an antibody that recognizes an isoform of tissue-non-specific ALP (TNALP) [21]. STRO-4 identifies the beta isoform of heat shock protein-90 (Hsp90-β) [22]. STRO-1 mAb is still the antibody with the highest affinity and efficiency for isolating all clonogenic MSCs as a stand-alone reagent [23]. However, the epitope recognized by STRO-1 remains unidentified.

More recently, CD146 (MCAM), which is a surface marker expressed by smooth muscle, endothelium, myofibroblasts, and pericytes, has been reportedly expressed by MSCs in the bone marrow [24] and in many other tissues [25]. Furthermore, Russell et al. have proposed that greater cell amplification, colony-forming efficiency, and colony diameter for tri-lineage versus uni-lineage potential clones suggest that MSC proliferation may be a function of potency and that CD146 may be a marker of this multi-potency [26]. Two novel CD markers, CD200 and CD271, have also been identified and used to isolate bone-marrow-derived MSCs [27, 28]. However, these markers do not distinguish between multi-potent MSCs versus more lineage-restricted MSCs.

In another approach to identify surface markers of MSCs, global quantitative mass spectrometry-based proteomics have been used to identify novel plasma-membrane-associated protein makers [11]. These global methods have provided many novel candidate marker genes and proteins but need further verification.

Multipotent stem cells from bone marrow have been isolated based on the concept of a cellular hierarchy in MSC populations analogous to that in HSC. For example, Reyes et al. isolated a multipotent MSC population (termed multipotent adult progenitor cells, MAPCs) from CD45-/glycoprotein A-depleted bone-marrow-derived mononuclear cell fraction that selectively adhered to laminin-coated cell culture plastic plates under low serum conditions [29], and in several publications by the same group, an extensive plasticity of murine MAPC has been reported [30]. Murine side population cells, isolated from bone marrow based on their Hoechest dye exclusion, can develop into MSCs (and HSCs) and thus it may represent an earlier, more primitive population of bone marrow stem cells [30].

In vitro growth of MSCs

The classical method for culturing MSCs in vitro is in serum-containing media. However, some investigators have described the development of chemically defined culture conditions [31], or the culture of MSCs in human plasma [32]. The addition of basic fibroblast growth factor (FGF-2) can enhance the in vitro growth of MSCs [33]. Irrespective of the culture method, MSCs exhibit limited expansion during long-term in vitro culture known as "in vitro replicative senescence" [34]. MSCs obtained from young donors can grow to 40 population doublings (PD) whereas only to 25 PD when obtained from elderly donors [2, 34]. Replicative senescence is caused by several mechanisms including progressive telomere shortening during continuous subculture in vitro [34] owing to absence of telomerase activity in MSCs [35, 36]. As an approach to abolish the senescence-phenotype of MSCs, we demonstrated that over-expression of human telomerase reverse transcriptase gene (*hTERT*) in MSC restores telomerase activity [35]. These telomerized cells exhibit an extended lifespan and maintain their "stemness" [10], making these cells an attractive candidate in regenerative medicine and tissue engineering applications [37]. Unfortunately, extensive cell proliferation of telomerized cells in vitro led to genetic instability and transformation after approximately 250 PD in culture [38], thus limiting the clinical use of this approach. Conditional over-expression of the *hTERT* gene or intermittent chemical stimulation of its expression may be a more appropriate approach. Trichostatin A treatment, which affects DNA chromatin structure, resulted in transient expression of the *hTERT* gene [39], demonstrating the feasibility of using chemicals (or small molecules) to stimulate *hTERT* expression with controlled and beneficial biological effects.

Molecular mechanisms orchestrating MSC fate and cellular programming

Adult tissue-derived stem cells differ from embryonic stem cells which arise from the inner cell mass of the blastocyst and give rise to all of the cells of the organism. MSCs are adult stem cells (or somatic stem cells) defined as undifferentiated cells among the differentiated cells in a tissue or organ that self-renew and differentiate to form some or all of the specialized cells of that tissue or organ.

The characterization of MSCs by their functional properties accompanied by cell surface expression does not represent a pattern of unique stem cell markers [40]. On the other hand, there is a list of stem cell markers associated with human embryonic stem cells such as the transcription factors Oct4 (Pou5f1), Nanog, SOX2, and cell-surface antigens SSEA-3 and -4, among others [41]. Many studies have shown that adult human stem cells, including MSCs, can express some embryonic stem cell markers: SSEA-4 expression has been detected in bone marrow [42, 43] and dental pulp stem cells [44]; Oct4 expression has been reported in bone marrow [43, 45] and adipose tissue-derived stem cells [46], peripheral blood mononuclear cells [47], dental pulp stem cells [44], heart, and liver cells [48]; Nanog expression has been found in bone marrow, heart, and liver MSCs [45]. The expression of SOX2 has been detected in bone marrow, neural tissues, and sensory epithelia from the early stages of development [45, 49, 50]. In support of these findings, a recent side-by-side comparison of different MSC sources showed that human bone marrow MSCs expressed the embryonic stem cell markers Oct4, Nanog, alkaline phosphatize (ALP), and SSEA-4. Adipose tissue and dermis MSCs expressed Oct4, Nanog, SOX2, ALP and SSEA-4, whereas heart MSCs expressed Oct4, Nanog, SOX2, and SSEA-4 [51].

MSC-mediated immunosuppression

The potent immunosuppressive effects of MSCs have been widely demonstrated [52, 53]. In contrast to classical immune tolerance, MSC-induced unresponsiveness is not cognate dependent as the expression of major histocompatibility complex (MHC) molecules on the surface is not required. In fact, the immunosuppressive activity on MHC class I-restricted CD8$^+$ T cells can still be observed using MSCs deleted for the genes encoding MHC class I molecules [54]. Furthermore, the use of MSCs from third-party donors fully mismatched for the MHC haplotype of the responder T cells is similarly effective [55]. MSC-induced unresponsiveness also lacks selectivity, because MSCs are equally effective at inhibiting the proliferation of memory and naïve T cells [54], do not preferentially affect CD4$^+$ or CD8$^+$ subsets [56] and have similar effects on B-cell proliferation.

The characterization of the anergic T cells generated by MSCs has helped to elucidate mechanisms underlying MSC-mediated immunosuppression; molecular mediators of this are discussed below. T cells, stimulated in the presence of MSCs, are arrested at the G0/G1 phase of cell cycle as a result of inhibition of cyclinD2 [56]. Because the effector functions are only partly impaired, MSCs induce an unresponsive T cell profile that is fully consistent with division arrest anergy [57, 58]. As the T cells are only temporarily inhibited in their proliferative/functional capacity, MSCs are unlikely to cause cell death and can actually protect from activation-induced cell death in murine T cells [40, 59], despite engaging the inhibitory molecule programmed death 1 (PD-1) pathway in the arrest of cell proliferation [60]. The prominent role of indoleamine 2,3-dioxygenase (IDO) in the T-cell–MSC interactions may help explain why MSCs inhibit T-cell proliferation by inducing the apoptosis of activated T cells, but have no effect on resting T cells [61].

The immunosuppressive effects of MSCs are not confined to T cells. MSC inhibit interleukin-2 (IL-2)-induced proliferation of resting natural killer (NK) cells and prevent the induction of effector functions although they only partly interfere with proliferation of activated NK cells [62, 63]. However, MSCs are not resistant to NK-cell-mediated killing provided that the NK cells have been pre-activated with IL-2.

Human MSCs can also inhibit B-cell function as demonstrated by impaired immunoglobulin production. Additionally, the expression of certain chemokine receptors and their response to the specific chemokines is negatively affected by MSCs [64]. However, later studies examining the influence of bone marrow-derived MSCs on highly purified B-cell subsets demonstrated the proliferation and differentiation of B cells into immunoglobulin-secreting cells when stimulated with an agonist of Toll-like receptor 9 in the absence of B-cell receptor triggering. Under these conditions, MSCs enhanced proliferation and differentiation into plasma cells of memory B-cell populations

[65]. These results suggest that MSC immunosuppressive activity is regulated and not necessarily indiscriminate. Additionally, MSCs contribute to the bone marrow reticular niche, where mature B cells and long-lived plasma cells are maintained [66] and in the thymus they exert a similar activity [67].

The immunosuppressive properties of MSCs can also target antigen-presenting cells (APCs). MSCs inhibit the differentiation of dendritic cells, impair their APC function [68–70], and induce dendritic cells to acquire regulatory features. Human MSCs induce the generation of dendritic cells producing large amounts of interleukin-10. Therefore, the direct inhibitory activity on immune effectors is accompanied by the recruitment of regulatory networks with T cell suppressive properties [71, 72]. The mechanisms affecting these MSC properties involve several molecules. Using neutralizing monoclonal antibodies, it was shown that transforming growth factor-$\beta 1$ (TGF-β) and hepatocyte growth factor play a significant role [73], and recently TGF-β has been implicated in the beneficial effects mediated by MSCs in suppressing allergic responses [74].

MSC use IDO, among other factors, for their immunosuppressive activity. IDO, an intracellular enzyme that initiates tryptophan breakdown along the kynurenine pathway, was shown to mediate immune privilege and prevent rejection of the allogeneic fetus during pregnancy. Tryptophan depletion causes a rise in the level of uncharged transfer RNA (tRNA) in T cells, resulting in activation of the amino-acid-sensitive general control non-depressible 2 (GCN2) stress kinase pathway with consequent cell cycle arrest and anergy [75, 76]. The functional phenotype of T cells exposed to IDO is remarkably similar to that described in T cells after contact with MSCs [56]. Moreover, IDO production is highly sensitive to the presence of interferon-γ (IFN-γ), which plays a prominent role in promoting the immunosuppressive activity of MSCs. It should be noted that most of this work has been performed in human cells and evidence that it has an equal function in murine MSCs is contradictory [77]. It should also be noted that other mechanisms of MSC-mediated immunosuppression have been reported that involve interleukin-6 (IL-6) [78] or the production of insulin growth factor binding protein independently of IDO [79].

A further mechanism mediating immune tolerance during gestation is HLA-G. HLA-G is a non-classic class I MHC molecule that functions as a tolerogenic molecule with restricted tissue expression [80]. HLA-G is constitutively expressed in MSCs and anti-HLA-G blocking antibodies partly abolish the inhibitory activity of MSCs on lymphocyte proliferation [81]. It was observed that the soluble form of HLA-G protected target cells from cytotoxic T-cell-mediated lysis [82] and triggers the expansion of CD4(+)CD25(high)FOXP3(+) regulatory T cells [83]. Like IDO, HLA-G has an important role in immunological tolerance to the fetus, thus suggesting that MSC-mediated immunosuppressive activity should be considered as a modality of "innate tolerance", a function shared by other cells of different ontogenetic origin rather than a function of a specific cell type.

Murine MSCs are reported to use nitric oxide (NO) [84] by which they suppress Stat5 phosphorylation and proliferation in T cells. NO at high concentrations is known to inhibit T-cell responses [85] but, because of its rapid diffusion, the active form must be available in close proximity to the target cell. The induction of inducible NO synthase (iNOS) was readily detected in MSCs, and specific inhibitor of iNOS reversed the suppression of T-cell proliferation [77]. Heme oxygenase-1 (HO-1), a mediator of NO that has anti-inflammatory and immunosuppressive activities, has been proposed as a further arbitrator of MSC-mediated immunosuppression [86], as demonstrated in vivo by administration of HO-1; and iNOS inhibitors reversed the ability of MSC to prolong cardiac allograft survival in a rat model [87].

A further mediator reported in several studies is prostaglandin E2 (PGE$_2$). Human MSCs produce elevated levels of PGE$_2$ when cultured with immune cells, and PGE$_2$ inhibitors partly restore MSC immune modulation on T71 and NK cells [63]. MSCs can reprogram macrophages by releasing PGE$_2$ that interact with the prostaglandin EP2 and EP4 receptors on macrophages [88]. When MSCs were administered to a mouse model of acute sepsis, macrophage recruitment, which was observed to follow MSC infusions, was demonstrated to be fundamental for the beneficial effect [88].

MSC immunosuppressive activity requires "licensing"

The immunosuppressive properties of MSCs are not constitutive, but rather require a "licensing" step; a step likely to involve the production of soluble factors. We have shown that only supernatants obtained from cultures where MSCs were incubated with activated T cells displayed an immunosuppressive effect when added to secondary cultures in which T cells were induced to proliferate [40]. This suggests that T cells provide molecules necessary for MSC functions to be enacted.

There is evidence that the nature of the "licensing" signals is related to inflammation. In vitro, IFN-γ is necessary to promote MSC-mediated immunosuppression, and the suppressive activity of MSC on CD4$^+$ and CD8$^+$ T cells can be reversed after the addition of anti-IFN-γ receptor neutralizing antibodies to the cultures [89]. These data are consistent with the fact that IFN-γ is a potent inducer of IDO. Similar findings were also observed in mice whereby the "licensing" signal was identified as a combination of IFN-γ, tumor necrosis factor-α (TNF-α) and interleukin-1β (IL-1β) [90].

Although much attention has been paid to the acquirement of immunosuppressive activities, the concept of "licensing" should be considered more widely. In fact, early studies observed that, although high numbers of MSCs suppress alloreactive T cells, very low numbers stimulate lymphocyte proliferation [55]. The ability to inhibit or stimulate T-cell alloresponses seems to be independent of the MHC identity between MSC and the responding lymphocyte population. It is therefore possible that MSC immunological properties can be "polarized" either toward an immunosuppressive/anti-inflammatory or an immunostimulating/pro-inflammatory phenotype. Among the molecular mechanisms involved in immune polarization is the engagement of Toll-like receptors (TLRs). TLR-2 ligands have been demonstrated to inhibit MSC differentiation while not affecting their immunosuppressive effect [91]. On the contrary, ligation of TLR3 and TLR4 inhibit the ability of MSCs to suppress T-cell responses, without influencing their differentiation potential [92]. TLR activation combined with IFN-γ priming seems to increase the efficiency of MSCs to function as APCs [93]. In the presence of CpG (TLR9 ligand), MSCs stimulate B-cell proliferation and immunoglobulin production [65], whereas the presence of IFN-γ enables MSCs to inhibit B-cell proliferation [92].

Therefore, MSCs are constitutively immunologically neutral but can acquire pro- or anti-inflammatory properties depending on the surrounding environment. The in vivo implications are crucial and will be discussed in the section on the therapeutic use of MSCs.

MSCs boost immunoregulation

One of the reasons why MSC-mediated immunosuppression is so vigorous is that it is not confined to direct action on the effector cells but also involves the recruitment of other immunoregulatory networks. In particular, MSCs inhibit the differentiation of monocytes into dendritic cells and impair their ability to stimulate allogeneic T cells [70]. It has also been shown that MSCs confer APCs of different types (dendritic cells and macrophages) to acquire tolerogenic activity, thus becoming an active part in a generalized immunosuppressive effect.

There are several lines of evidence supporting the notion that MSCs activate and expand regulatory T cells (T_{reg}), although T_{reg} themselves are not required as a unique component to effect MSC immunosuppressive activity [56, 71]. MSC-mediated T_{reg} expansion has been widely documented in several in vivo systems, including experimental arthritis [94], breast cancer [95], asthma [74], diabetes [96], and experimental autoimmune encephalomyelitis [97]. The nature of the molecules produced by MSCs, like TGF-β, IDO, or HLA-G, is fully consistent with this notion because these molecules directly activate and expand T_{regs} and activate cellular networks that actively engage T_{regs}.

Functions of MSCs: cytoprotection and tissue engineering

The first evidence that MSCs could exert an immunosuppressive activity was derived from an in vivo model of skin grafting in non-human primates [98]. With their immunomodulatory and regenerative potential, MSCs have shown promising results in preclinical and clinical studies for a variety of conditions, such as Alzheimer's disease, spinal cord injury, stroke, burns, diabetes, graft-versus-host disease (GvHD), Crohn's disease, osteogenesis imperfecta, acute cardiovascular disease and myocardial infarction, and osteo-arthritis and rheumatoid arthritis [99, 100].

Over the past decade, MSCs have been used in the treatment of myocardial infarction, although whether these cells directly contribute to myocyte regeneration or provide paracrine factors remains controversial [101]. The myogenic potential of MSCs has been reported following the delivery of bone marrow MSCs into muscle tissues, especially the myocardium, in animal models [102–104]. Enrichment of MSC populations for STRO-1 has been shown to increase the efficacy of MSC therapy in cardiovascular injury [105]. Despite promising findings in animal models, the success of this approach has been varied in humans [106]. It remains to be elucidated whether most of the benefit achieved from MSC infusion stems from their integration and differentiation to repair injured tissue, or if their profound immunoregulatory ability ameliorates the tissue damage process and promotes an environment suitable for tissue repair. Because MSCs have been reported to reduce endotoxemia-induced myocardial injury and dysfunction [107], it seems likely that the latter or a combination of the two contributions of MSCs would explain these findings.

In rodent models of brain and spinal cord injury and Parkinson's disease, MSCs have been tested for their ability to differentiate into astrocytes and, potentially, neurons after transplantation [108] as well as facilitating functional recovery of damaged brain or spinal cord in rats [109, 110]. However, more recently in a murine model of Parkinson's disease, the therapeutic effects of MSC were attributed to the production of SDF-1 and not to a direct cellular contribution by MSC [111]. Clinical trials where granulocyte macrophage colony-stimulating factors were administered with MSCs appeared to improve the conditions for acute and sub-acute spinal cord injuries, but not chronic injury [112].

The loss of cartilage and bone is a debilitating consequence of joint diseases such as arthritis. This can be approached in two ways: grow new cartilage in the laboratory and reintroduce it with MSC to aid the formation of scar tissue, or inject the MSC directly to the site of injury. In osteoarthritis, a primary concern is to replace lost or damaged cartilage. To this end, MSCs have been used by direct injection into the cartilage or by growth on hyaluronan scaffolds [113]. In the murine model of rheumatoid arthritis,

CASE STUDY 16.1

Effects of MSCs on mesenchymal tissue repair

MSCs are progenitor cells capable of differentiating into chondrocytes, osteocytes, and adipocytes with obvious implication in regenerative medicine.

A 21-year-old rugby player was referred to the orthopedic surgeon for a painful knee. Investigations disclosed a cartilage defect related to repeated microfractures. The patient underwent a bone marrow aspirate from which autologous MSCs were generated and expanded. The patient was subject to arthroscopy, and MSCs were administered during the procedure by using a high concentration of MSCs embedded in a matrix preparation. The procedure was repeated twice over a month and the cartilage defect showed a remarkable improvement with beneficial effects on pain.

Conclusions

1. There is very little experience with cases like these but it seems important that MSCs are delivered at high concentrations and that they remain at the site of the lesion for as long as possible.
2. For tissue regeneration, it is important to deliver MSCs in a proper scaffold.

collagen-induced arthritis, the administration of MSCs can either improve disease scores or have a deleterious effect on disease outcome depending on the time of administration (JR Timoshanko, unpublished results). Other researchers have found that MSCs do not alter the course of collagen-induced arthritis, despite in vitro inhibition of T cell proliferation [114], whereas others report beneficial effects of MSC with on overall reduction in inflammatory cytokine production [115].

There has been considerable debate about the capacity of MSCs to undergo transdifferentation, i.e., differentiation into cell types outside their restricted lineage [116]. MSC have been reported to transdifferentiate spontaneously into neural cells [117], pancreatic cells [118], hepatocytes [119], and cardiomyocytes [120], although this remains controversial. However, encouraging results have been shown with MSCs transduced to express transcription factors for specific cell lineages. Functional insulin-producing cells were reported following the overexpression of pancreatic β-cell-specific transcription factor, pancreatic duodenal homeobox 1 (PDX1) [121, 122]. Similarly, expression of the proneural transcription factor nerogenin 1 (Ngn1) or LMX1a have been found to promote neuronal differentiation of MSCs [123, 124]. This kind of targeted approach is growing in favor.

CASE STUDY 16.2

Effects of MSCs on non-mesenchymal tissue repair

There is some evidence that MSCs can be differentiated into tissues of non-mesenchymal origin, thus giving rise to the possibility that they can be harnessed to repair virtually every tissue of the body.

A 62-year-old gentleman affected by late-onset diabetes mellitus arrives to the hospital with chest pain and a diagnosis of myocardial infarction is made at ECG and angiogram. During his stay in hospital, his renal function tests show a progressive impairment (creatinine 747 mmol) suggesting acute kidney injury. The patient receives the intravenous infusion of MSC from a third-party donor that was prepared in a central facility and stocked at the National Blood Service. After a week, creatinine is much reduced (350 mmol). A kidney biopsy, performed to assess the nature of the transient renal failure, does not detect any sign of donor cells at chimerism analysis.

Conclusions (this is a hypothetical situation based on pre-clinical models only)

1. MSCs can be effective at repairing tissues of non-mesenchymal origin.
2. MSCs do not directly intervene in the generation of new tissue but boost the capacity of the residual host stem cells to recover and repair the lesion.
3. It also appears that, for tissue repair activity, MSCs are not required to be autologous or fully matched for histocompatibility antigens.

Clinical experience: MSC-mediated immunomodulation for therapeutics

In the field of MSC clinical applications, many therapeutic uses of these cells have preceded more basic scientific investigations and proof of principle experiments in animal models. After the first promising report describing the efficacious treatment of a young boy affected by severe steroid-resistant GvHD [125], a later phase II multicenter clinical trial demonstrated that MSCs administered to 55 patients with steroid-resistant acute GvHD produced complete remission in 30 and measurable improvement in a further nine [126]. In contrast, a previous multicenter study where patients received MSCs as a prophylaxis of GvHD failed to show any difference in the incidence or severity of GvHD [127]. These apparently discordant findings may be explained by the need for appropriate stimulation to implement MSC "licensing" in vivo as MSC infused at the time of transplant would not encounter the inflammatory environment that is generated during full-blown GvHD [128].

CASE STUDY 16.3

Effects of MSCs on immune-mediated diseases

MSCs have been shown to exhibit a potent immunosuppressive activity. Therefore, an important therapeutic application would be in immune-mediated diseases resistant to aggressive immunosuppressive treatments.

A 10-year-old girl was diagnosed with acute leukemia and referred for an allogeneic HSC transplant. The only donor available was her haplo-identical mother. The transplant went well but after three weeks the patient developed a severe graft-versus-host disease characterized by extensive exfoliating dermatitis and copious diarrhea (6 litres a day) that proved resistant to high-dose steroids and monoclonal antibodies against interleukin-2 receptor. After two weeks, a third-party donor, different from the original HSC donor, provided a bone marrow sample to generate MSCs that were infused into the patient. After five days the diarrhea resolved and after further 10 days the severity of her dermatitis was much reduced. Neither bacterial infections nor viral reactivations were detectable. Three years after the MSC infusion, the patient remained leukemia- and GvHD-free.

Conclusions

1. MSCs exhibit a potent immunosuppressive effect that appears to be confined to the site of the inflammatory lesions.
2. The beneficial effects are durable.
3. MSCs do not need to be of the same MHC identity as the recipient.

The clinical use of MSCs in HSC transplantation was reported even before these dramatic effects on GvHD. The first published multicenter clinical trial with MSC was conducted in North America and enrolled 28 patients with breast cancer who received culture-expanded autologous MSC while undergoing autologous HSC transplantation. MSC infusions at the time of transplant produced a faster hematopoietic recovery than historical controls [129]. The mechanisms accounting for the clinical improvement are thought to be related to the anti-proliferative and anti-apoptotic activity [130] that favors the reconstitution of hematopoiesis in the recipient [24]. A recent study in a pediatric cohort of patients confirms that the immunosuppressive and graft facilitating effects can be effectively combined as transplantation of donor MSCs improved the engraftment of HLA-disparate hemopoietic stem cells [131].

Despite the expectations that MSC immunomodulatory properties might change the outcome of solid organ transplantation, very few initiatives are currently being pursued, possibly because of the contrasting results summarized in the previous section [132]. Patients with autoimmune diseases are also potential candidates for MSC therapies although the ethics of treating patients during the active phase of the disease remain questionable. The use of MSCs to control systemic inflammation in Crohn's disease could be promising but commercial studies have failed to provide supporting evidence. Encouraging results came from attempts to treat complex perianal fistula [133]. Very recently, a small study reported on the use of allogeneic MSCs in four patients with treatment-refractory systemic lupus erythematosus. All patients responded with a stable 12–18-month clinical remission of disease and an improvement in serologic markers and renal function [134].

What does the future hold for the therapeutic uses of MSC?

Concerns that transplanted, culture-expanded MSCs may undergo spontaneous transformation [135] are based mainly on extrapolation from studies performed on murine MSCs. Murine MSCs accumulate chromosomal aberrations and exhibit a spontaneous malignant transformation during long-term culture [136]. However, human MSC differ from murine MSC as they exhibit replicative senescence and are limited to 30–50 population doublings [34]. Bernardo and colleagues [137] performed extensive genetic characterizations using comparative genomic hybridization, karyotyping, sub-telomeric fluorescent in situ hybridization analysis, and telomerase activity, as well as assessing the alternative lengthening of telomeres at different stages of long-term culture. They found no evidence for transformation of human MSCs. Although Rubio et al. reported that cultured adipose-tissue-derived MSCs from young children exhibited a spontaneous transformation in long-term culture [138], this was shown to be due to contamination with an osteosarcoma cell line in the laboratory [139]. Another evolving area of interest and concern is the possible role of administered MSCs in promoting the growth of a latent tumor. Some studies have demonstrated that MSCs can be recruited to the stroma of developing tumors when systemically infused in animal models for glioma, colon carcinoma, ovarian carcinoma, Kaposi's sarcoma, and melanoma [140]. Conversely, transplanted bone marrow contains MSCs and these cells have been used clinically for decades without recognizing adverse effects on tumor growth and formation. Hence, the relevance of these experimental studies for MSC-based cell therapies is unclear. The information available allows us to conclude that human MSCs obtained from healthy individuals do not readily transform in culture; however, further studies are needed to develop a set of safety criteria predicting normal behavior of MSCs used in clinical programs.

Another aspect that should be considered in MSC therapy is whether an off-the-shelf preparation from third-party donors is feasible. Prominent immunosuppressive activities suggest that MSCs might represent an immunoprivileged cell type. Unfortunately, it does not seem to be the case. It has been shown that MSCs exhibit phagocytic properties and, in the presence of low levels of IFN-γ, upregulate MHC class II molecules. Under these circumstances MSCs can function as APCs and stimulate CD4$^+$ T cells to recall antigens [141]. It has been shown that human MSCs can process and present HLA class I-restricted virus- or tumor-encoded antigens to CD8$^+$ cytotoxic T cells (CTL) [82] and MSC immunogenicity has also been demonstrated in vivo in several experimental models [69, 142]. Hence, despite the clinical successes in GvHD using third-party MSCs, the use of these cells may be limited in diseases requiring long-term reconstitution of MSC function.

CASE STUDY 16.4

Effects of MSCs on hemopoietic reconstitution

One of the therapeutic potential treatments with MSCs is based on their ability to support hemopoiesis in the bone marrow as constituents of the HSC niche. Therefore, the co-administration of MSCs with HSC should expedite hemopoietic recovery after myeloablative regimes. Furthermore, this notion could also be applied to improve hemopoietic repopulation in bone marrow failure syndromes like aplastic anemia, where an autoimmune response is primarily responsible for the disease.

A 26-year-old gentleman was diagnosed with a severe aplastic anemia and treated with conventional immunosuppressive therapies obtaining only a transient response. He then received three allogeneic HSC transplants following reduced or fully myeloablative regimens that resulted in graft failure. A fourth transplant was planned with HSC and MSC isolated from a third-party donor. This last attempt produced sustained hemopoietic engraftment. MSCs were isolated from the patient's bone marrow before and after the transplant but no signs of donor MSCs were detected. This is in accord with most studies showing that donor MSCs do not engraft/persist in the recipient.

Conclusions

1. MSC potently inhibit immune responses and in combination with HSC have a direct effect on hemopoietic recovery.
2. The therapeutic effects are not associated with MSC engraftment, thus suggesting a paracrine mechanism.
3. The therapeutic effects are durable despite the lack of MSC persistence.

MSCs in tissue engineering

Tissue engineering may provide alternative ways for obtaining tissues and organs needed for transplantation because of lack of sufficient numbers of organ donors and limitations attributable to immunologic rejection and mismatch of physical dimensions. It allows harvesting of the patient's own cells and seeding them on biodegradable scaffolds that induce formation of a particular tissue needed for repair of tissue defects due to disease or trauma. Also, tissue engineering may allow ex vivo engineering of tissue by means of three-dimensional bio-scaffolds seeded with mature cells or stem cells and cultivated in bioreactors that lead to the formation of tissues or organs, for example liver, hearts, cartilage, or kidneys [143]. MSCs are good candidates for use in tissue engineering protocols [143]. Several scaffolds are currently available and may be classified as either biologically derived polymers isolated from extracellular matrix, plants and seaweed, for example collagen type I or fibronectin, alginate from brown algae or synthetic, for example hydroxyapatite (HA), tri-calcium phosphate (TCP) ceramics, polylactide and polyglycolide and a combination of these in the form of poly-DL-lactic-co-glycolic acid (PLGA). Animal experiments have shown the success of using this approach, for example for treatment of large bone defects in animal models [144]. The development of "functionalized" scaffold i.e., scaffolds containing biological material in the form of microRNA (miRNA), short interfering RNA (siRNA), or growth factors, provides an innovative approach for the in vivo control of stem cell differentiation after implantation. The clinical usefulness of tissue engineering has been reported as a "proof of concept" study in humans. A titanium mesh scaffold filled with bone mineral blocks that were infiltrated with bone morphogenic protein-7 (BMP7) and cells from the bone marrow successfully produced large amounts of bone tissue for the reconstruction of a mandibular defect in a patient [145].

MSCs for off-the-shelf use: implications for banking

For MSCs to be useful for therapeutic purposes, these cells must be able to: reproducibly proliferate in order to obtain sufficient quantities, differentiate into the desired cell types, survive in the recipient after transplant, integrate into the surrounding tissue, and function appropriately without harming the recipient in any way. MSCs are also being evaluated as potential vehicles for cell- and gene-specific therapy against disease because of their ability to home to sites of injury.

Bone marrow MSCs are the most extensively studied stromal stem cell population [6, 146–148]. Because harvesting bone marrow MSCs can result in donor site pain and morbidity as well as low cell numbers, alternative sources of MSCs have been sought. MSCs have been isolated from other organs including peripheral blood [149], umbilical cord blood [150], synovial membrane [151], adipose tissue [152], lung [153], fetal liver [154], dental pulp [155], and deciduous teeth [156]. In particular, adipose-tissue-derived MSCs cultured from fat aspirates obtained during liposuction are relevant from the perspective of clinical applications because of the availability of clinical samples [157]. It is important to note that MSCs obtained from different tissues may share some basic morphological and differentiation characteristics, but these cells are not identical and differences in their "genetic signature" as determined by global analysis of their transcriptome have been reported [158–161]. Also, the current phenotypic assay used to compare different cell populations may not be optimal and there is a need for the development of in vivo models that assay the functionality of different cell populations in a clinically relevant fashion. An example of the difference of in vivo functional ability of different MSC populations has been reported. MSCs obtained from synovial tissue and bone marrow have been reported to be more effective in repair of cartilage defects of the knee of rabbits than muscle- or adipose-tissue-derived MSCs [162].

Concluding remarks

The identification of MSC immunosuppressive properties has catalyzed the interests of many groups to characterize and better understand this phenomenon. Current data indicate that MSCs use several synergistic mechanisms to control immune responses non-specifically and activate further immunosuppressive circuits to boost MSC action. The dramatic results obtained in GvHD have not yet been evaluated in other conditions that have a higher prevalence in the population. The main reason is that these conditions (like multiple sclerosis, arthritis, inflammatory bowel disease) are not generally associated with a mortality rate sufficient to justify ethically the use of an experimental and thus potentially harmful treatment. Nevertheless, there is plenty of pre-clinical evidence to support the hypothesis that MSC treatment could improve disease outcome, at least in selected patients. These expectations have ignited several initiatives from National Health Service entities and companies to expand and cryopreserve MSC in banks for easy availability in case of need. The outstanding problem in this approach is validation of the cell product because there are no assays at the moment capable of predicting the clinical efficacy of a cell preparation. A further complication is that MSC immunosuppressive activity is acquired in vivo when MSCs reach the site of the tissue lesion, and thus a suitable inflammatory environment must be produced by the lesion to "license" MSC immunosuppression. These questions do not yet have answers, but there is active progress in the field with a variety of contributions from specialists in different areas including those driven by the biotechnology sector and big pharmaceutical companies. The full realization of the diverse capabilities of MSCs in immunomodulation and tissue repair is only just around the corner.

KEY LEARNING POINTS

- Mesenchymal stromal cells are stem cell populations that are capable of multi-lineage differentiation into mesoderm-type cells such as osteoblasts, adipocytes, and chondrocytes and, possibly but still controversially, other non-mesodermal cell types.

- The properties of MSCs make them suitable for the modulation of immune responses and in the treatment of autoimmune disorders, as well as giving them their potential in the arena of tissue repair.

- Although MSCs are usually defined by their ability to differentiate into osteoblastic, adipocytic, and chondrocytic cells (i.e., multipotentiality) in vitro, it is their ability to form stromal tissue such as bone upon transplantation subcutaneously in immune-deficient mice that is considered to be the "gold standard" for the stem cell potential of MSCs.

- MSCs are constitutively immunologically neutral but can be turned to acquire pro- or anti-inflammatory properties depending on the surrounding environment.

- Concerns that transplanted, culture-expanded MSCs may undergo spontaneous transformation are based mainly on extrapolations from studies performed on murine MSCs.

- The information available allows us to conclude that human MSCs obtained from healthy individuals do not readily transform in culture; however, further studies are needed to develop a set of safety criteria predicting the normal behavior of MSCs used in clinical programs.

- Current data indicate that MSCs use several synergistic mechanisms to control immune responses non-specifically and activate further immunosuppressive circuits to boost MSC action. This has therapeutic potential however many diseases that might benefit from these properties may not be severe enough to warrant the introduction of experimental therapies.

References

1. Dominici M, et al. Minimal criteria for defining multipotent mesenchymal stromal cells. The International Society for Cellular Therapy position statement. Cytotherapy 2006;8:315–7.
2. Bianco P, Riminucci M, Gronthos S, Robey PG Bone marrow stromal stem cells: nature, biology, and potential applications. Stem Cells 2001;19:180–92.
3. Dezawa M, et al. Specific induction of neuronal cells from bone marrow stromal cells and application for autologous transplantation. J Clin Invest 2004;113: 1701–10.

4. Luk JM, Wang PP, Lee CK, Wang JH, Fan ST. Hepatic potential of bone marrow stromal cells: development of in vitro co-culture and intra-portal transplantation models. J Immunol Methods 2005;305:39–47.

5. Dexter TM. Haemopoiesis in long-term bone marrow cultures. A review. Acta Haematol 1979;62:299–305.

6. Friedenstein AJ, Gorskaja JF, Kulagina NN. Fibroblast precursors in normal and irradiated mouse hematopoietic organs. Exp Hematol 1976;4:267–74.

7. Owen M. Marrow stromal stem cells. J Cell Sci Suppl 10, 63–76 (1988).

8. Friedenstein AJ, Chailakhjan RK, Lalykina KS. The development of fibroblast colonies in monolayer cultures of guinea-pig bone marrow and spleen cells. Cell Tissue Kinet 1970;3:393–403.

9. Luria EA, Panasyuk AF, Friedenstein AY. Fibroblast colony formation from monolayer cultures of blood cells. Transfusion 1971;11:345–9.

10. Abdallah BM, et al. Maintenance of differentiation potential of human bone marrow mesenchymal stem cells immortalized by human telomerase reverse transcriptase gene despite [corrected] extensive proliferation. Biochem Biophys Res Commun 2005;326:527–38.

11. Foster LJ, et al. Differential expression profiling of membrane proteins by quantitative proteomics in a human mesenchymal stem cell line undergoing osteoblast differentiation. Stem Cells 2005;23:1367–77.

12. Abdallah BM, Ditzel N, Kassem, M. Assessment of bone formation capacity using in vivo transplantation assays: procedure and tissue analysis. Methods Mol Biol 2008;455:89–100.

13. Kassem, M, Mosekilde, L & Eriksen, EF. 1,25-dihydroxyvitamin D3 potentiates fluoride-stimulated collagen type I production in cultures of human bone marrow stromal osteoblast-like cells. J Bone Miner Res 1993;8:1453–8.

14. Rickard DJ, et al. Isolation and characterization of osteoblast precursor cells from human bone marrow. J Bone Miner Res 1996;11:312–24.

15. Kuznetsov SA, et al. Single-colony derived strains of human marrow stromal fibroblasts form bone after transplantation in vivo. J Bone Miner Res 1997; 12:1335–47.

16. Larsen KH, Frederiksen CM, Burns JS, Abdallah BM, Kassem, M. Identifying a molecular phenotype for bone marrow stromal cells with in vivo bone forming capacity. J Bone Miner Res 2010;25:796–808.

17. Post S, Abdallah BM, Bentzon JF, Kassem, M. Demonstration of the presence of independent pre-osteoblastic and pre-adipocytic cell populations in bone marrow-derived mesenchymal stem cells. Bone 2008;43:32–9.

18. Haynesworth SE, Baber MA, Caplan AI. Cell surface antigens on human marrow-derived mesenchymal cells are detected by monoclonal antibodies. Bone 1992; 13:69–80.

19. Bruder, SP, Horowitz, MC, Mosca, JD, Haynesworth, SE. Monoclonal antibodies reactive with human osteogenic cell surface antigens. Bone 1997;21:225–35.

20. Zannettino, AC, Harrison, K, Joyner, CJ, Triffitt, JT, Simmons, PJ. Molecular cloning of the cell surface antigen identified by the osteoprogenitor-specific monoclonal antibody, HOP-26. J Cell Biochem 2003;89:56–66.

21. Gronthos S, et al. A novel monoclonal antibody (STRO-3) identifies an isoform of tissue nonspecific alkaline phosphatase expressed by multipotent bone marrow stromal stem cells. Stem Cells Dev 2007;16:953–63.

22. Gronthos S, et al. Heat shock protein-90 beta is expressed at the surface of multipo-tential mesenchymal precursor cells: generation of a novel monoclonal antibody, STRO-4, with specificity for mesenchymal precursor cells from human and ovine tissues. Stem Cells Dev 2009;18:1253–62.

23. Gronthos S, Graves SE, Ohta S, Simmons PJ. The STRO-1+ fraction of adult human bone marrow contains the osteogenic precursors. Blood 1994;84:4164–73.

24. Sacchetti B, et al. Self-renewing osteoprogenitors in bone marrow sinusoids can organize a hematopoietic microenvironment. Cell 2007;131:324–36.

25. Crisan M, et al. A perivascular origin for mesenchymal stem cells in multiple human organs. Cell Stem Cell 2008;3:301–13.

26. Russell KC, et al. In vitro high-capacity assay to quantify the clonal heterogeneity in trilineage potential of mesenchymal stem cells reveals a complex hierarchy of lineage commitment. Stem Cells 2010;28:788–98.

27. Buhring HJ, et al. Novel markers for the prospective isolation of human MSC. Ann N Y Acad Sci 2007;1106:262–71.

28. Delorme B, et al. Specific plasma membrane protein phenotype of culture-amplified and native human bone marrow mesenchymal stem cells. Blood 2008;111: 2631–5.

29. Reyes, M, et al. Purification and ex vivo expansion of postnatal human marrow mesodermal progenitor cells. Blood 2001;98;2615–25.

30. Jiang Y, et al. Pluripotency of mesenchymal stem cells derived from adult marrow. Nature 2002;418:41–9.

31. Ng F, et al. PDGF, TGF-beta, and FGF signaling is important for differentiation and growth of mesenchymal stem cells (MSCs): transcriptional profiling can identify markers and signaling pathways important in differentiation of MSCs into adipo-genic, chondrogenic, and osteogenic lineages. Blood 2008;112:295–307.

32. Kasten P, et al. Influence of platelet-rich plasma on osteogenic differentiation of mesenchymal stem cells and ectopic bone formation in calcium phosphate ceram-ics. Cells Tissues Organs 2006;183:68–79.

33. Sotiropoulou PA, Perez SA, Salagianni M, Baxevanis CN, Papamichail M. Charac-terization of the optimal culture conditions for clinical scale production of human mesenchymal stem cells. Stem Cells 2006;24:462–71.

34. Stenderup K, Justesen J, Clausen C, Kassem, M. Aging is associated with decreased maximal life span and accelerated senescence of bone marrow stromal cells. Bone 2003;33:919–26.

35. Simonsen JL, et al. Telomerase expression extends the proliferative life-span and maintains the osteogenic potential of human bone marrow stromal cells. Nat Bio-technol 2002;20:592–6.

36. Zimmermann S, et al. Lack of telomerase activity in human mesenchymal stem cells. Leukemia 2003;17:1146–9.

37. McKee JA, et al. Human arteries engineered in vitro. EMBO Rep 2003;4: 633–8.

38. Serakinci N, et al. Adult human mesenchymal stem cell as a target for neoplastic transformation. Oncogene 2004;23:5095–8.

39. Serakinci N, Hoare SF, Kassem M, Atkinson SP, Keith WN. Telomerase promoter reprogramming and interaction with general transcription factors in the human mesenchymal stem cell. Regen Med 2006;1:125–31.

40. Jones S, Horwood N, Cope A, Dazzi, F. The antiproliferative effect of mesenchymal stem cells is a fundamental property shared by all stromal cells. J Immunol 2007; 179:2824–31.

41. Adewumi O, et al. Characterization of human embryonic stem cell lines by the International Stem Cell Initiative. Nat Biotechnol 2007;25:803–16.

42. Gang EJ, Bosnakovski D, Figueiredo CA, Visser JW, Perlingeiro RC. SSEA-4 identifies mesenchymal stem cells from bone marrow. Blood 2007;109:1743–51.

43. Pozzobon M, et al. Mesenchymal stromal cells can be derived from bone marrow CD133+ cells: implications for therapy. Stem Cells Dev 2009;18:497–510.

44. Kerkis I, et al. Isolation and characterization of a population of immature dental pulp stem cells expressing OCT-4 and other embryonic stem cell markers. Cells Tissues Organs 2006;184:105–16.

45. Greco SJ, Liu K, Rameshwar, P. Functional similarities among genes regulated by OCT4 in human mesenchymal and embryonic stem cells. Stem Cells 2007; 25:3143–54.

46. Lin G, et al. Defining stem and progenitor cells within adipose tissue. Stem Cells Dev 2008;17:1053–63.

47. Kotoula V, Papamichos SI, Lambropoulos, AF. Revisiting OCT4 expression in peripheral blood mononuclear cells. Stem Cells 2008;26:290–1.

48. Beltrami AP, et al. Multipotent cells can be generated in vitro from several adult human organs (heart, liver, and bone marrow). Blood 2007;110:3438–46.

49. Kim JB, et al. Pluripotent stem cells induced from adult neural stem cells by reprogramming with two factors. Nature 2008;454:646–50.

50. Lengler J, Bittner T, Munster D, Gawad Ael D, Graw J. Agonistic and antagonistic action of AP2, Msx2, Pax6, Prox1 AND Six3 in the regulation of Sox2 expression. Ophthalmic Res 2005;37:301–9.

51. Riekstina U, et al. Embryonic stem cell marker expression pattern in human mesenchymal stem cells derived from bone marrow, adipose tissue, heart and dermis. Stem Cell Rev 2009;5:378–86.

52. Wing K, Sakaguchi S. Regulatory T cells exert checks and balances on self tolerance and autoimmunity. Nat Immunol 2010;11, 7–13.

53. Mantovani A, Sica A, Allavena P, Garlanda C, Locati M. Tumor-associated macrophages and the related myeloid-derived suppressor cells as a paradigm of the diversity of macrophage activation. Hum Immunol 2009;70:325–30.

54. Krampera M, et al. Bone marrow mesenchymal stem cells inhibit the response of naive and memory antigen-specific T cells to their cognate peptide. Blood 2003;101:3722–9.

55. Le Blanc K, Tammik L, Sundberg B, Haynesworth SE, Ringden O. Mesenchymal stem cells inhibit and stimulate mixed lymphocyte cultures and mitogenic responses independently of the major histocompatibility complex. Scand J Immunol 2003; 57:11–20.

56. Glennie S, Soeiro I, Dyson PJ, Lam EW, Dazzi F Bone marrow mesenchymal stem cells induce division arrest anergy of activated T cells. Blood 2005;105: 2821–7.

57. Ramasamy R, Tong CK, Seow HF, Vidyadaran S, Dazzi F. The immunosuppressive effects of human bone marrow-derived mesenchymal stem cells target T cell proliferation but not its effector function. Cell Immunol 2008;251:131–6.

58. Beyer M, et al. Cancer vaccine enhanced, non-tumor-reactive CD8(+) T cells exhibit a distinct molecular program associated with "division arrest anergy". Cancer Res 2009;69:4346–54.

59. Benvenuto F, et al. Human mesenchymal stem cells promote survival of T cells in a quiescent state. Stem Cells 2007;25:1753–60.

60. Augello A, et al. Bone marrow mesenchymal progenitor cells inhibit lymphocyte proliferation by activation of the programmed death 1 pathway. Eur J Immunol 2005;35:1482–90.

61. Plumas J, et al. Mesenchymal stem cells induce apoptosis of activated T cells. Leukemia 2005;19:1597–604.

62. Spaggiari GM, Capobianco A, Becchetti S, Mingari MC, Moretta L. Mesenchymal stem cell-natural killer cell interactions: evidence that activated NK cells are capable of killing MSCs, whereas MSCs can inhibit IL-2-induced NK-cell proliferation. Blood 2006;107:1484–90.

63. Spaggiari GM, et al. Mesenchymal stem cells inhibit natural killer-cell proliferation, cytotoxicity, and cytokine production: role of indoleamine 2,3-dioxygenase and prostaglandin E2. Blood 2008;111:1327–33.

64. Corcione A, et al. Human mesenchymal stem cells modulate B cell functions. Blood 2006;107:367–72.

65. Traggiai E, et al. Bone marrow-derived mesenchymal stem cells induce both polyclonal expansion and differentiation of B cells isolated from healthy donors and systemic lupus erythematosus patients. Stem Cells 2008;26:562–69.

66. Manz RA, Thiel A, Radbruch A. Lifetime of plasma cells in the bone marrow. Nature 1997;388:133–4.

67. Anderson G, Jenkinson EJ. Lymphostromal interactions in thymic development and function. Nat Rev Immunol 2001;1:31–40.

68. Jiang XX, et al. Human mesenchymal stem cells inhibit differentiation and function of monocyte-derived dendritic cells. Blood 2005;105:4120–6.

69. Nauta AJ, et al. Donor-derived mesenchymal stem cells are immunogenic in an allogeneic host and stimulate donor graft rejection in a nonmyeloablative setting. Blood 2006;108:2114–20.

70. Ramasamy R, et al. Mesenchymal stem cells inhibit dendritic cell differentiation and function by preventing entry into the cell cycle. Transplantation 2007;83:71–6.

71. Aggarwal S, Pittenger MF. Human mesenchymal stem cells modulate allogeneic immune cell responses. Blood 2005;105:1815–22.

72. Beyth S, et al. Human mesenchymal stem cells alter antigen-presenting cell maturation and induce T-cell unresponsiveness. Blood 2005;105:2214–9.

73. Di Nicola M, et al. Human bone marrow stromal cells suppress T-lymphocyte proliferation induced by cellular or nonspecific mitogenic stimuli. Blood 2002;99:3838–43.

74. Nemeth K, et al. Bone marrow stromal cells use TGF-beta to suppress allergic responses in a mouse model of ragweed-induced asthma. Proc Natl Acad Sci U S A 2010;107:5652–7.

75. Munn DH, et al. Inhibition of T cell proliferation by macrophage tryptophan catabolism. J Exp Med 1999;189:1363–72.

76. Munn DH, et al. GCN2 kinase in T cells mediates proliferative arrest and anergy induction in response to indoleamine 2,3-dioxygenase. Immunity 2005;22:633–42.

77. Sato K, et al. Nitric oxide plays a critical role in suppression of T-cell proliferation by mesenchymal stem cells. Blood 2007;109, 228–34.

78. Djouad F, et al. Mesenchymal stem cells inhibit the differentiation of dendritic cells through an interleukin-6-dependent mechanism. Stem Cells 2007;25:2025–32.

79. Gieseke F, et al. Human multipotent mesenchymal stromal cells inhibit proliferation of PBMCs independently of IFNgammaR1 signaling and IDO expression. Blood 2007;110:2197–200.

80. Carosella ED, Moreau P, Lemaoult J, Rouas-Freiss N. HLA-G: from biology to clinical benefits. Trends Immunol 2008;29:125–32.

81. Nasef A, et al. Immunosuppressive effects of mesenchymal stem cells: involvement of HLA-G. Transplantation 2007;84:231–7.

82. Morandi F, et al. Immunogenicity of human mesenchymal stem cells in HLA-class I-restricted T-cell responses against viral or tumor-associated antigens. Stem Cells 2008;26:1275–87.

83. Selmani Z, et al. Human leukocyte antigen-G5 secretion by human mesenchymal stem cells is required to suppress T lymphocyte and natural killer function and to induce CD4+CD25highFOXP3+ regulatory T cells. Stem Cells 2008;26:212–22.

84. Oh I, et al. Interferon-gamma and NF-kappaB mediate nitric oxide production by mesenchymal stromal cells. Biochem Biophys Res Commun 2007;355:956–62.

85. Niedbala W, Cai B, Liew FY. Role of nitric oxide in the regulation of T cell functions. Ann Rheum Dis 2006;65 (Suppl 3):37–40.

86. Bach FH. Heme oxygenase-1: a therapeutic amplification funnel. FASEB J 19, 1216–9 (2005).

87. Chabannes, D, et al. A role for heme oxygenase-1 in the immunosuppressive effect of adult rat and human mesenchymal stem cells. Blood 2007;110:3691–4.

88. Nemeth K, et al. Bone marrow stromal cells attenuate sepsis via prostaglandin E(2)-dependent reprogramming of host macrophages to increase their interleukin-10 production. Nat Med 2009;15:42–9.

89. Krampera M, et al. Role for interferon-gamma in the immunomodulatory activity of human bone marrow mesenchymal stem cells. Stem Cells 2006;24:386–98.

90. Ren G, et al. Mesenchymal stem cell-mediated immunosuppression occurs via concerted action of chemokines and nitric oxide. Cell Stem Cell 2008;2:141–50.

91. Pevsner-Fischer M, et al. Toll-like receptors and their ligands control mesenchymal stem cell functions. Blood 2007;109:1422–32.

92. Liotta F, et al. Toll-like receptors 3 and 4 are expressed by human bone marrow-derived mesenchymal stem cells and can inhibit their T-cell modulatory activity by impairing Notch signaling. Stem Cells 2008;26:279–89.

93. Romieu-Mourez R, et al. Cytokine modulation of TLR expression and activation in mesenchymal stromal cells leads to a proinflammatory phenotype. J Immunol 2009;182:7963–73.

94. Gonzalez MA, Gonzalez-Rey E, Rico L, Buscher D, Delgado M. Treatment of experimental arthritis by inducing immune tolerance with human adipose-derived mesenchymal stem cells. Arthritis Rheum 2009;60:1006–19.

95. Patel SA, et al. Mesenchymal stem cells protect breast cancer cells through regulatory T cells: role of mesenchymal stem cell-derived TGF-β. J Immunol 2010;184:5885–94.

96. Madec AM, et al. Mesenchymal stem cells protect NOD mice from diabetes by inducing regulatory T cells. Diabetologia 2009;52:1391–9.

97. Zappia E, et al. Mesenchymal stem cells ameliorate experimental autoimmune encephalomyelitis inducing T-cell anergy. Blood 2005;106:1755–61.

98. Bartholomew A, et al. Mesenchymal stem cells suppress lymphocyte proliferation in vitro and prolong skin graft survival in vivo. Exp Hematol 2002;30:42–8.

99. Dazzi F, Horwood NJ. Potential of mesenchymal stem cell therapy. Curr Opin Oncol 2007;19:650–5.

100. Newman RE, Yoo D, LeRoux MA, Danilkovitch-Miagkova A. Treatment of inflammatory diseases with mesenchymal stem cells. Inflamm Allergy Drug Targets 2009;8:110–23.

101. Song H, et al. Interrogating functional integration between injected pluripotent stem cell-derived cells and surrogate cardiac tissue. Proc Natl Acad Sci U S A 2010;107:3329–34.

102. Barbash IM, et al. Systemic delivery of bone marrow-derived mesenchymal stem cells to the infarcted myocardium: feasibility, cell migration, and body distribution. Circulation 2003;108:863–8.

103. Ferrari, G, et al. Muscle regeneration by bone marrow-derived myogenic progenitors. Science 1998;279:1528–30.

104. Shake JG, et al. Mesenchymal stem cell implantation in a swine myocardial infarct model: engraftment and functional effects. Ann Thorac Surg 2002;73:1919–25; discussion 1926.

105. Psaltis, PJ, et al. Enrichment for STRO-1 expression enhances the cardiovascular paracrine activity of humanbone marrow-derived mesenchymal cell populations. J Cell Physiol 2010;223:530–40.

106. Segers VF, Lee RT. Stem-cell therapy for cardiac disease. Nature 2008;451: 937–42.

107. Weil BR, et al. Mesenchymal stem cells attenuate myocardial functional depression and reduce systemic and myocardial inflammation during endotoxemia. J Surg Res 2010;148:2.

108. Kopen GC, Prockop DJ, Phinney DG. Marrow stromal cells migrate throughout forebrain and cerebellum, and they differentiate into astrocytes after injection into neonatal mouse brains. Proc Natl Acad Sci U S A 1999;96:10711–6.

109. Chen J, et al. Therapeutic benefit of intracerebral transplantation of bone marrow stromal cells after cerebral ischemia in rats. J Neurol Sci 2001;189: 49–57.

110. Hofstetter CP, et al. Marrow stromal cells form guiding strands in the injured spinal cord and promote recovery. Proc Natl Acad Sci U S A 2002;99:2199–204.

111. Wang F, et al. Intravenous administration of mesenchymal stem cells exerts therapeutic effects on parkinsonian model of rats: Focusing on neuroprotective effects of stromal cell-derived factor-1alpha. BMC Neurosci 2010;11:52.

112. Yoon SH, et al. Complete spinal cord injury treatment using autologous bone marrow cell transplantation and bone marrow stimulation with granulocyte macrophage-colony stimulating factor: Phase I/II clinical trial. Stem Cells 2007; 25:2066–73.

113. Grigolo B, et al. Osteoarthritis treated with mesenchymal stem cells on hyaluronan-based scaffold in rabbit. Tissue Eng Part C Methods 2009;15, 647–58.

114. Schurgers E, Kelchtermans H, Mitera T, Geboes L, Matthys P. Discrepancy between the in vitro and in vivo effects of murine mesenchymal stem cells on T-cell proliferation and collagen-induced arthritis. Arthritis Res Ther 2010;12:R31.

115. Mao F, et al. Immunosuppressive effects of mesenchymal stem cells in collagen-induced mouse arthritis. Inflamm Res 2010;59:219–25.

116. Herzog EL, Chai L, Krause DS. Plasticity of marrow-derived stem cells. Blood 2003;102:3483–93.

117. Zhao, LX, et al. Modification of the brain-derived neurotrophic factor gene: a portal to transform mesenchymal stem cells into advantageous engineering cells for neuroregeneration and neuroprotection. Exp Neurol 2004;190:396–406.

118. Tang DQ, et al. In vivo and in vitro characterization of insulin-producing cells obtained from murine bone marrow. Diabetes 2004;53:1721–32.

119. Sato Y, et al. Human mesenchymal stem cells xenografted directly to rat liver are differentiated into human hepatocytes without fusion. Blood 2005;106: 756–63.

120. Toma C, Pittenger MF, Cahill KS, Byrne BJ, Kessler PD. Human mesenchymal stem cells differentiate to a cardiomyocyte phenotype in the adult murine heart. Circulation 2002;105, 93–8.

121. Karnieli O, Izhar-Prato Y, Bulvik S, Efrat S. Generation of insulin-producing cells from human bone marrow mesenchymal stem cells by genetic manipulation. Stem Cells 2007;25:2837–44.

122. Li Y, et al. Generation of insulin-producing cells from PDX-1 gene-modified human mesenchymal stem cells. J Cell Physiol 2007;211:36–44.

123. Barzilay R, Ben-Zur T, Bulvik S, Melamed E, Offen D. Lentiviral delivery of LMX1a enhances dopaminergic phenotype in differentiated human bone marrow mesenchymal stem cells. Stem Cells Dev 2009;18:591–601.

124. Kim SS, et al. Neural induction with neurogenin1 increases the therapeutic effects of mesenchymal stem cells in the ischemic brain. Stem Cells 2008;26: 2217–28.

125. Le Blanc K, et al. Treatment of severe acute graft-versus-host disease with third party haploidentical mesenchymal stem cells. Lancet 2004;363:1439–41.

126. Le Blanc K, et al. Mesenchymal stem cells for treatment of steroid-resistant, severe, acute graft-versus-host disease: a phase II study. Lancet 2008;371:1579–86.

127. Lazarus HM, et al. Cotransplantation of HLA-identical sibling culture-expanded mesenchymal stem cells and hematopoietic stem cells in hematologic malignancy patients. Biol Blood Marrow Transplant 2005;11:389–398.

128. Dazzi F, Marelli-Berg FM. Mesenchymal stem cells for graft-versus-host disease: close encounters with T cells. Eur J Immunol 2008;38:1479–82.

129. Koc ON, et al. Rapid hematopoietic recovery after coinfusion of autologous-blood stem cells and culture-expanded marrow mesenchymal stem cells in advanced breast cancer patients receiving high-dose chemotherapy. J Clin Oncol 2000;18: 307–16.

130. Dazzi F, Ramasamy R, Glennie S, Jones SP, Roberts I. The role of mesenchymal stem cells in haemopoiesis. Blood Rev 2006;20:161–71.

131. Ball LM, et al. Cotransplantation of ex vivo expanded mesenchymal stem cells accelerates lymphocyte recovery and may reduce the risk of graft failure in haploidentical hematopoietic stem-cell transplantation. Blood 2007;110:2764–67.

132. Vanikar AV, et al. Effect of co-transplantation of mesenchymal stem cells and hematopoietic stem cells as compared to hematopoietic stem cell transplantation alone in renal transplantation to achieve donor hypo-responsiveness. Int Urol Nephrol 2010;43: 225–32.

133. Garcia-Olmo D, et al. Expanded adipose-derived stem cells for the treatment of complex perianal fistula: a phase II clinical trial. Dis Colon Rectum 2009;52: 79–86.

134. Sun L, et al. Mesenchymal stem cell transplantation reverses multiorgan dysfunction in systemic lupus erythematosus mice and humans. Stem Cells 2009;27: 1421–32.

135. Lepperdinger G, Brunauer R, Jamnig A, Laschober G, Kassem M. Controversial issue: is it safe to employ mesenchymal stem cells in cell-based therapies? Exp Gerontol 2008;43:1018–23.

136. Zhou YF, et al. Spontaneous transformation of cultured mouse bone marrow-derived stromal cells. Cancer Res 2006;66:10849–54.

137. Bernardo ME, et al. Human bone marrow derived mesenchymal stem cells do not undergo transformation after long-term in vitro culture and do not exhibit telomere maintenance mechanisms. Cancer Res 2007;67:9142–9.

138. Rubio D, et al. Spontaneous human adult stem cell transformation. Cancer Res 2005;65:3035–9.

139. Garcia S, et al. Pitfalls in spontaneous in vitro transformation of human mesenchymal stem cells. Exp Cell Res 2010;316: 1648–50.

140. Lazennec G, Jorgensen C. Concise review: adult multipotent stromal cells and cancer: risk or benefit? Stem Cells 2008;26:1387–94.

141. Chan JL, et al. Antigen-presenting property of mesenchymal stem cells occurs during a narrow window at low levels of interferon-gamma. Blood 2006;107: 4817–24.

142. Eliopoulos N, Stagg J, Lejeune L, Pommey S, Galipeau J Allogeneic marrow stromal cells are immune rejected by MHC class I- and class II-mismatched recipient mice. Blood 2005;106:4057–65.

143. Bianco P, Robey PG. Stem cells in tissue engineering. Nature 2011;414:118–21.

144. Kon E, et al. Autologous bone marrow stromal cells loaded onto porous hydroxyapatite ceramic accelerate bone repair in critical-size defects of sheep long bones. J Biomed Mater Res 2000;49:328–37.

145. Warnke PH, et al. Growth and transplantation of a custom vascularised bone graft in a man. Lancet 2004;364:766–70.

146. Caplan AI. Mesenchymal stem cells. J Orthop Res 1991;9:641–50.

147. Pittenger MF, et al. Multilineage potential of adult human mesenchymal stem cells. Science 1999;284:143–7.

148. Prockop DJ. Marrow stromal cells as stem cells for nonhematopoietic tissues. Science 1997;276:71–4.

149. Kuznetsov SA, et al. Circulating skeletal stem cells. J Cell Biol 2001;153: 1133–40.

150. Rosada C, Justesen J, Melsvik D, Ebbesen P, Kassem M. The human umbilical cord blood: a potential source for osteoblast progenitor cells. Calcif Tissue Int 2003; 72:135–42.

151. De Bari C, Dell'Accio F, Tylzanowski P, Luyten FP. Multipotent mesenchymal stem cells from adult human synovial membrane. Arthritis Rheum 2001;44: 1928–42.

152. Gronthos S, et al. Surface protein characterization of human adipose tissue-derived stromal cells. J Cell Physiol 2001;189:54–63.

153. in 't Anker PS, et al. Mesenchymal stem cells in human second-trimester bone marrow, liver, lung, and spleen exhibit a similar immunophenotype but a heterogeneous multilineage differentiation potential. Haematologica 2003;88:845–52.

154. Campagnoli C, et al. Identification of mesenchymal stem/progenitor cells in human first-trimester fetal blood, liver, and bone marrow. Blood 2001;98:2396–402.

155. Gronthos S, et al. Stem cell properties of human dental pulp stem cells. J Dent Res 2002;81:531–5.

156. Miura, M, et al. SHED: stem cells from human exfoliated deciduous teeth. Proc Natl Acad Sci U S A 2003;100:5807–12.

157. Bunnell BA, Flaat M, Gagliardi C, Patel B, Ripoll C. Adipose-derived stem cells: isolation, expansion and differentiation. Methods 2008;45:115–20.

158. Djouad F, et al. Transcriptional profiles discriminate bone marrow-derived and synovium-derived mesenchymal stem cells. Arthritis Res Ther 2005;7:R1304–15.

159. Wagner W, et al. Comparative characteristics of mesenchymal stem cells from human bone marrow, adipose tissue, and umbilical cord blood. Exp Hematol 2005;33:1402–16.

160. Kern S, Eichler H, Stoeve J, Kluter H, Bieback K. Comparative analysis of mesenchymal stem cells from bone marrow, umbilical cord blood, or adipose tissue. Stem Cells 2006;24:1294–301.

161. Noel D, et al. Cell specific differences between human adipose-derived and mesenchymal-stromal cells despite similar differentiation potentials. Exp Cell Res 2008;314:1575–84.

162. Koga H, et al. Comparison of mesenchymal tissues-derived stem cells for in vivo chondrogenesis: suitable conditions for cell therapy of cartilage defects in rabbit. Cell Tissue Res 2008;333:207–15.

17 Embryonic or Neural Stem Cells in Neurodegenerative Disease of the Central Nervous System (with Relevance to PD, HD, AD, MS, SCI, and Stroke)

Stephen B. Dunnett[1], Cesar V. Borlongan[2], and Paul R. Sanberg[2]
[1]Cardiff University, Cardiff, UK
[2]University of South Florida College of Medicine, Tampa, FL, USA

Past: functional cell transplantation in the adult central nervous system

For most of the twentieth century, cell transplantation in the brain was widely considered not to be possible, alongside the *Zeitgeist* that once it reaches adulthood the mammalian central nervous system (CNS) loses all capacity for neurogenesis, regeneration, and plasticity [1]. This view has changed over recent decades: first, with the realization that even adult neurons retain a capacity for sprouting, axon growth and reorganization of connections [2]; second, with the demonstration that both peripheral and central neurons can survive transplantation into the adult brain so long as they are provided with an appropriate environment in which to thrive [3, 4]; and third, with the demonstration that although most neurones are born early in development there remain progenitor cells located in particular niches within the adult brain that retain the capacity to generate new neurons in at least modest numbers throughout life [5]. With this change in perspective, the past 40 years has seen a dramatic increase in our

Tissue and Cell Clinical Use: An Essential Guide, First Edition. Edited by Ruth M. Warwick and Scott A. Brubaker.
© 2012 Blackwell Publishing Ltd. Published 2012 by Blackwell Publishing Ltd.

understanding of how to replace neurons lost through aging, trauma, or disease, to repair brain damage to varying degrees, and to achieve significant functional recovery in a variety of models of human neurodegenerative disease.

Principles of primary fetal cell transplantation

The earliest experimental attempts at cell transplantation were undertaken as early as the 1890s, and clear evidence of survival was first reported in 1917 [1]. Then, throughout the 1930s, 1940s, and 1950s, several noted anatomists – including Le Gros Clark, Glees, Windle, and Clemente – used cell transplantation with growing success, in particular to explore principles of normal and tumor cell growth in the developing and adult nervous system [1]. However, the modern era is generally dated from 1971 when Das and Altman first used ^{3}H-thymidine labeling of newborn cerebellar neurons successfully to label and identify grafted cerebellar cells from neonatal rat pups implanted into the cerebellums of host rats of the same age [1, 3, 6].

At about the same time, Olson and colleagues started their pioneering studies using the in oculo transplantation method, which has provided one of the most powerful tools to identify donor factors underlying successful cell transplantation in the nervous system [7, 8]. What these studies first clarified is that diverse neural cell types can readily survive transplantation into the adult nervous system if they are harvested at an appropriate stage in development. Critically, CNS neurons need to be collected from a restricted time window in embryonic or neonatal development that corresponds within a couple of days before or after the initial birth dates of the target cells: any earlier and the cell fate is not yet fully specified in the developing embryo; any later and the neurons have matured and developed extensive processes that cannot sustain the traumas of dissection and temporary anoxia involved in the transplantation process. The anterior eye chamber provides a highly vascularized, immunologically isolated site that is suitable for receiving the grafted cells, akin to an in vivo cell culture, in which the survival and growth of a wide variety of different cell preparations can then be explored both anatomically and physiologically. Indeed a distinctive feature of this model is that graft survival and growth can be directly observed in vivo through the transparent cornea. The studies of the Olson group demonstrated that newborn neurons survive transplantation and continue to develop and express their normal transmitter phenotypes (including grafts of embryonic cortex, hippocampus, striatum; brainstem dopaminergic, adrenergic, and serotonergic neurons; and peripheral neurons of the sympathetic, parasympathetic, sensory ganglia, and neuroendocrine glands). Moreover, neurons that survive the surgical translocation continue to develop, extend extensive axon networks that make connections with appropriate target populations of co-grafted cells, and attract axonal connections not only from other grafted embryonic neurons but also from sprouting adult peripheral neurons that innervate the host iris [7, 9]. Although the in oculo model system may appear esoteric, it has provided the fundamental insights into the key donor characteristics necessary to achieve functional cell replacement and repair of neurons in the adult brain.

The third set of studies to establish cell transplantation as a feasible experimental method was the recognition that an additional key to graft survival in the brain is the need to provide an appropriate nutritive environment in which the transplanted cells can thrive. These methods were pioneered by Björklund and Stenevi, who first showed that natural vascular-rich sites lining the ventricles could support transplantation in the brain [10], then introducing methods to generate new vascular-rich cavities that could sustain grafts implanted at other sites remote from the ventricular system [11], and finally introducing a cell suspension method that at last allowed the total flexibility of stereotaxic implantation of cell deposits at will into any deep location within the host parenchyma [12]. Early studies using these intracerebral transplantation techniques used primarily anatomical measures to study the principles that underlay the organization and development of axon pathways in the CNS [13], but it soon became apparent that the new transplantation techniques allowed a new approach to functional repair, initially observed using electrophysiological recording methods [14, 15], but rapidly transferring to behavioral studies in animal models of disease.

Functional cell transplantation

The first functional studies were conducted in rats treated with the catecholamine toxin, 6-hydroxydopamine (6-OHDA). When injected unilaterally into the medial forebrain bundle, this toxin induces massive unilateral depletion of forebrain dopamine and a marked motor and sensorimotor impairment affecting the contralateral side of the body. Grafts of embryonic dopamine neurons readily survive implantation into the striatum on the side of the lesion and provide a rich dopaminergic reinnervation of the denervated forebrain areas [11, 16]. Moreover, such grafts are effective in alleviating the marked motor asymmetry of the host animals which is made manifest in amphetamine and apomorphine rotation tests [11, 16]. Such grafts are immensely potent, and indeed can completely alleviate the motor asymmetry with no more than a few hundred surviving dopamine neurons in the grafts (2–5% of normal) [17]. This is in part due to the compensatory capacity of dopamine neurons per se [18], but also to the fact that to be effective the grafted cells have to be placed accurately [19]. The striatum has a complex topographic organization related to the connectivity of discrete zones with different areas of cerebral cortex, and the positioning of the grafts and their local dopaminergic innervation determines which of a diverse range of striatal functions are affected [20]. Consequently, on the one hand, grafts in different placements will have different functional effects, even when the underlying lesion is common; on the other hand, multiple graft deposits can be used to achieve additive profiles of functional recovery [20]. In addition, these studies highlight the importance of selecting an appropriate panel of tests to evaluate the extent to which any transplantation paradigm is effective. It can be as easy to achieve evidence of dramatic recovery (but only on a very restrictive range of symptoms) as it is to conclude that a graft is quite without functional benefit (but completely missing marked positive effects in a different domain); either conclusion misrepresents a complex profile of partial recovery, which can only be corrected by using a test battery of appropriate breadth for the system under investigation.

The observation of functional recovery from the symptoms induced by selective CNS lesions by cell replacement of the appropriate cell populations, led during the following decade to a proliferation of studies exploring cell transplantation in animal models of a wide variety of neurodegenerative diseases. Thus, for example, a variety of neuroendocrine disorders can be traced to a loss of hypothalamic neurons releasing signaling hormones acting through the pituitary gland, with resultant neuroendocrine deficits. Two models in particular attracted attention. One was the demonstration that the diabetic hyperdiuretic symptoms in the vasopressin-deficient mutant Brattleboro rat can be significantly alleviated by hypothalamic tissue grafts rich in vasopressin neurons [21]. The other was that the loss of sexual behaviors and reproductive capacity associated with genetic deficiency of the gonadotrophin releasing hormone (GnRH) in mice can be corrected by transplantation into the third ventricle of hypothalamic grafts containing GnRH neurons [22]. Most remarkably, grafts restore not only the normal sexual behavioral of both male and female GnRH-deficient mice, but render infertile mice capable of conception and bearing litters [23, 24]. Whereas these studies suggest that it may be sufficient for grafted cells to alleviate deficits by restoration of deficient neurohormonal secretion, in fact in each of the models grafted embryonic neurons have been seen to develop neuronal connections with appropriate targets [25, 26], so the necessary and sufficient conditions for functional recovery are not immediately clear.

These early studies of functional recovery using grafts rich in dopamine, vasopressin and GnRH neurons to replace selective patterns of cell loss, presaged the first wave of new models during the 1980s focused on other diseases and conditions where replacement of a single lost or dysfunctional neuronal cell type may be effective. Thus, for example, cholinergic cell replacement was seen to be remarkably effective in alleviating spatial learning and memory impairments not only in animals with selective cholinergic denervations of the hippocampus and neocortex [27, 28], but also in aged animals [29]. This fitted well with the prevailing hypothesis that age-related memory impairment may reflect a selective cholinergic deficiency [30], but fell out of favor with the realization that frank dementia, whether associated with Alzheimer's or multi-infarct disease, is likely to involve far more wide-spread cellular pathology than can be effectively treated with enhancement of a single afferent brainstem regulatory system as provided by the ascending forebrain cholinergic projections [31]. Of more interest, however, was the use of the power of the selective cell transplantation paradigms to parse the complementary role of cholinergic, serotonergic and noradrenergic regulation separately and together in mediating the normal physiology, neuro-chemistry and behavioral function of hippocampal processes underlying spatial memory [32–35].

With the extent of success achieved with loss and replacement of single neuronal cell types, subsequent studies have taken up the challenge of seeking restoration of more complex networks comprising mixed populations of nuclei. Although it has been possible to achieve long-distance growth and connectivity of cortical tissues [36], any functional repair in such precisely organized laminar and columnar structures has proved difficult [37]. Similarly in the cerebellum [38], early claims of functional recovery have been criticized as artefactual. Greater success has been achieved in the striatal system which, like the hippocampus, is involved in important forms of learning [39] and retains a significant degree of plasticity throughout life [40]. Striatal grafts have emerged as a particularly remarkable system for study of circuit repair in the nervous system. After intrinsic striatal lesions, implanted striatal neurons establish extensive afferent and efferent connections with the host brain [41] sufficient to restore a full cortico-striato-pallidal relay of information through an integrated graft/host circuitry [42]. Moreover, not only do they alleviate a range of simple and more complex motor behaviors [43, 44], they restore a capacity for motor learning that seems to be mediated within the grafted striatum [45], and is indeed mirrored by synaptic plasticity, both long-term potentiation and long-term depression as appropriate, at the (host) cortico-striatal synapse onto medium spiny neurons within the graft [46]. Thus, striatal grafts provide probably the clearest evidence of true circuit repair by implanted cells into the damaged brain. Nevertheless, even here, restoration of connections and normalization of physiological signalling remains incomplete [47, 48].

Note should be made of the several other model systems that have been similarly well explored, including neuronal transplantation in the retina, retinotectal systems, spinal cord, in response to focal or global stroke, and transplantation of glial cells for remyelination (see Table 17.1 and associated references), but for which space is insufficient to allow further elaboration here.

Clinical trials

At the time of the very first demonstration of functional transplantation in nigral grafted rats, Perlow and colleagues speculated that these results might presage clinical application in human Parkinson's disease (PD) [16], and

Table 17.1 Clinical trials of CNS transplantation

Disease	Transplant	Target	Outcome	Refs
PD	Adrenal grafts	DA depleted striatum	Modest effects on Parkinsonian symptoms, not long lasting, not associated with significant graft survival, and with significant morbidity and mortality	[53,56,110]
PD	Fetal VM	DA depleted striatum	Clear long-term graft survival, functional reinnervation, and clinical benefit in some patients, limited benefit in others; some patients exhibit dyskinetic side effects	[69,74,111]
HD	Fetal striatal	Atrophied striatum	Suggestion of alleviation of symptoms in motor cognitive and psychiatric domains in some patients lasting up to five years; surgical risks in advanced patients	[78,82,112]
SCI	Fetal SC; OECs	Spinal cavity or cyst	Primary, progenitor and stem cell grafts may have modest benefit by blocking lesion progression; clinically beneficial repair demonstrated by remyelination	[113–115]
ALS	ENC/eng xeno	Ventral horn		[116]
Stroke	hNT cells	Infracted striatum	Modest effects in stroke patients; specific cell survival and mechanism not known.	[87]
AD	Omentum	Parietal/temporal Ctx	Non-neuronal tissues claimed to promote plasticity; not yet convincingly shown.	[117]
MS	hESC	CNS plaques	Trials believed to be in preparation	
Retinal	RGCs or RPE	Intraocular	Improvement of visual acuity in patients with retinitis pigmentosa and with macular degeneration	[118]
Other	MSCs, OECs	Peripheral or central	There is a growing literature on commercial exploitation of peripheral and central "adult stem cell" transplantation for a wide range of neurodegenerative conditions, generally without proper experimental validation or evaluation	[84, 119, 120]

ALS, amyotrophic lateral sclerosis; DA, dopamine; AD, Alzheimer's disease; Ctx, neocortex; HD, Huntington's disease; hESC, human embryonic stem cells; hNT, human neuroteratoma cell line; MSCs, mesenchymal stem cells; OECs, olfactory ensheathing cells; PD, Parkinson's disease; RGCs, retinal ganglion cells; RPE, retinal pigment epithelium; SCI, spinal cord injury; VM, ventral mesencephalon.

indeed work progressed very rapidly to clinical trial. To avoid the use of human fetal cells, and reasoning that a peripheral source of dopamine-secreting neuroendocrine cells might provide a suitable alternative, William Freed and colleagues showed that intraventricular transplants of catecholamine-secreting adrenal medulla tissues could alleviate Parkinsonian-like deficits in apomorphine rotation in the unilateral 6-OHDA lesion rat model [49] as effectively as they had seen for embryonic nigral transplants [16, 50]. This then paved the way for the first clinical trials involving harvest of one of the two adrenal glands from patients with PD, separation of the medullary chromaffin cells and autotransplantation of the cells back into the patient's own brain [51]. This was without significant clinical benefit in the first Swedish trial using a stereotaxic transplantation method [52], but was rapidly followed by report of a more positive result using a different open ventricular approach for implantation of adrenal medulla in two patients with PD from Mexico City [53]. The dramatic benefit claimed in this latter report stimulated replications in many centers worldwide, in particular in the USA, where there was a systematic collation of data from multiple centers in large scale neurological and neurosurgical registries [54, 55]. For a period of five years the results were heavily disputed, but finally reached a consensus conclusion that the adult adrenal autografts survived only poorly in most patients, providing at best limited and short-lasting clinical benefit, and accompanied by significant side effects, morbidity, and occasional mortalities, resulting not least from the need for abdominal surgery in elderly and frail patients in order to harvest the graft tissue [55, 56]. Any benefits simply did not outweigh the costs, and the adrenal autotransplantation approach has now largely fallen out of favor.

The alternative strategy in Parkinson's disease was to return to techniques that appeared to provide the best results in experimental animals, both in terms of experimental repair and functional recovery, namely using fetal nigral tissues for transplantation. Although use of human fetal tissues raises a range of ethical concerns, a consortium of European transplantation labs established a first consensus code of practice for donation and use of human fetal tissues in clinical transplantation trials [57], which provided a foundation for the diverse national and international ethical reviews (e.g., [58]) that now provides the regulatory and legislative framework for present trials. In essence, the use of human fetal tissues derived from elective abortion for research or therapy is considered not to be unethical provided that: the donation is subject to fully informed consent; and procedures are established to ensure that the consent, timing and procedure for the termination of pregnancy is entirely independent of any subsequent use of the tissue [57, 59]. Lindvall and colleagues [60] provided the first clear evidence that fetal nigral tissues can survive transplantation in the PD brain, restore dopamine turnover as demonstrated by positron emission tomography (PET) imaging

[61, 62], and provide a significant alleviation of Parkinsonian symptoms – in particular the rigidity and bradykinesia, less so the tremor – that can be long lasting for at least 10–15 years [60, 62]. These clear benefits have been replicated in many patients subsequently, both in the Swedish series [63], and in other open label studies in France, Canada, and the USA [64–68].

Nevertheless, two double-blind trials challenged this consensus, not only finding rather variable and limited functional benefits in comparison to sham-operated controls, but also reporting significant side-effects in grafted patients involving dyskinetic movements that were not resolved even with complete withdrawal of concomitant L-dopa medication ("runaway dyskinesia") [69, 70]. These two trials have resulted in a moratorium on further trials pending resolution of three key issues, which have been actively addressed in the intervening eight years. Firstly, intensive study of the dyskinesias, both by retrospective analysis in transplanted patients [71] and in newly developed animal models [72] have identified a combination of factors predisposing to graft-induced dyskinesias, including the requirement for extensive priming with L-dopa before transplantation, inclusion of serotonin cells within the grafts, and focal graft placements ("hotspots") in widely denervated background [73]. Secondly, retrospective analysis of patients that have received grafts has yielded credible hypotheses of the factors that differentiate patients showing a clear and sustained clinical response from those that receive little benefit after transplantation, which again relate to the preexisting profiles of denervation and the extent to which the grafts are effective in providing broad and extensive reinnervation [74]. Thirdly, there are significant practical constraints on the availability of sufficient suitable donor tissue of the correct age, and appropriate quality, which is exacerbated by the requirement for multiple donor embryos for each graft. The last decade has seen significant improvements in preparation to increase cell yields [75], and to prolong the period of storage in hibernation [76, 77], although the logistics of adequate supply are likely to ensure that fetal cell transplantation remains an experimental therapy for the foreseeable future. Nevertheless, we are now in a position to design new clinical trials in PD addressing factors of patient selection, pre-transplantation medication, graft preparation, and placement with the potential to yield significant benefit to a larger proportion of patients, and without incurring the side effects associated with graft-induced dyskinesia. A multi-national clinical trial sponsored by the European Union Framework 7 program ("TRANS-EURO") is now in preparation to test this hypothesis.

Following the progress achieved in translating experimental transplantation methods to clinical trials in Parkinson's disease, translational programs are in active development for a range of other neurodegenerative diseases (Table 17.1). Trials in Huntington's disease have shown a similar trajectory to those in PD, whereby the transplantation methods have been shown to be safe and feasible [78–80], and to produce modest functional benefit in both motor and cognitive domains in some patients [78, 81], but where the reliability of the grafts and healthy long-term survival has been challenged [82, 83]. As in PD, a large-scale, multicenter French-language trial is currently in progress in an open, delayed start, placebo-controlled paradigm, the results of which are eagerly anticipated. Further trials have started in stroke [87], Alzheimer's disease, retinal degeneration, spinal cord trauma, amyotrophic lateral sclerosis, and focal demyelination (see Table 17.1), but in each case the results are too early to determine functional efficacy. Although the efficacy of grafts is still unproven, it is important to emphasize that all such studies should be undertaken within well-controlled experimental contexts if we are to refine present techniques and achieve optimal outcomes. Studies like that recently reported from China [84] of olfactory ensheathing cell implants in 1255 patients with conditions varying from spinal cord injury, amyotrophic lateral sclerosis, chronic pain, cerebral palsy, stroke, ataxia, yet without any systematic evaluation and follow-up in any of them, are uninformative if the goal is to advance evidence-based medicine.

Mechanisms of graft function

The search to develop effective clinical cell therapies highlights the need to incorporate an analysis of the mechanisms of graft function in order to design effective reparative treatments on a rational basis. Initially, when observing that recovery on motor symptoms in Parkinsonian rats was associated with reinnervation of the host brain by the grafts, it was natural to assume that recovery was simply attributable to cell replacement and reconstruction of connections. However, the observation that different graft tissues could yield differing profiles of functional recovery on similar tests (e.g., comparison between the effects of adrenal, nigral, and striatal grafts in the striatum) clearly suggested that grafts could exert functional effects on the behavior of the host animals via a variety of conceptually different mechanisms (see Table 17.2) [85]. Subsequent analysis of recovery in different model systems has indicated that the question: "how do grafts work?" is misplaced; rather, there are clear examples where each of the prospective mechanisms – involving non-specific, pharmacological, neurotrophic, neuroprotective, neuroregenerative, and reconstructive processes – can and does apply in certain circumstances [86]. When developing an alternative cell source for transplantation, it is therefore necessary not only to establish whether the cells survive, differentiate, connect and integrate into the host brain, but also to ask what level of influence or mechanism of action is required to alleviate the particular class(es) of symptoms of particular concern in the target disease, and to design the cell therapy protocol according to relevant criteria for the specific application.

Table 17.2 Mechanisms of functional action

Mechanisms	Description	Example(s)	References
Trauma	Grafts cause adverse effects through damage, interference or noise	Graft tissue overgrowth; expansion of non-neural tissues within grafts	[121]
Non-specific	Surgical damage providing compensation	Pallidal or thalamic lesions in PD; DBS	[122,123]
Trophic-protective	Grafts release trophic molecules that protect neurons against disease progression	Engineered cells, Sertoli cells, etc., protect in model HD, SCI, PD	[124–126]
Trophic-restorative	Grafts release trophic molecules that stimulate endogenous plasticity, sprouting & reorganization	Adrenal grafts stimulate regenerative sprouting in partial DA lesions	[109,127,128]
Pharmacological	Diffuse release of deficient neurochemicals (as a "biological minipump")	Neuroendocrine secretory grafts	[21;22]
Bridges	Grafts provide substrates to stimulate and direct axon growth to remote targets	PNS bridges allow CNS regeneration across spinal transection	[129–132]
Neuronal reinnervation	Grafted neurons reinnervate host brain and restore locally regulated transmitter release	Ectopic VM grafts provide local DA reinnervation and reactivation of denervated striatum under local feedback regulation	[85,108]
Circuit integration	Grafts establish reciprocal connections with host brain so that grafted cells integrate in host circuit	Homotopic striatal grafts establish reciprocal connections with host brain and restore cortico-striatal loops	[42,46,133]
Full reconstruction	Full repair of complex host brain circuits	Not (yet) achieved	

DA, dopamine; DBS, deep brain stimulation; HD, Huntington's disease; PD, Parkinson's disease; SCI, spinal cord injury; VM, ventral mesencephalon.

Present: stem cells as alternative sources of cells for transplantation

So far, most clinical cell transplantation studies have used cells and tissues derived from human fetal donors. Although taking donor tissues from developing embryos – when the neurons are newly born, fully specified, and entering a phase of active directed neurite outgrowth – has proved optimal in experimental studies, a dependence on human fetal donor tissues is severely constraining for the development of cell transplantation therapies, as follows.

(1) Use of human fetal tissues remains ethically sensitive, irrespective of whether for research or therapeutic application, and although permitted subject to strict guidelines and rigid legislation in some countries (e.g., UK, Scandinavia), it is difficult (e.g., Spain, USA) or impossible (e.g., Ireland) under other jurisdictions.
(2) Even when tissue donation from elective termination of pregnancies is approved, supply of tissues of suitable donor age and quality is extremely limited.
(3) Tissue availability is further hampered by the requirement that tissues must be implanted within 4–6 hours of collection to yield viable grafts, a logistic challenge that has only be partly resolved by the introduction of short-term hibernation protocols [76, 77]. And
(4) At a fundamental level, tissues derived from elective terminations can never be subject to the level of standardization and quality control that should be expected of any medicinal product for widespread distribution and use.

Thus, there has emerged a compelling imperative need to identify alternative sources of cells and tissues that might provide a suitable, efficient, effective, and quality-assured replacement for primary fetal cells (see Chapter 16).

The leading candidates for new cell therapies are stem cells. Stem cells are defined by two primary features: self-replication, the capacity for symmetric and asymmetric division which will allow both indefinite expansion and differentiation into progeny; and pluripotency, the capacity to generate multiple different cell phenotypes from an initial undifferentiated cell.

If the expansion and differentiation can be fully controlled in the laboratory, stem cells promise the prospect of having unlimited supplies of cells that can be expanded indefinitely, banked, fully characterized for purposes of safety, standardization and quality control, and delivered "off the shelf" for differentiation into specific cell phenotypes required for single or multiple different applications on demand. The availability of such validated cells would transform the future potential of restorative cell therapies, and offers a tantalizing promise for an idealized future. However, to achieve that goal, we must do the following: identify suitable sources of stem cells; understand how to expand them stably in vitro but switch off their proliferative capacity in vivo; determine how to achieve reliable differentiation into defined terminal phenotypes required for each specific application; establish the limits of immunological privilege of the brain to allografts and establish appropriate standards of histocompatibility matching; and achieve the whole process under medicinal grade (good manufacturing practice) conditions. These are the challenges for the future.

Cells harvested from bone marrow, peripheral blood, and adipose tissue are derived from adult donors, raising a concern that they may exhibit only limited multipotency and/or a limited capacity for stable long-term expansion, as required to produce an adequate renewable supply of neural stem or progenitor cells, whether for research or therapeutic application. In addition, the time required to process stem/progenitor cells from procurement to transplant-ready status may take weeks, suggesting that allogeneic transplantation instead of autologous grafting is indicated for such adult cell therapy. To this end, immature donors may offer a better source of stem cells.

Umbilical-cord blood (UCB) has been demonstrated to provide a rich source of immature stem cells that exhibit a significantly lower immune response than those derived from bone marrow [88]. Transplantation of UCB cells in animal models of CNS injury has been proven safe and effective [89–91]. In particular, intracerebral or intravenous UCB transplantation into stroke rats, created using the routine middle carotid artery occlusion model, reversed many of the motor and neurological symptoms associated with this disease [92–96]. That functional recovery occurred without the need for direct cell deposition into the stroke brain [97, 98] suggests that therapeutic benefits of UCB cells are likely to be mediated by bystander effects rather than by a direct cell replacement mechanism. Of note, the observed beneficial effects in UCB-transplanted stroke animals were detected despite lack of migration of the grafted cells into the ischemic brain. These observations indicate that the mechanism of action of UCB transplantation in stroke is through the release of therapeutic molecules, such as trophic factors and anti-inflammatory agents [98, 99]. Nonetheless, the UCB dose is critical in affording the regenerative process in stroke, in that a dose-dependent effect is seen with the reduction of cerebral infarcts [100]. Moreover, the heterogenous stem/progenitor cell populations residing within UCB may synergistically promote their functional benefits [95]. Compared with the current pharmacologic treatment of tissue plasminogen activator for stroke that has a very narrow therapeutic window of three hours, UCB transplantation displays an extended efficacy profile, even up to a few days after stroke onset [94]. On the other hand, when transplantation of UCB is initiated immediately after stroke, therapeutic benefits are not apparent, probably because of the disease-induced inflammatory response creating a hostile microenvironment to the grafted cells. Of particular interest, the preclinical finding that UCB transplantation could ameliorate the neurological deficits of cerebral palsy in a rat model [101] has recently been translated into clinical practice, and even extended to anoxic and traumatic brain injury cases in pediatric patients, apparently with encouraging results [102].

Based on the positive results of the laboratory studies on UCB, related cord tissues have been similarly examined as potent sources of stem cells, including Wharton jelly, amnion tissue and fluid, and other distinct regions of the placenta [103–106].

In March 2009, the new US administration reversed the moratorium on stem cell research funding, noting the potential of these cells in treating human disorders for which no reliable treatment methods have been established by other routes. Around the same time, the US Food and Drug Administration allowed the first clinical trials of human embryonic stem cells for spinal cord injury. Thereafter, the National Institutes of Health (NIH) released the Guidelines for Human Stem Cell Research, which became effective on July 7, 2009. As further evidence of this change in sentiment towards stem cell research, a recent case of tumor formation was recognized in a patient that received stem cells [107], but the response to this stem cell setback from the public, government and scientific community – while still critical – seems to have been tempered by cautious optimism.

Future: functional stem cell therapies in neurodegenerative disease

So, there is now a renewed energy and optimism for rapid development of stem cell therapies taking place in many centers in most of the advanced economies. And yet, although the range of therapeutic targets is large, the number and scale of clinical trials are still extremely limited. In particular, the optimism that the new cellular, molecular and genetic technologies will lead rapidly to a new era of off-the-shelf cell therapies "on demand" has had to be tempered by the realization that, notwithstanding a range of promising "proofs-of-principle," the technical and biological as well as the regulatory challenges to be overcome have turned out to be far more complex than originally envisaged. For stem cell therapies to achieve their full potential, the challenges still to be overcome fall under several different headings:

1. Directed differentiation

The greatest outstanding technical problem with all pluripotential stem cells, whether embryonic stem cells, adult, or induced pluripotent stem (iPS) cells is achieving full control of directed differentiation to the specific and precise phenotype required for each particular cell replacement application. The complex cascade of developmental switches in achieving the terminal phenotype in all cases remains incompletely understood, and in most cases we do not have full knowledge of the exact specification required nor adequate markers to determine if it has been achieved.

2. Genetic stability

The potential power of stem cell sources for transplantation resides in their capacity for indefinite expansion, with the prospect of providing unlimited supply of fully characterized and quality-assured cells, on demand. However, there is now abundant evidence for a non-trivial level of chromosomal instability and genetic drift through successive passaging of expanding populations of stem cell derived lines. A rigorous process of establishing master banks and standardized working banks of cells for therapeutic application is required to ensure that the cells delivered to the clinic are indeed identical to those characterized during the processes of recurrent quality control.

3. In vivo stability

Grafts of stem cells (of whatever source) into the brain typically show a rapid and progressive reduction in the numbers of surviving graft-derived neurons and expansion in the proportions of glial phenotypes, over one to two months after implantation, even when the cells have been fully differentiated to a neuronal fate before implantation. Whether this is due to selective cell death or an ongoing process of de-differentiation and re-specification following transplantation remains unknown. Clearly this is critical for functional efficacy when the hypothesized mode of graft function involves neuronal replacement and integration into the host circuitry. Even where the hypothesized mode of graft function is trophic or protective, and a neuronal phenotype is not specifically required, precise control over cell fate and cell numbers is likely to be an important regulatory requirement.

4. Cell integration

When the hypothesized mechanism is neuronal repair, then the function of the grafted cells will be critically dependent upon their establishing appropriate reciprocal connections with the host brain, and the degree to which they integrate into the host neuronal circuitry. Although it is well established that developing primary embryonic cells have such a capacity to recognize, express, and respond to the necessary precise development guidance clues in the adult brain, the extent to which in vitro expanded and directed stem cells have a similar capacity remains poorly demonstrated.

5. Safety

Given that a defining feature of stem cells is their capacity for self renewal, the frequent observation of neoplasia and tissue overgrowth raises significant issues of safety and regulatory concern. The predominant strategy is to seek ways to ensure full differentiation of cells into terminal phenotypes before transplantation, but it remains extremely difficult to ensure that not a single cell is retained in a proliferative state. Alternative strategies of engineering suicide genes have been developed that are effective in experimental models, but the additional burden of adding genetic manipulation on top of stem cell derivation for regulatory approval is widely considered as impractical.

6. In vivo assessment

Standard PET and magnetic resonance imaging modalities have been reasonably successful in demonstrating the survival of large grafts of primary neurons in PD and Huntington's disease, and the capacity to track cell fate has proved to be an important component both in assessing outcome experimentally, and in the ongoing medical care and management of transplantation patients. However, imaging of single cells or small cell clusters of cells, determining their phenotypic differentiation, and identification of any inflammatory or immunological tissue reactions, remains challenging with existing imaging technologies. This is particularly true for stem cell derived grafts, which frequently exhibit a greater capacity for cell migration than do grafted primary neurons. There is an urgent need to identify better imaging modalities and novel ligands that can track the fate of grafted cells with better spatial and phenotypic resolution, and this must be achieved in the absence of pre-labelling which, although useful experimentally, is unacceptable in the prospective regulatory and safety environments.

7. Immunology

Although the brain is an "immunologically privileged" transplantation site, that privilege is only relative to other peripheral organ and tissue transplantation; there remain significant issues of potential immunogenicity, inflammatory reactions, etc. Three potential strategies are plausible. The dominant contemporary approach is to use rigorous but time-limited immunosuppression prophylactically over 6–12 months after transplant surgery. Second, it is estimated that as few as 100–200 stem cell lines may be sufficient to provide good HLA tissue matching for most recipients, making feasible the prospect of establishing banks of multiple stem cell lines for matched allografting. One of the constraints of this approach is that, although we understand so little about the precise factors controlling differentiation, different stem cell lines have their own individual characteristics of stability, expandability, and ease of differentiation to alternative fates. Consequently, the present option of selecting a line most suitable for a particular fate and application would be lost if selection needed to be governed by immunological compatibility instead. A third strategy is to develop the options for autologous cell transplantation. This had widely been considered to be infeasible based on human embryonic stem (hES) cell approaches, but has changed dramatically with the recent development of iPS technology. Engineering cell lines from donor somatic cells is rapidly becoming routine within a research and disease-modeling context. However, the likely demands of developing and undertaking full characterization and quality control of one-off lines from individual patients for autologous therapy are likely to prove extremely costly, time limiting, and potentially quite unreliable.

8. Regulatory

Regulatory factors are increasingly determining manufacturing, safety, and quality control environments under which all experimental cell fates are undertaken. To this is added the additional challenges associated with ethical concerns related to the sourcing, consent and derivation of stem cells for therapeutic application that dominate our societies. Academic and clinical scientists are increasingly recognizing the need to work closely with industry – both biotechnology and the large-scale pharmaceutical industry (also known as "big pharma") – which alone has the expertise and resources to implement translational operations within complex regulatory environments.

9. Business model

A final challenge for recruiting industrial investment and involvement in stem cell therapies relates to a widely perceived absence of a viable business model, with concerns about loss of recurrent income from one-off treatments, issues of patentability of human cells, and problems of distribution and marketing when the cells require extensive further post-distribution processing before implantation. Until recently, "big pharma" has shied away from involvement, leaving the field to small biotechnology companies. This situation is now changing, with larger companies increasingly seeing the business opportunities in cell processing technologies rather than in the cells themselves. This can only help to promote the opportunities for scale-up, technical efficiency, and quality standards involved in translating novel cell therapies not only into clinical trials but their subsequent development and distribution as reliable, available, and effective therapies for patients.

All of these remain to be solved. However, from our current perspective (in 2012), all the issues – biological, clinical, commercial, and regulatory – appear soluble, with an appropriate technical focus and skilled effort. We are optimistic in anticipating rapid progress of stem cell technologies from their present status as an interesting but challenging experimental opportunity, to realizing the opportunities for delivering new therapies that are safe, reliable and widely available to patients with a wide range of both acute and progressive neurodegenerative conditions.

Acknowledgments

We acknowledge the support of the following funding agencies for their own studies in this area. S.B.D.: the Medical Research Council, the Welsh Assembly Government, and the European Union Framework 6 and 7 programs.

P.R.S. is a shareholder of Cryo-Cell International Inc. and co-founder of Saneron CCEL Therapeutics Inc. C.V.B. is a consultant for Saneron. C.V.B. is supported by National Institutes of Health grant R01 5R01NS071956-02, James and Esther King Biomedical Program Grant 1KG01-33966, SanBio Inc., Celgene Cellular Therapeutics, and NeuralStem Inc.

KEY LEARNING POINTS

- The adult mammalian CNS is a permissive site for cell transplantation, although the immune privilege is only partial not complete, and raises distinctive challenges for clinical transplantation.
- Newly differentiated embryonic neurons survive transplantation and integrate functionally into the adult mammalian host CNS.
- The most effective stem cell sources for CNS transplantation have been derived from embryonic stem cells, but raise as yet unsolved challenges for safety and control of tumorigenesis.
- Fetal neural progenitors can survive transplantation but long-term maintenance of differentiation and integration has been disappointing.
- Stem/precursor cells from the adult, whether from brain or peripheral sources, do not at present offer a feasible alternative to embryonic and fetal derived stem cells.
- Use of human fetal tissues remains ethically sensitive.

References

1. Dunnett SB. History of neurology: neural transplantation. Handb Clin Neurol 2010;95:885–912.
2. Raisman G, Field PM. A quantitative investigation of the development of collateral reinnervation after partial deafferentation of the septal nuclei. Brain Res 1973; 50:241–64.
3. Das GD, Altman J. Transplanted precursors of nerve cells: their fate in the cerebellums of young rats. Science 1971;173:637–8.
4. Olson L. Fluorescence histochemical evidence for axonal growth and secretion from transplanted adrenal medullary tissue. Histochemie 1970;22:1–7.
5. Reynolds BA, Weiss S. Generation of neurons and astrocytes from isolated cells of the adult mammalian central nervous system. Science 1992;255:1707–10.
6. Das GD, Altman J. Studies on the transplantation of developing neural tissue in the mammalian brain. I. Transplantation of cerebellar slabs into the cerebellum of neonate rats. Brain Res 1972;38:233–49.
7. Olson L, Malmfors T. Growth characteristics of adrenergic nerves in the adult rat. Fluorescence histochemical and 3H-noradrenaline uptake studies using tissue

transplantation to the anterior chamber of the eye. Acta Physiol Scand Suppl 1970;348:1–112.

8. Olson L, Seiger Å, Strömberg I. Intraocular transplantation in rodents: a detailed account of the procedure and examples of its use in neurobiology with special reference to brain tissue grafting. Adv Cell Neurobiol 1983;4: 407–42.

9. Olson L, Björklund H, Hoffer BJ. Camera bulbi anterior: new vistas on a classical locus for neural tissue transplantation. In: Sladek JR, Gash DM, editors. Neural Transplants: Development and Function. New York: Plenum Press, 1984: 125–65.

10. Stenevi U, Björklund A, Svendgaard N-A. Transplantation of central and peripheral monoamine neurons to the adult rat brain: techniques and conditions for survival. Brain Res 1976;114:1–20.

11. Björklund A, Stenevi U. Reconstruction of the nigrostriatal dopamine pathway by intracerebral transplants. Brain Res 1979;177:555–60.

12. Dunnett SB. Neural transplantation. In: Finger S, Boller F, Tyler K, editors. Handbook of Clinical Neurology. Vol. 95 (3rd Series), History of Neurology. Amsterdam & New York: Elsevier, 2009: 887–914.

13. Björklund A, Stenevi U, Svendgaard N-A. Growth of transplanted monoaminergic neurones into the adult hippocampus along the perforant path. Nature 1976; 262:787–90.

14. Hoffer BJ, Seiger Å, Ljungberg T, Olson L. Electrophysiological and cytological studies of brain homografts in the anterior chamber of the eye: maturation of cerebellar cortex in oculo. Brain Res 1974;79:165–84.

15. Björklund A, Segal M, Stenevi U. Functional reinnervation of rat hippocampus by locus coeruleus implants. Brain Res 1979;170:409–26.

16. Perlow MJ, Freed WJ, Hoffer BJ, Seiger Å, Olson L, Wyatt RJ. Brain grafts reduce motor abnormalities produced by destruction of nigrostriatal dopamine system. Science 1979;204:643–7.

17. Nakao N, Frodl EM, Duan WM, Widner H, Brundin P. Lazaroids improve the survival of grafted rat embryonic dopamine neurons. Proc Natl Acad Sci USA 1994;91:12408–12.

18. Zigmond MJ, Abercrombie ED, Berger TW, Grace AA, Stricker EM. Compensations after lesions of central dopaminergic neurons: some clinical and basic implications. Trends Neurosci 1990;13:290–96.

19. Dunnett SB, Björklund A, Stenevi U, Iversen SD. Grafts of embryonic substantia nigra reinnervating the ventrolateral striatum ameliorate sensorimotor impairments and akinesia in rats with 6-OHDA lesions of the nigrostriatal pathway. Brain Res 1981;229:209–17.

20. Dunnett SB, Björklund A, Schmidt RH, Stenevi U, Iversen SD. Intracerebral grafting of neuronal cell suspensions. IV. Behavioral recovery in rats with unilateral 6-OHDA lesions following implantation of nigral cell suspensions in different forebrain sites. Acta Physiol Scand suppl 1983;522:29–37.

21. Gash DM, Sladek JR, Sladek CD. Functional development of grafted vasopressin neurons. Science 1980;210:1367–9.

22. Krieger DT, Perlow MJ, Gibson MJ, Davies TF, Zimmerman EA, Ferin M, et al. Brain grafts reverse hypogonadism of gonadotropin releasing hormone deficiency. Nature 1982;298:468–71.

23. Gibson MJ, Krieger DT, Perlow MJ, Davies TF, Zimmerman EA, Ferin M, et al. Hypothalamic brain transplants reverse hypogonadism in male mutant mice with gonadotropin-releasing hormone deficiency. Trans Assoc Am Physicians 1982; 95:188–95.

24. Gibson MJ, Krieger DT, Charlton HM, Zimmerman EA, Silverman AJ, Perlow MJ. Mating and pregnancy can occur in genetically hypogonadal mice with preoptic area brain grafts. Science 1984;225:949–51.

25. Kokoris GJ, Silverman AJ, Zimmerman EA, Perlow MJ, Gibson MJ. Implantation of fetal preoptic area into the lateral ventricle of adult hypogonadal mutant mice: the pattern of gonadotropin-releasing hormone axonal outgrowth into the host brain. Neuroscience 1987;22:159–67.

26. Boer GJ, Griffioen HA. Developmental and functional aspects of grafting of the suprachiasmatic nucleus in the brattleboro and the arhythmic rat. Eur J Morphol 1990;28:330–45.

27. Dunnett SB, Low WC, Iversen SD, Stenevi U, Björklund A. Septal transplants restore maze learning in rats with fornix-fimbria lesions. Brain Res 1982;251: 335–48.

28. Dunnett SB, Toniolo G, Fine A, Ryan CN, Björklund A, Iversen SD. Transplantation of embryonic ventral forebrain neurons to the neocortex of rats with lesions of nucleus basalis magnocellularis. 2. Sensorimotor and learning impairments. Neuroscience 1985;16:787–97.

29. Gage FH, Björklund A, Stenevi U, Dunnett SB, Kelly PAT. Intrahippocampal septal grafts ameliorate learning impairments in aged rats. Science 1984;225: 533–6.

30. Bartus RT, Dean RL, Beer B, Lippa AS. The cholinergic hypothesis of geriatric memory dysfunction. Science 1982;217:408–17.

31. Dunnett SB. Neural transplants as a treatment for Alzheimer's disease? Psychol Med 1991;21:825–30.

32. Buzsaki G, Gage FH, Czopf J, Björklund A. Restoration of rhythmic slow activity (theta) in the subcortically denervated hippocampus by fetal CNS transplants. Brain Res 1987;400:334–47.

33. Nilsson OG, Kalén P, Rosengren E, Björklund A. Acetylcholine release from intra-hippocampal septal grafts is under control of the host brain. Proc Natl Acad Sci USA 1990;87:2647–51.

34. Nilsson OG, Brundin P, Björklund A. Amelioration of spatial memory impairment by intrahippocampal grafts of mixed septal and raphe tissue in rats with combined cholinergic and serotonergic denervation of the forebrain. Brain Res 1990; 515:193–206.

35. Björklund A, Nilsson OG, Kalén P. Reafferentation of the subcortically denervated hippocampus as a model for transplant-induced functional recovery in the CNS. Prog Brain Res 1990;83:411–26.

36. Gaillard A, Prestoz L, Dumartin B, Cantereau A, Morel F, Roger M, et al. Reestablishment of damaged adult motor pathways by grafted embryonic cortical neurons. Nat Neurosci 2007;10:1294–9.

37. Sofroniew MV, Dunnett SB, Isacson O. Remodeling of intrinsic and afferent systems in neocortex with cortical transplants. Prog Brain Res 1990;82:313–320.

38. Wallace RB, Das GD. Behavioral effects of CNS transplants in the rat. Brain Res 1982;243:133–9.

39. McDonald RJ, White NM. A triple dissociation of memory systems: hippocampus, amygdala, and dorsal striatum. Behav Neurosci 1993;107:3.

40. Calabresi P, Centonze D, Gubellini P, Marfia GA, Pisani A, Sancesario G, et al. Synaptic transmission in the striatum: from plasticity to neurodegeneration. Prog Neurobiol 2000;61:231–65.

41. Wictorin K, Clarke DJ, Bolam JP, Brundin P, Gustavii B, Lindvall O, et al. Extensive efferent projections of intra-striatally transplanted striatal neurons as revealed by a species-specific neurofilament marker and anterograde axonal tracing. Prog Brain Res 1990;82:391–399.

42. Clarke DJ, Dunnett SB. Synaptic relationships between cortical and dopaminergic inputs and intrinsic GABAergic systems within intrastriatal striatal grafts. J Chem Neuroanat 1993;6:147–158.

43. Dunnett SB, Isacson O, Sirinathsinghji DJS, Clarke DJ, Björklund A. Striatal grafts in rats with unilateral neostriatal lesions. III. Recovery from dopamine-dependent motor asymmetry and deficits in skilled paw reaching. Neuroscience 1988;24: 813–20.

44. Isacson O, Dunnett SB, Björklund A. Graft-induced behavioral recovery in an animal model of Huntington disease. Proc Natl Acad Sci USA 1986;83:2728–32.

45. Brasted PJ, Watts C, Robbins TW, Dunnett SB. Associative plasticity in striatal transplants. Proc Natl Acad Sci USA 1999;96:10524–29.

46. Mazzocchi-Jones D, Döbrössy MD, Dunnett SB. Synaptic plasticity in striatal grafts. Eur J Neurosci 2009;30:2134–42.

47. Rutherford A, Garcia-Muñoz M, Dunnett SB, Arbuthnott GW. Electrophysiological demonstration of host cortical inputs to striatal grafts. Neurosci Lett 1987;83: 275–81.

48. Xu ZC, Wilson CJ, Emson PC. Synaptic potentials evoked in spiny neurons in rat neostriatal grafts by cortical and thalamic stimulation. J Neurophysiol 1991; 65:477–43.

49. Freed WJ, Morihisa JM, Spoor E, Hoffer BJ, Olson L, Seiger Å, et al. Transplanted adrenal chromaffin cells in rat brain reduce lesion-induced rotational behavior. Nature 1981;292:351–2.

50. Freed WJ, Perlow MJ, Karoum F, Seiger Å, Olson L, Hoffer BJ, et al. Restoration of dopaminergic function by grafting of fetal rat substantia nigra to the caudate nucleus: long term behavioral, biochemical, and histochemical studies. Ann Neurol 1980;8:510–9.

51. Backlund EO, Granberg PO, Hamberger B, Knutsson E, Mårtensson A, Sedvall G, et al. Transplantation of adrenal medullary tissue to striatum in parkinsonism. First clinical trials. J Neurosurg 1985;62:169–73.

52. Lindvall O, Backlund EO, Farde L, Sedvall G, Freedman R, Hoffer B, et al. Transplantation in Parkinson's disease: 2 cases of adrenal medullary grafts to the putamen. Ann Neurol 1987;22:457–68.

53. Madrazo I, Drucker-Colín R, Díaz V, Martínez-Mata J, Torres C, Becerril JJ. Open microsurgical autograft of adrenal medulla to the right caudate nucleus in two patients with intractable Parkinson's disease. N Engl J Med 1987;316: 831–4.

54. Bakay RAE, Allen GS, Apuzzo MLJ, Borges LF, Bullard DE, Ojemann GA, et al. Preliminary report on adrenal medullary grafting from the American Association of Neurological Surgeons graft project. Prog Brain Res 1990;82:603–10.

55. Goetz CG, Stebbins GT, Klawans HL, Koller WC, Grossman RG, Bakay RAE, et al. United Parkinson Foundation neurotransplantation registry on adrenal medullary transplants: presurgical, and 1-year and 2-year follow up. Neurology 1991;41: 1719–22.

56. Quinn NP. The clinical application of cell grafting techniques in patients with Parkinson's disease. Prog Brain Res 1990;82:619–25.

57. Boer GJ. Ethical guidelines for the use of human embryonic or fetal tissue for experimental and clinical neurotransplantation and research. J Neurol 1994; 242:1–13.

58. Redmond DE, Freeman TB. The American Society for Neural Transplantation and Repair: Considerations and guidelines for studies of human subjects. Cell Transplant 2001;10:661–4.

59. Polkinghorne J, Hoffenberg R, Kennedy I, Macintyre S. Review of the Guidance on the Research Use of Fetuses and Fetal Material. London: HMSO, 1989.

60. Lindvall O, Brundin P, Widner H, Rehncrona S, Gustavii B, Frackowiak R, et al. Fetal brain grafts and Parkinson's disease – response. Science 1990;250: 1435.

61. Lindvall O, Sawle G, Widner H, Rothwell JC, Björklund A, Brooks DJ, et al. Evidence for long-term survival and function of dopaminergic grafts in progressive Parkinson's disease. Ann Neurol 1994;35:172–80.

62. Piccini P, Brooks DJ, Björklund A, Gunn RN, Grasby PM, Rimoldi O, et al. Dopamine release from nigral transplants visualised *in vivo* in a Parkinson's patient. Nat Neurosci 1999;2:1137–40.

63. Lindvall O. Clinical experiences with dopamine neuron replacement in Parkinson's disease: what is the future? In: Iversen LL, Iversen SD, Dunnett SB, Björklund A, editors. New York: Oxford University Press, 2010: 478–488.

64. Hauser RA, Freeman TB, Snow BJ, Nauert M, Gauger L, Kordower JH, et al. Long-term evaluation of bilateral fetal nigral transplantation in Parkinson disease. Arch Neurol 1999;56:179–87.

65. Mendez I, Vinuela A, Astradsson A, Mukhida K, Hallett P, Robertson H, et al. Dopamine neurons implanted into people with Parkinson's disease survive without pathology for 14 years. Nat Med 2008;14:507–9.

66. Mendez I, Dagher A, Hong M, Hebb A, Gaudet P, Law A, et al. Enhancement of survival of stored dopaminergic cells and promotion of graft survival by exposure of human fetal nigral tissue to glial cell line-derived neurotrophic factor in patients with Parkinson's disease – Report of two cases and technical considerations. J Neurosurg 2000;92:863–9.

67. Rémy P, Samson Y, Hantraye P, Fontaine A, Defer G, Mangin JF, et al. Clinical correlates of [^{18}F]fluorodopa uptake in five grafted Parkinsonian patients. Ann Neurol 1995;38:580–8.

68. Levivier M, Dethy S, Rodesch F, Peschanski M, Vandesteene A, David P, et al. Intracerebral transplantation of fetal ventral mesencephalon for patients with advanced Parkinson's disease – Methodology and 6-month to 1-year follow-up in 3 patients. Stereotact Funct Neurosurg 1997;69:99–111.

69. Freed CR, Greene PE, Breeze RE, Tsai WY, DuMouchel W, Kao R, et al. Transplantation of embryonic dopamine neurons for severe Parkinson's disease. N Engl J Med 2001;344:710–9.

70. Olanow CW, Goetz CG, Kordower JH, Stoessl AJ, Sossi V, Brin MF, et al. A double-blind controlled trial of bilateral fetal nigral transplantation in Parkinson's disease. Ann Neurol 2003;54:403–14.

71. Hagell P, Piccini P, Björklund A, Brundin P, Rehncrona S, Widner H, et al. Dyskinesias following neural transplantation in Parkinson's disease. Nat Neurosci 2002;5:627–8.

72. Lane EL, Winkler C, Brundin P, Cenci MA. The impact of graft size on the development of dyskinesia following intrastriatal grafting of embryonic dopamine neurons in the rat. Neurobiol Dis 2006;22:334–46.

73. Lane EL, Björklund A, Dunnett SB, Winkler C. Unraveling the mechanisms underlying graft-induced dyskinesia. Prog Brain Res 2010;184:295–309.

74. Piccini P, Pavese N, Hagell P, Reimer J, Björklund A, Oertel WH, et al. Factors affecting the clinical outcome after neural transplantation in Parkinson's disease. Brain 2005;128):2977–86.

75. Brundin P, Karlsson J, Emgård M, Schierle GS, Hansson O, Petersén Å, et al. Improving the survival of grafted dopaminergic neurons: a review over current approaches. Cell Transplant 2000;9:179–95.

76. Sauer H, Brundin P. Effects of cool storage on survival and function of intrastriatal ventral mesencephalic grafts. Restor Neurol Neurosci 1991;2:123–35.

77. Hurelbrink CB, Tyers P, Armstrong RJE, Dunnett SB, Barker RA, Rosser AE. Long-term hibernation of human fetal striatal tissue does not adversely affect its differentiation *in vitro* or graft survival: implications for clinical trials in Huntington's disease. Cell Transplant 2003;12:687–95.

78. Bachoud-Lévi AC, Rémy P, Nguyen JP, Brugières P, Lefaucheur JP, Bourdet C, et al. Motor and cognitive improvements in patients with Huntington's disease after neural transplantation. Lancet 2000;356:1975–9.

79. Rosser AE, Barker RA, Guillard J, Harrower T, Watts C, Pickard J, et al. Unilateral transplantation of human primary fetal tissue in four patients with Huntington's disease: NEST-UK safety report (ISRCTN no 36485475). J Neurol Neurosurg Psychiat 2002;73:678–85.

80. Freeman TB, Cicchetti F, Hauser RA, Deacon TW, Li XJ, Hersch SM, et al. Transplanted fetal striatum in Huntington's disease: phenotypic development and lack of pathology. Proc Natl Acad Sci USA 2000;97:13877–82.

81. Reuter I, Tai YF, Pavese N, Chaudhuri KR, Mason S, Polkey CE, et al. Long-term clinical and positron emission tomography outcome of fetal striatal transplantation in Huntington's disease. J Neurol Neurosurg Psychiat 2008;79: 948–51.

82. Hauser RA, Furtado S, Cimino CR, Delgado H, Eichler S, Schwartz S, et al. Bilateral human fetal striatal transplantation in Huntington's disease. Neurology 2002; 58:687–95.

83. Cicchetti F, Saporta S, Hauser RA, Parent M, Saint-Pierre M, Sanberg PR, et al. Neural transplants in patients with Huntington's disease undergo disease-like neuronal degeneration. Proc Natl Acad Sci USA 2009;106:12483–8.

84. Huang H, Chen L, Xi H, Wang O, Zhang J, Liu Y, et al. Olfactory ensheathing cells transplantation for central nervous system diseases in 1,255 patients (in Chinese). Chinese journal of reparative and reconstructive surgery 2009; 23(1):14–20.

85. Björklund A, Lindvall O, Isacson O, Brundin P, Wictorin K, Strecker RE, et al. Mechanisms of action of intracerebral neural implants – studies on nigral and striatal grafts to the lesioned striatum. Trends Neurosci 1987;10:509–16.

86. Dunnett SB, Björklund A. Mechanisms of function of neural grafts in the injured brain. In: Dunnett SB, Björklund A, editors. Functional Neural Transplantation. New York: Raven Press, 1994: 531–67.

87. Kondziolka D, Wechsler L, Goldstein S, Meltzer C, Thulborn KR, Gebel J, et al. Transplantation of cultured human neuronal cells for patients with stroke. Neurology 2000;55:565–9.

88. Sanberg PR, Park DH, Kuzmin-Nichols N, Cruz E, Hossne NA, Jr., Buffolo E, et al. Monocyte transplantation for neural and cardiovascular ischemia repair. J Cell Mol Med 2010;14:553–63.

89. Park DH, Borlongan CV, Willing AE, Eve DJ, Sanberg PR. Human umbilical cord blood cell grafts for stroke. Cell Transplant 2009;18:985–98.

90. Yasuhara T, Hara K, Maki M, Xu L, Yu G, Ali MM, et al. Mannitol facilitates neurotrophic factor upregulation and behavioral recovery in neonatal hypoxic–ischemic rats with human umbilical cord blood grafts. J Cell Mol Med 2010;14: 914–21.

91. Garbuzova-Davis S, Klasko SK, Sanberg PR. Intravenous administration of human umbilical cord blood cells in an animal model of MPS III B. J Comp Neurol 2009;515:93–101.

92. Sanberg PR, Eve DJ, Willing AE, Garbuzova-Davis S, Tan J, Sanberg CD, et al. The treatment of neurodegenerative disorders using umbilical cord blood and menstrual blood-derived stem cells. Cell Transplant 2011;20:85–94.

93. Ou Y, Yu S, Kaneko Y, Tajiri N, Bae EC, Chheda SH, et al. Intravenous infusion of GDNF gene-modified human umbilical cord blood CD34+ cells protects against cerebral ischemic injury in spontaneously hypertensive rats. Brain Res 2010;1366: 217–25.

94. Newcomb JD, Ajmo CT, Jr., Sanberg CD, Sanberg PR, Pennypacker KR, Willing AE. Timing of cord blood treatment after experimental stroke determines therapeutic efficacy. Cell Transplant 2006;15:213–23.

95. Xiao J, Nan Z, Motooka Y, Low WC. Transplantation of a novel cell line population of umbilical cord blood stem cells ameliorates neurological deficits associated with ischemic brain injury. Stem Cells Dev 2005;14:722–33.

96. Chen J, Sanberg PR, Li Y, Wang L, Lu M, Willing AE, et al. Intravenous administration of human umbilical cord blood reduces behavioral deficits after stroke in rats. Stroke 2001;32:2682–8.

97. Willing AE, Lixian J, Milliken M, Poulos S, Zigova T, Song S, et al. Intravenous versus intrastriatal cord blood administration in a rodent model of stroke. J Neurosci Res 2003;73:296–307.

98. Borlongan CV, Hadman M, Sanberg CD, Sanberg PR. Central nervous system entry of peripherally injected umbilical cord blood cells is not required for neuroprotection in stroke. Stroke 2004;35:2385–9.

99. Newman MB, Willing AE, Manresa JJ, Sanberg CD, Sanberg PR. Cytokines produced by cultured human umbilical cord blood (HUCB) cells: implications for brain repair. Exp Neurol 2006;199:201–8.

100. Vendrame M, Cassady J, Newcomb J, Butler T, Pennypacker KR, Zigova T, et al. Infusion of human umbilical cord blood cells in a rat model of stroke

dose-dependently rescues behavioral deficits and reduces infarct volume. Stroke 2004;35):2390–5.

101. Meier C, Middelanis J, Wasielewski B, Neuhoff S, Roth-Haerer A, Gantert M, et al. Spastic paresis after perinatal brain damage in rats is reduced by human cord blood mononuclear cells. Pediatr Res 2006;59:244–9.

102. Kurtzberg J. Update on umbilical cord blood transplantation. Curr Opin Pediatr 2009;21:22–9.

103. Yu SJ, Soncini M, Kaneko Y, Hess DC, Parolini O, Borlongan CV. Amnion: a potent graft source for cell therapy in stroke. Cell Transplant 2009;18:111–8.

104. de Coppi P, Bartsch G, Jr., Siddiqui MM, Xu T, Santos CC, Perin L, et al. Isolation of amniotic stem cell lines with potential for therapy. Nat Biotechnol 2007; 25:100–6.

105. Weiss ML, Anderson C, Medicetty S, Seshareddy KB, Weiss RJ, VanderWerff I, et al. Immune properties of human umbilical cord Wharton's jelly-derived cells. Stem Cells 2008;26):2865–74.

106. Parolini O, Alviano F, Bergwerf I, Boraschi D, De Bari C, De Waele P, et al. Toward cell therapy using placenta-derived cells: Disease mechanisms, cell biology, pre-clinical studies, and regulatory aspects at the round table. Stem Cells Dev 2010;19:143–54.

107. Amariglio N, Hirshberg A, Scheithauer BW, Cohen Y, Loewenthal R, Trakhtenbrot L, et al. Donor-derived brain tumor following neural stem cell transplantation in an ataxia telangiectasia patient. PLoS Med 2009;6:e29.

108. Björklund A, Dunnett SB, Stenevi U, Lewis ME, Iversen SD. Reinnervation of the denervated striatum by substantia nigra transplants: functional consequences as revealed by pharmacological and sensorimotor testing. Brain Res 1980;199: 307–3.

109. Bohn MC, Cupit L, Marciano F, Gash DM. Adrenal grafts enhance recovery of striatal dopaminergic fibers. Science 1987;237:913–6.

110. Barker RA, Dunnett SB. The biology and behaviour of intracerebral adrenal transplants in animals and man. Rev Neurosci 1993;4:113–46.

111. Lindvall O, Brundin P, Widner H, Rehncrona S, Gustavii B, Frackowiak R, et al. Grafts of fetal dopamine neurons survive and improve motor function in Parkinson's disease. Science 1990;247:574–7.

112. Dunnett SB, Rosser AE. Cell transplantation for Huntington's disease. Should we continue? Brain Res Bull 2007;72:132–47.

113. Wirth ED, Reier PJ, Fessler RG, Thompson FJ, Uthman B, Behrman A, et al. Feasibility and safety of neural tissue transplantation in patients with syringomyelia. J Neurotrauma 2001;18:911–29.

114. Mackay-Sim A, Feron F, Cochrane J, Bassingthwaighte L, Bayliss C, Davies W, et al. Autologous olfactory ensheathing cell transplantation in human paraplegia: a 3-year clinical trial. Brain 2008;131:2376–86.

115. Sharp J, Frame J, Siegenthaler M, Nistor G, Keirstead HS. Human embryonic stem cell-derived oligodendrocyte progenitor cell transplants improve recovery after cervical spinal cord injury. Stem Cells 2009;28:152–163.

116. Aebischer P, Pochon NA, Heyd B, Déglon N, Joseph JM, Zurn AD, et al. Gene therapy for amyotrophic lateral sclerosis (ALS) using a polymer encapsulated xenogenic cell line engineered to secrete hCNTF. Hum Gene Ther 1996;7: 851–60.

117. Shankle WR, Hara J, Bjornsen L, Gade GF, Leport PC, Ali MB, et al. Omentum transposition surgery for patients with Alzheimer's disease: a case series. Neurol Res 2008;30:313–25.

118. Radtke ND, Aramant RB, Petry HM, Green PT, Pidwell DJ, Seiler MJ. Vision improvement in retinal degeneration patients by implantation of retina together with retinal pigment epithelium. Am J Ophthalmol 2008;146:172–82.

119. Tian ZM, Chen T, Zhong N, Li ZC, Yin F, Liu S. Clinical study of transplantation of neural stem cells in therapy of inherited cerebellar atrophy. Beijing Da Xue Xue Bao 2009;41:456–8.

120. Lee PH, Kim JW, Bang OY, Ahn YH, Joo IS, Huh K. Autologous mesenchymal stem cell therapy delays the progression of neurological deficits in patients with multiple system atrophy. Clin Pharmacol Ther 2008;83:723–30.

121. Folkerth RD, Durso R. Survival and proliferation of non-neural tissues, with obstruction of cerebral ventricles, in a parkinsonian patient treated with fetal allografts. Neurology 1996;46(5):1219–25.

122. Meyers R. The modification of alternating tremors, rigidity and festination by surgery of basal ganglia. Assoc Nerv Ment Dis Proc 1942;21:602–65.

123. Hallett M, Litvan I, Task Force Surg Parkinsons Dis. Evaluation of surgery for Parkinson's disease – A report of the therapeutics and technology assessment subcommittee of the American Academy of Neurology. Neurology 1999;53:1910–21.

124. Isacson O, Frim DM, Galpern WR, Tatter SB, Breakefield XO, Schumacher JM. Cell-mediated delivery of neurotrophic factors and neuroprotection in the neostriatum and substantia nigra. Restor Neurol Neurosci 1995;8:59–61.

125. Åkerud P, Canals JM, Snyder EY, Arenas E. Neuroprotection through delivery of glial cell line-derived neurotrophic factor by neural stem cells in a mouse model of Parkinson's disease. J Neurosci 2001;21:8108–18.

126. Borlongan CV, Cameron DF, Saporta S, Sanberg PR. Intracerebral transplantation of testis-derived Sertoli cells promotes functional recovery in female rats with 6-hydroxydopamine-induced hemiparkinsonism. Exp Neurol 1997;148:388–92.

127. Bankiewicz KS, Mandel RJ, Sofroniew MV. Trophism, transplantation, and animal models of Parkinson's disease. Exp Neurol 1993;124:140–9.

128. Georgievska B, Carlsson T, Lacar B, Winkler C, Kirik D. Dissociation between short-term increased graft survival and long-term functional improvements in Parkinsonian rats overexpressing glial cell line-derived neurotrophic factor. Eur J Neurosci 2004;20:3121–30.

129. David S, Aguayo AJ. Axonal elongation into peripheral nervous system "bridges" after central nervous system injury in adult rats. Science 1981;214:931–3.

130. Dunnett SB, Rogers DC, Richards SJ. Nigrostriatal reconstruction after 6-OHDA lesions in rats: combination of dopamine-rich nigral grafts and nigrostriatal bridge grafts. Exp Brain Res 1989;75:523–35.

131. Guest JD, Rao A, Olson L, Bunge MB, Bunge RP. The ability of human Schwann cell grafts to promote regeneration in the transected nude rat spinal cord. Exp Neurol 1997;148:502–22.

132. Reier PJ, Bregman BS, Wujek JR. Intraspinal transplantation of embryonic spinal cord tissue in neonatal and adult rats. J Comp Neurol 1986;247:275–96.

133. Dunnett SB, Nathwani F, Björklund A. The integration and function of striatal grafts. Prog Brain Res 2000;127:345–80.

18 Pancreatic Islet Cells

Katie Kinzer[1], Patrick Salmon[2], and Jose Oberholzer[1]
[1]University of Illinois at Chicago, Chicago, Illinois, USA
[2]Centre Médical Universitaire, Geneva, Switzerland

The past

Clinical

The clinical potential for islet transplantation in the treatment of patients with type 1 diabetes was first suggested over one century ago. In 1894 Dr Williams, at the Bristol Infirmary in England, transplanted three pieces of freshly slaughtered sheep's pancreas into the subcutaneous tissues of a young boy dying from diabetic ketoacidosis [1]. Improvement in glucosuria was initially noted; however, the boy died three days after the procedure. This rudimentary pancreatic tissue transplant, almost three decades before the discovery of insulin therapy, marked the origin from which modern clinical islet transplantation would develop.

The first record of human pancreatic tissue transplantation came in 1924 when Charles Pybus, an English surgeon, transplanted fragments of cadaveric pancreatic tissue into patients with diabetes with unsuccessful results [2]. Refinement of this procedure began with the use of collagenase for pancreas digestion and isolation of insulin-producing β cells. A method was first developed to isolate islets from the guinea pig pancreas by Moskalewski in 1965 and from the rat pancreas by Lacy and Kostianovsky two years later. After the establishment of a method to isolate islet cells, Ballinger and Lacy performed the first islet transplantation in rats in 1972 and Mirkovitch and Campiche performed the first successful islet transplant in dogs in 1976.

Evidence of the reversal of chemically induced diabetes in rodent and canine models propelled islet transplantation forward into the clinical realm.

Tissue and Cell Clinical Use: An Essential Guide, First Edition. Edited by Ruth M. Warwick and Scott A. Brubaker.
© 2012 Blackwell Publishing Ltd. Published 2012 by Blackwell Publishing Ltd.

Najarian and Sutherland at the University of Minnesota attempted the first clinical trials in 1977; however, the first successful clinical trials, with well-documented cases of insulin independence, did not occur until Ricordi et al. developed a method to isolate functional islets from the human pancreas in 1988 [3]. In this method, islets are concentrated and separated from exocrine tissue by density-gradient centrifugation after enzymatic digestion of the pancreas with collagenase and mechanical dissociation in a temperature-controlled digestion chamber. Several other technical advances in the 1990s that enhanced the functional quality of the harvested islets included the development and implementation of controlled pancreas perfusion with collagenase, the COBE® cell processor for large-scale islet purification, and more purified enzymes with higher digestion efficacy [4].

Despite these advances, early clinical trials of islet transplantation remained largely unsuccessful. In the 353 cases of islet transplantation in type 1 diabetic recipients recorded by the International Islet Transplant Registry from 1974 to 1999, less than 10% attained insulin independence for over one year (http://www.med.uni-giessen.de/itr/). Furthermore, long-term C-peptide secretion by the transplanted β cells was observed only in a few cases. In contrast, early attempts to prevent the onset of diabetes after surgical pancreatectomy through autologous transplantation proved more successful. In the 114 reported cases of islet autografts from 1990 to 1998, 50% of all recipients and 70% of the recipients who received more than 300,000 IEQ (islet equivalent) remained insulin independent for over one year. In this early period, reports that autologous transplantation could prevent diabetic onset for over seven years provided the biological proof-of-principle for long-term, stable glucose control by transplanted islets.

Early factors impeding success

Although momentous preclinical studies were successfully conducted in both small and large mammal models in the early 1970s, translation to the human population was significantly limited until 2000. Comprehensive review of the clinical trials up until 1999 reveals that early failures in islet transplantation can be attributed largely to two factors: primitive manufacturing and ineffective immunosuppression. As a result of early limitations in the manufacturing process, both islet mass and potency were inadequate for successful transplantation outcomes.

Regardless of improvements in both the quantity and quality of the isolated islets, early clinical outcomes remained poor owing to the ineffective immunosuppression regimen. The use of toxic, diabetogenic immunosuppression that was ineffective against graft rejection by both allo- and autoimmune pathways prevented function and survival of islet grafts. Immunosuppressive problems in the early stages were especially highlighted by reports of long-term insulin independence after autologous islet

CASE STUDY 18.1

Long-term insulin independence: first islet transplant case to pass the 10-year mark

Adapted from Berney et al. [37].

Background. This clinical case represents the longest reported period of insulin independence after allogeneic islet transplantation. After a 27-year history of type 1 diabetes, this patient was able to discontinue insulin within 3 months of transplantation and remained off insulin for over 12 years. Before islet transplantation, this patient had presented with severe hypoglycemia, lack of awareness, and had required a low mean insulin dose of 16 units per day with poor metabolic control (HbA1c at 11.2%). Additionally, this patient had severe peripheral and autonomic neuropathy, a history of panretinal photocoagulation, blindness in the left eye, 60% visual acuity in the right eye, and had received two kidney transplants for end-stage diabetic nephropathy.

Procedure. The patient received a single islet-after-kidney graft of 8800 insulin equivalents per kilogram, pooled from two donors at the University of Geneva in Switzerland. The pancreas was digested with crude collagenase and transplanted intraportally under local anesthesia by the transhepatic percutaneous approach. The patient received immunosuppressive induction with equine antithymocyte globulin for 10 days and maintenance immunosuppression was achieved with ciclosporin A microemulsion, prednisone, and azathioprine. One year after transplantation, azathioprine was switched to mycophenolate mofetil.

Outcome. Insulin administration was discontinued within three months posttransplantation. HbA1c normalized to 4.8% and has never been higher than 5.8% since. C-peptide levels remained within the normal range (Figure 18.1). Previous microangiopathy complications remained stable after islet transplantation and kidney function remained remarkably stable, most likely owing to proper glycemic control.

Conclusions. The authors explore the unique features that may have been critical determinants of success in this patient. Of the many possibilities, they propose that low metabolic demand, the immunosuppressive regimen, and low immune responsiveness, owing to excellent HLA donor–recipient matching with a high circulating regulatory T cells count, may have been important factors in the long-term islet graft survival.

Significance. This case clearly demonstrates that long-term insulin independence after allogeneic islet transplantation is a valid, achievable target. The resulting persistent, normal metabolic control was achieved with a single islet infusion of a marginal islet mass (less than 10,000 insulin equivalents per kilogram). As the first report of insulin independence for a post-transplantation period of over a decade, this case represents the first of many patients who were transplanted since the turn of the century who will achieve the symbolic 10 years of

(Continued)

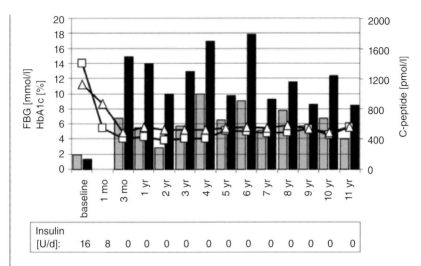

Figure 18.1 Follow-up of major metabolic parameters before and after islet transplantation. Left axis, HbA1c (%) is represented as open triangles, and fasting blood glucose (mmol/L) is represented as open squares. Right axis, basal, fasting C-peptide (pmol/L) is represented as gray histograms, and glucagon-stimulated C-peptide is represented as black histograms. Daily insulin requirements (U/day) are marked below the graph for each time point.

insulin independence. It is difficult to conclude which are the key determinants of long-term success from this single case, but the availability of a larger cohort to reach 10 years of independence of insulin administration in the near future will enable a more thorough examination of the critical factors for successful outcomes. This analysis will be important for reproducing long-term successful outcomes on a larger scale.

transplantation. Limitations associated with the early protocol restricted the application of this procedure mainly to patients whose clinical history already necessitated immunosuppressive drugs, such as those who had previously received another organ transplant.

Transition to the modern era of islet transplantation: the Edmonton protocol

Amid variable reports and unpredictable outcomes of islet allotransplantation emerged a pilot trial in seven patients from the University of Alberta in 2000 that dramatically affected the clinical course of islet transplantation. Implementation of this method, which became known as the Edmonton protocol, resulted in insulin independence and restoration of blood glucose

Table 18.1 Summary of the history of islet transplantation

Important steps in the development of clinical islet transplantation	
1960s	Methods for islet isolation developed in rodent models
1972	First successful islet transplantation in rats
1976	First successful islet transplantation in canines
1988	Method for human islet isolation and purification developed
1989	First successful human islet transplant
2000	Edmonton protocol developed

levels to a narrow physiological range in all seven patients for an average follow up of one year. The success of this clinical trial was attributed mainly to two factors: transplantation of an adequate number of high-quality islets and a glucocorticoid-free immunosuppressive protocol. To obtain a mean islet transplant mass of approximately 11,500 islet equivalents (IE) per kilogram recipient body weight, each recipient received islets from at least two donor pancreata. Additionally, to protect this infused islet mass more effectively from both allo- and autoimmune rejection and to minimize the diabetogenic effects of the immunosuppressant drugs, a glucocorticoid-free protocol of sirolimus, low-dose tacrolimus, and daclizumab (an anti-IL-2 mAb) was implemented. This significant trial in Edmonton became the ground from which the modern era of islet transplantation would emerge.

A summary of the history of islet transplantation is given in Table 18.1.

The present

Clinical

Since the Edmonton protocol marked the beginning of pancreatic islet transplantation as a viable treatment for type 1 diabetes, the original findings have been both replicated and expanded at clinical centers worldwide. The success of the Edmonton procedure resulted in series of multicenter clinical programs, such as the Immune Tolerance Network (ITN) Clinical Islet Transplant Trial [5] and the National Center for Research Resources (NCRR)-supported Islet Cell Resource Centers [6]. Additionally, the Collaborative Islet Transplant Registry (CITR) was established in 2001 to collect, analyze, and annually distribute data from islet programs (http://www.citregistry.org). Stringent regulations, imposed by the US Food and Drug Administration (FDA) and equivalent organizations in other countries, that define islets as a biological drug and islet transplantation as an experimental somatic cellular therapy currently limit clinical trials. However, both collaborative and single-center trials have improved upon previous results and continue to augment knowledge concerning the multiple facets of islet transplantation.

Overall, the ITN trial exhibited procedural safety and standardization across nine international centers under the Edmonton protocol, from pancreas selection to post-transplantation care. In 2006, this trial reported that 58% of recipients became insulin independent and that 44% retained insulin independence for one year. A dependence on center experience in islet isolation and immunosuppressant protocol was indicated, as three of the most experienced centers reported a 90% insulin independence rate [5]. Around this same time, the Edmonton five-year follow-up revealed that 80% of the patients maintained graft-derived C-peptide biosynthesis, but only 10% maintained insulin independence [7]. Despite evidence of a temporal decline of transplant function, with most recipients returning to insulin therapy by 5 years, the demonstration that insulin independence could be maintained over a longer time course in a small group of patients was promising.

In parallel with the ITN trial, substantial efforts were made in the USA to begin a network of clinical centers. In 2004, the NIH funded the Islet Resource Centers to specialize in the isolation, purification, and characterization of human islet cells for approved clinical or research protocols. Although many islets were shipped to numerous researchers, clinical application remained modest at best, mostly because of the high costs of the procedure and follow-up treatment and the low number of suitable organs available for transplantation. Clinical trials have been conducted at single centers, such as the University of Minnesota [8] and the University of Illinois at Chicago [9], using slightly different protocols aimed at improving clinical outcomes. In 2008, there were a total of 15 active islet transplant centers reported in the USA (http://www.citregistry.com).

According to the 2009 CITR report, 412 patients have received islet transplants from 1999 to 2008 at 37 medical centers, 347 of which were islet transplants alone and 65 of which were islet after kidney transplants. Donor and recipient characteristics, as well as methods, are fully described in the CITR report (http://www.citregistry.com). Briefly, recipients had to be between 18 and 65 years of age, with type 1 diabetes longer than five years poor diabetes control, including episodes of severe hypoglycemia and hypoglycemia unawareness, wide swings of blood glucose levels, or consistently high HbA1c levels (>8%). Overall, 70% of the recipients reached insulin independence, of which 70% remained free from exogenous insulin one year later. The percentage of recipients with HbA1c less than 6.5% and the absence of severe hypoglycemic episodes increased from 2% before transplant to approximately 60% at year one after the last islet infusion.

Consistent with reports from the ITN and Edmonton follow-up, a temporal trend of decreasing insulin independence is observed. However, this decline is substantially less drastic than that observed in the past (Table 18.2). Furthermore, these data include all transplant centers, even those that are no longer in practice. In contrast to the overall low rate of long-term insulin

Table 18.2 Comparison of past (1974–1999) and current (1999–2008) reports of the percentage of all recipients who are insulin independent across a period of four years after the last islet infusion. Reported transplants from 1974 to 1999 (n = 353) were recorded by the International Islet Transplant Registry at the University of Giessen and reported transplants from 1999 to 2008 (n = 347) were recorded by the CITR.

	1974–1999	1999–2008
6 months	10%	55%
12 months	8%	47%
24 months	5%	36%
36 months	2%	27%
48 months	<1%	16%

independence, single centers have observed insulin independence in over 50% of islet graft recipients five years after transplantation. Additionally, confirming reports from the ITN trial and Edmonton five-year follow-up, islet function even without insulin independence provides protection from severe hypoglycemia and can improve levels of glycosylated hemoglobin. The reason for the progressive loss of islets and graft function over time is not entirely understood; however, contributing factors include chronic allograft rejection, recurrence of autoimmunity, β-cell toxicity from immunosuppressive drugs, and immunosuppression-related loss of β-cell regenerative capacity [4].

As concluded from the current clinical trials, islet transplantation is a safe treatment that consistently demonstrates short-term benefits of insulin independence, stabilization of glucose metabolism, normal or near normal HbA1c levels, a significant decrease in severe hypoglycemic episodes, and a restoration of hypoglycemic awareness. Importantly, the wide-scale collection and distribution of data has enabled the analysis of procedural safety, risk factors important for potential recipients, and key determinants of success. Long-term primary efficacy, immunosuppression safety, and effects on secondary complications are not as well understood; however, these continue to be an important area of study and avenue for improvement.

Current transplant procedure and adverse events

The most common method for transplantation involves intraportal infusion of the isolated islets via percutaneous transhepatic portal vein catheterization with subsequent embolization in the liver [10]. The liver site has been extensively characterized; however, it remains unclear if this is the optimal transplant site. It is estimated that only 25–50% of the infused islet mass engrafts in the recipient, as a result of the initial islet mass loss due to the resulting instant blood-mediated inflammatory reaction (IBMIR) and hypoxia before neovascularization. Despite the implementation of heparin

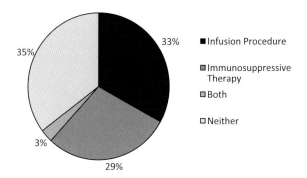

Figure 18.2 Breakdown of the serious adverse events reported to the CITR within year one after islet transplantation. Of the total islet recipients, 44% reported one or more serious adverse events. Most reported adverse events were attributed to the infusion procedure and/or immunosuppression therapy.

in clinical trials to reduce the initial clotting process, IBMIR-induced cell death, which involves leukocyte infiltration of the islets, continues to limit optimal β-cell function. Furthermore, it is estimated that a neovascular capillary network of host origin is not well established until 10–14 days after islet transplant and, therefore, islets are susceptible to death by hypoxia [11]. Additional sites have been proposed, but not extensively explored.

As a minimally invasive surgery, islet transplantation has a lower morbidity rate than whole organ pancreas transplantation. The occurrence of death caused by adverse events was reported as 1.5% by the CITR in the 412 islet graft recipients from 1999 to 2008. Despite a relatively low mortality rate, adverse side effects exist. Most serious adverse side effects are related to the infusion procedure and/or immunosuppression therapy (Figure 18.2). The potential complications of an infusion into the liver include bleeding, portal vein thrombosis, and portal hypertension. Reported adverse effects of sirolimus and tacrolimus include painful oral ulceration, diarrhea, peripheral edema, proteinuria, anemia, neutropenia, hypertension, and hypercholesterolaemia [4]. Approximately 82% of reported events have resolved with no residual effects. Overall, this minimally invasive surgery presents few adverse side effects independent from immunosuppression-related side effects typically associated with solid organ transplantation.

What currently impedes success?

1. Donor factors
Currently the demand for human islets significantly exceeds the supply of human pancreatic tissue. In the USA alone, type 1 diabetes accounts for 5–10% of all diagnosed cases of diabetes in persons aged 20 years or older,

which is estimated at approximately 18 million, with an additional 1.6 million new cases diagnosed each year (http://www.niddk.nih.gov). In contrast, there are approximately 6000 multi-organ donor per year in the USA, of whom only about 40% are suitable as a pancreas donor. This large discrepancy between supply and demand inherently limits the clinical applicability of this treatment worldwide.

Underscoring the prevalent and pervasive problem of donor shortage is the issue of donor factors specific to islet isolation and transplant outcome. Donor factors have been extensively researched and include body mass index, age, cause of death, hemodynamic stability, and surgical technique. Low islet yields have been associated with donor factors such as low body mass index, age below 20 years, uncontrolled hyperglycemia, duration of cardiac arrest, cold ischemia time, prolonged hypotensive episodes, pancreas capsular damage, and elevated serum creatinine levels [12]. One factor with a particularly detrimental effect on islet isolation outcome is cold ischemia time; more than eight hours of cold storage before human islet isolation significantly reduces islet yield and functional viability [13]. Despite attempts to optimize organ procurement and preservation, the variability of donor factors prevents consistent isolation success. Donor factors, for the most part, are not subject to change and can be influenced only by adequate donor selection. In consideration of the dependence of transplant outcome on islet yield and function, optimal donor selection is critical to maximize efficient use of this limited resource and minimize wasteful transplants.

2. Manufacturing

During the manufacturing process, even the highest-grade preparations only recover about 20–50% of the potential islet mass and less than half of the processed pancreata yield a transplantable islet mass [4]. In consideration of the donor shortage, extraneous variables other than pancreas quality that lead to inconsistent outcomes in the manufacturing of islets are particularly concerning. Even at leading centers, the rate of successful islet isolations varies widely. Despite intensified efforts to increase procedural standardization, many factors, such as lot-to-lot enzyme variability and temporal deterioration of enzyme quality and strength [14], remain challenging obstacles that contribute to inconsistent isolation outcomes both between centers and within individual centers. Owing to the low success rate of islet isolations that yield sufficient islets for transplantation, most cases require the use of multiple donors. Typically, two or three infusions of islets isolated from a total of two to four donors have been required for recipients to achieve insulin independence (Figure 18.3).

In the past few years, advances in the field have enabled successful transplantation outcomes using islets isolated from a single donor. For instance, clinical trials from Minnesota [8] and the University of Illinois at Chicago

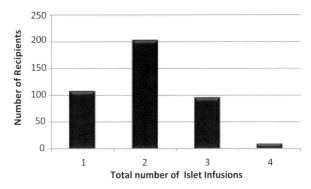

Figure 18.3 Total number of islet infusion procedures per recipient, as reported to the CITR. After the first infusion, 74% of recipients are re-infused. A total of 905 donors were required for the 412 islet transplant recipients from 1999 to 2008.

[9] suggest that use of etanercept, a tumor-necrosis factor (TNF)-α receptor antagonist, facilitates the achievement of insulin independence with fewer islets through its anti-inflammatory effects. In addition to increasing the number of patients who can be transplanted, advantages of single-donor islet transplantation include decreasing both the expense, by limiting organ acquisition costs, and risk of immunological sensitization, by avoiding exposure to multiple donors. However, the use of single donors is not consistent or widespread.

CASE STUDY 18.2

This patient presented with multiple autoimmune diseases, including type I diabetes mellitus, hypothyroidism, vitiligo, and lupus with arthritis. The patient received a total of three islet infusions as part of the University of Illinois at Chicago phase 1/2 islet transplant clinical study. At the time of the first transplantation, the patient had been diagnosed with type 1 diabetes for over 40 years, from the age of seven years, and required 35–38 units per day of insulin. The first two transplants of 877,000 EIN and 481,000 EIN, respectively, occurred within an eight-month period. After both of these transplants, insulin could be discontinued for a period of less than four months, but insulin therapy had to be resumed because of declining islet graft function. Both islet transplants had been performed under induction therapy with a humanized, monoclonal anti-IL-2 receptor antibody, tacrolimus, and sirolimus. The first two transplants showed suboptimal graft function, despite excellent quality islet preparations infused. Both transplants eventually ceased functioning.

In the presence of multiple autoimmune diseases and the limited success of two previous islet transplants, the patient was given more potent immunosuppression for her third transplant by using rabbit polyclonal anti-thymocyte antibody. The third transplantation was completed more than two years after the second transplant, and yielded a remarkable success. Insulin was discontinued less than four weeks after infusion of 474,000 EIN and this patient has remained insulin independent for over a year, with normal HbA1c and with completely normal oral glucose tolerance. The patient has near-normal insulin secretory reserves during intravenous glucose challenge, which is hardly ever achieved after islet transplantation.

The reason for success after the third transplant may be attributed to the change in immunosuppressive induction. However, this patient had an additional, distinct, concomitant treatment that was started by her rheumatologist a few weeks after the third transplant for intractable arthritic pain. She received an IL1 receptor antagonist. Interestingly, IL-RA had been previously shown to increase islet function in patients with type II diabetes. It is difficult to conclude from a single case whether IL-RA had any role in the observed outcome, but this report shows that modern immunosuppression can achieve excellent islet transplant outcomes even in patients with very reactive immune systems. The role of various cytokines and the clinical effects of their blockade in islet graft function is an area that deserves further clinical investigation.

Variability in isolation and, subsequently, transplant outcome is exacerbated by the fact that pre-transplant measures used to determine islet cell quality are not consistently predictive of transplant outcome. Currently accepted tests include DNA-binding dye exclusion, dithizone (DTZ) staining, and in vitro glucose-stimulated insulin release. The use of low quality islet preparations that remain undetected by current assessment techniques may be a factor at centers that have reported difficulty replicating the Edmonton results [15]. The in vivo assessment of isolated islets, by transplantation into immunodeficient mice, provides predictive value for islet function [16]; however, the time required for this test renders it impractical for application in clinical settings. Processing of islet cells is also covered in the sister tissue and cell book to this one (Fehily D, Brubaker SA, Kearney JN, Wolfinbarger L (eds). *Tissue and Cell Processing: An Essential Guide*. Blackwell Publishing Ltd. 2012).

3. Chronic immunosuppression

Although recent changes in the immunosuppressive protocol have dramatically improved clinical outcomes, the need to balance potent drugs with serious adverse effects persists. The requirement of chronic immunosuppression, to control both donor allo- and autoimmunity, limits this treatment to patients with severe glycemic lability and hinders its application to a broader proportion of the type 1 diabetic population. For instance, the estimated 15,000 youth in the USA who are annually diagnosed with type 1 diabetes (http://www.niddk.nih.gov), in which early prevention of the many devastating long-term complications would be of significant medical and economic benefit, are excluded from this treatment.

CASE STUDY 18.3

This patient, as part of the University of Illinois at Chicago phase 1/2 islet transplant clinical study, received two islet infusions of 404,000 equivalent islet number (EIN) and 560,000 during a six-week period. The patient's past medical history included the diagnosis of type 1 diabetes in his twenties, coronary artery disease, chronic venous insufficiency in both legs, and hypertension. At the time of islet transplantation, he had been diagnosed with type 1 diabetes for 37 years. He became insulin independent two months after his last transplant and displayed consistently normal glycemic control for five years, but at that stage was admitted after complaints of malaise and fevers for three weeks, with concurrent diarrhea, nausea, and vague abdominal pain. He was hospitalized for two weeks and was diagnosed with cytomegalovirus pneumonia. After diagnosis, he commenced gancicolvir, an antiviral agent, and his immunosuppression decreased. Cytomegalovirus resolved, but before immunosuppression could be increased again, he presented with elevated blood sugar levels and had to resume low-dose insulin administration. Currently, the patient still uses approximately half of the insulin (13–22 units per day) compared with pre-transplant (34–41 units per day).

This case exemplifies the dilemma of immunosuppression. At present, there are no reliable tests available that could help the clinician determine the immunosuppressive level required to prevent rejection without unduly increasing the risk for opportunistic infections. Post-transplantation, the patient presented with an opportunistic infection as a consequence of over-immunosuppression and, subsequently, presented with decreased graft function, probably owing to rejection from reduced immunosuppression. Finding a balance between the consequences of too much or too little immunosuppression is not a clinical challenge unique to islet transplantation, but rather represents one of the most difficult clinical problems in all areas of transplantation.

Modification of the immunosuppression protocol remains an important area of study to improve clinical safety and applicability. Substantial work has been conducted to improve long-term islet graft function, such as the successful use of antithymoglobulin and anti-CD3 monoclonal antibodies in the peri-transplant period in single-donor islet transplant protocols [8, 17]. In addition to modification of the current immunosuppressive protocol, attempts have been made to completely circumvent the need for chronic immunosuppression. Extensive research has been conducted concerning immune tolerance, which remains an elusive goal. Several immuno-isolation systems have been developed, including perfusion shunt devices anastomosed to the vascular system, diffusion chambers of macrocapsules, and microcapsules; none of these approaches has been successfully applied in patients.

One immuno-isolation method that has displayed promising clinical potential in the prevention of autoimmune destruction and graft rejection is microencapsulation. Since the first evidence that microencapsulated islets could regulate blood glucose in rats in 1980 [18], the ability of micro-encapsulated islets to reverse chemically induced diabetes has since been confirmed in small and large animal models, including monkeys and dogs. Calafiore et al. (2006) conducted the first clinical trial of microencapsulated islets in non-immunosuppressed patients with type 1 diabetes in Italy; however, the recipients were unable to withdraw from exogenous insulin [19]. More recent research and preclinical trials, such as the development of a novel five-component/three-membrane hybrid capsule system that enables sustained islet graft function in non-immunosuppressed diabetic dogs for up to seven months [20], have expanded interest in the clinical application of microencapsulated islets in the future. Until such technology becomes clinically available, however, the adverse effects of chronic immu-nosuppression, in relation to both patient health and islet graft function, remains a significant hindrance to the expansion of islet transplantation to a broader proportion of affected individuals. A summary of the current limitations associated with the multiple steps of islet transplantation is given in Plate 18.1.

Preclinical research

Results from clinical studies have provided the proof-of-principle that res-toration of a sufficient functional β-cell mass can alleviate and even elimi-nate symptoms of type 1 diabetes. The current limitations of this treatment, especially the restricted pool of high quality donor organs, have provided the impetus in the search for alternative sources of β cells. Major alternatives include the use of porcine islets for xenotransplantation and the creation of new human β cells. Under the latter alternative, three possibilities currently exist: the proliferation of existing β cells, the use of embryonic or adult stem cells, and cellular reprogramming of other cell types.

Xenotransplantation

The successful use of porcine insulin before the development of synthetic insulin demonstrates sufficient metabolic function in humans. Methods have already been developed to isolate high quantities of islets from porcine pancreata and substantial work has recently been dedicated to exploring the option of transplanting these porcine islets. Currently, 15 institutions have conducted 181 preclinical xenotransplants in non-human primates and mul-tiple groups have reported insulin independence for time periods greater than three months [21]. Recently the International Xenotransplantation Association has identified three main hurdles to overcome before consider-ing the clinical implementation of porcine xenotransplants: immunologic rejection, physiologic incompatibility, and risk of transmission of porcine pathogens [22]. Although pathogen-free breeding of pigs can prevent the transmission of most porcine microbes, porcine endogenous retroviruses (PERV), which are integrated in the pig genome and can infect human cells in vitro, remain a serious risk. The development of RNA interference technology to knockdown post-transcriptional gene expression offers promise in combating this issue. Indeed, preliminary studies have shown that a combination of nuclear transfer cloning and RNA interference can produce pigs that do not propagate PERV [23].

Evidence of success in preclinical studies provides a strong impetus for continued development of islet xenotransplantation in nonhuman primates. Xenotransplantation remains an important long-term option; however, serious epidemiological and ethical considerations have prompted many others to focus on the reproduction of human tissue to solve the problem of limited resources in the face of high demand.

Creation of new human β cells
1. Proliferation of existing β cells
Although β cells represent a highly differentiated cell type, it is evident that the adult population maintains its ability to divide and that this basal rate of proliferation is subject to modulation by a variety of intrinsic and extrinsic factors. For instance, β-cell mass is known to increase under certain conditions, such as during pregnancy and in an insulin-resistance state, and regenerate after certain circumstances of stress and injury [24]. Evidence suggests that proliferation of existing β cells may be the primary mode for both maintenance and expansion under normal adult homeostasis and regeneration after injury. As indicated by Dor et al. (2004), the major source of new β cells in the adult mouse pancreas is the proliferation of preexisting β cells [25]. Further research in this area by Nir et al. (2007) indicates that proliferation of surviving β cells is the primary mode for regeneration after specific and inducible destruction of β cells in transgenic mice [26]. In the human pancreas, there appears to be an age-related decreased capacity for plasticity; however, ongoing attempts of β-cell regeneration occur in aged adults, even in patients with long-standing type 1 diabetes [27].

Evidence that terminally differentiated β cells retain proliferative capacity and that certain physiological and pathological conditions can modulate this proliferation rate suggests the possibility to increase β-cell mass in vivo in patients with diabetes. Additionally, it may be possible to induce proliferation in vitro to create an unlimited source for transplant. Substantial efforts have been made to identify external stimuli that can expand primary β cells. A large-scale high throughput, cell-based screen by Wang et al. (2009) identified several small molecules that induce proliferation in growth-arrested, reversibly immortalized mouse β cells. The mechanisms underlying the regulation of β-cell mass and aspects of cell cycle regulation in relation to β-cell replication have been examined and other potential compounds to induce proliferation have been identified, such as HGF, human growth hormone, exendin-4, and high glucose concentration [28]. Whether these findings can be extended to human β cells remains unknown. Continued research on this topic will undoubtedly enhance knowledge on the cellular processes that control β-cell proliferation and the potential to create an unlimited source of human cells in vitro for islet transplantation.

2. Stem cells

Recent research in the field of developmental biology has increased our understanding of pancreatic development substantially, as well as the prospect of recreating this process in vitro to induce β-cell differentiation from stem cell sources. The knowledge that β cells normally arise from an endodermally derived, pancreas-specified precursor cell and that when transplanted these cells secrete insulin in a glucose-responsive manner has prompted attempts to create new β cells from embryonic stem cell sources [29]. Critical steps and necessary signaling molecules for proper β-cell formation have been identified in both mice and humans; this current knowledge of factors related to the emergence of endocrine β cells from pancreatic endoderm are extensively reviewed elsewhere [30]. Recently, several groups have been successful in generating endoderm and even insulin-producing cells with β-cell-like characteristics from embryonic stem cells [31]. However, these in vitro derived cells fail to adopt a normal β-cell fate completely. To design safe and effective clinical protocols, much work remains in understanding the processes that guide pancreatic specification, endocrine differentiation, and β-cell maturation.

Alternatively, induced differentiation of stem cells residing in the adult pancreas may present a source for new β cells. Contrary to past common belief that β-cell progenitors disappear during postnatal life, recent evidence suggests that the adult pancreas may retain the ability to activate progenitors under certain conditions. For instance, Ngn3 expression is induced in the mouse pancreas after partial duct ligation and can give rise to insulin-producing β cells [32]. It has been proposed that a resident stem/progenitor cell is the source of these Ngn3 positive cells. In support of this, Rovira et al. (2010) have recently identified a population of cells residing in a centroacinar/terminal ductal position in the adult mouse pancreas with the ability to form pancreatospheres that display glucose-responsive insulin secretion and have the capacity to differentiate into both endocrine and exocrine embryonic lineages [33]. It remains to be tested whether similar cells in the adult human pancreas can be isolated, expanded, and differentiated into glucose-responsive insulin-positive cells.

3. Reprogramming other mature cell types into β cells

Reprogramming, or the conversion of terminally differentiated existing cells into β cells, represents an alternative strategy to solve the current limited supply of β cells. This field has significantly expanded since 2006, when the demonstration that somatic cell nuclear transfer can reprogram differentiated adult cells into a totipotent state contradicted the previous belief that development is a one-way process. Recently, evidence for induced-pluripotent stem cells has immensely expanded the potential direction for cell-based therapy [34]. Under this option, induced-pluripotent stem cells may provide an alternative to embryonic stem cells for in vitro induced differentiation. This method would allow the generation of patient-specific β cells and, thus, would importantly circumvent the current limitation of the need for chronic immunosuppressive medication.

Alternatively, reprogramming without reversion to a pluripotent stem cell state constitutes a means to achieve the end β-cell fate. Specific to β cells, it has been shown that acinar cells from the exocrine pancreas of adult mice can be reprogrammed into endocrine, insulin-producing β cells [35]. This reprogramming by Zhou et al. (2008) was accomplished by in vivo adenoviral vector delivery of a combination of three key developmental transcription factors (Pdx1, Ngn3, and Mafa) and was sufficient to ameliorate hyperglycemia in diabetic mice. Reprogramming of alternative cells that are more abundant and easily accessible, such as fibroblasts or blood cells, may be more advantageous than reprogramming exocrine cells. Recent evidence by Yechoor et al. (2009) suggests that Ngn-3-induced β-cell neogenesis occurs through transdifferentiation from hepatic progenitor cells [36]. Here again, evidence that such phenomenon can occur and be exploited in human cells remains to be explored. Additionally, safer reagents to deliver instructive factors and extra measures to avoid the risk of teratomas need to be developed before clinical implementation can be considered.

The future

Although the concept of transplanting islets for the treatment of diabetes has existed for over a century, several technical and biological barriers have impeded clinical application of this approach. As a result of ongoing improvements in the past two decades, however, islet transplantation has moved forward from clinical potential to clinical reality and has now been demonstrated as a safe and effective therapy for select patients with type 1 diabetes. Indeed, the insulin independence rate one year after transplant has more than quadrupled since the Edmonton protocol was first implemented. Furthermore, recent advances in pre-isolation organ preservation and post-isolation islet cell preservation have expanded the degree to which regional islet processing centers and distant clinical islet transplant programs can collaborate. This provides a promising avenue for the immediate expansion of clinical trials, which is imperative in order to implement controlled new strategies for future improvements in islet transplantation.

Continued clinical trials that demonstrate safety and efficacy will be necessary to acquire a biologics license in the future. For islet transplantation to become an FDA-licensed therapy, a well-established islet preparation process and product manufacturing consistency will need to be demonstrated. To expand the impact of this promising treatment significantly, it will be necessary to explore further and use novel strategies in the areas of immunosuppressive therapy and alternative sources of β cells. Clinical trials for proof of concept of new immunosuppressive strategies that ameliorate the side effects and risks of immunosuppression will be important. For instance, the substitution of calcineurin inhibitors, such as tacrolimus, with more specific immunosuppressive drugs that have fewer side effects will be a desirable goal. Moreover, novel strategies will aim at promoting the engraftment and survival of transplanted islets to improve long-term graft function and insulin independence in transplant recipients. The ultimate goal is to eliminate the need for chronic immunosuppression, through promising technologies such as microencapsulation, to expand this treatment safely to a broader proportion of type 1 diabetics, such as the juvenile population and women who wish to become pregnant.

Additionally, ongoing efforts to find alternative β-cell sources offer promise for the widespread expansion of islet transplantation. Many possibilities exist, from xenotransplantation to the creation of new β cells through proliferation of existing β cells, cellular reprogramming of other cell types, and the reproducible and scalable differentiation of embryonic or pluripotent stem cells. Significant recent advances have been made in each area, although it remains unclear which option will be the most successful in the future. A better understanding of the proliferation and differentiation processes taking place in progenitor and fully differentiated β cells will undoubtedly facilitate the process of creating an unlimited transplant supply. Future challenges include improving the efficiency of differentiation into a stable mature β-cell phenotype and simultaneously eliminating the generation of unwanted cell types.

As the current limitations of islet transplantation are progressively overcome (Plate 18.1), the clinical application will greatly expand from a stringently regulated treatment, limited to controlled clinical research trials, to a licensed, more widely available cellular therapy that can be offered as a routine, alternative treatment for patients with type 1 diabetes. The ultimate goal of islet transplantation, to correct completely the diabetic state from an unlimited donor source without the need for chronic immunosuppressive therapy (Plate 18.2), remains a challenging, yet legitimate, prospect for the future.

KEY LEARNING POINTS

- The history of islet transplantation is given in Table 18.1.

- Present limitations that prevent more widespread clinical application include donor factors, variability in the manufacturing process, and the need for chronic immunosuppression.

- The islet manufacturing process involves (1) perfusion of the donor pancreas with digestive enzyme, (2) mechanical dissociation in a temperature-controlled digestion chamber, (3) collection of digested tissue, and (4) separation of islets from exocrine tissue by density-gradient centrifugation.

- After islet isolation from donor pancreas, the islets are infused into the portal vein and, subsequently engraft and form a neovascular capillary network in the liver. These transplanted islet cells produce insulin and maintain physiological glucose homeostasis.

- The reason for the progressive loss of islets and graft function over time is not entirely understood; however, contributing factors include chronic allograft rejection, recurrence of autoimmunity, β-cell toxicity from immunosuppressive drugs, and immunosuppression-related loss of β-cell regenerative capacity. In the area of immunosuppression, research is devoted to developing drugs that are more permissive for islet survival and technology, such as microencapsulation of islets, which would completely circumvent the need for chronic immunosuppression. Additionally, investigation of alternative β-cell sources to develop an unlimited supply of insulin-producing tissue (i.e. the stimulation of endogenous β cells, ex vivo differentiation of β cells from stem cells, cellular reprogramming, and xenotransplantation) represents an approach to prevent islet graft loss.

References

1. Williams PW. Notes on diabetes treated with grafts of sheep's pancreas. Br Med J 1894;2:1303.
2. Pybus F. Notes on suprarenal and pancreatic grafting. Lancet 1924;2:550–1.
3. Ricordi C, Lacy PE, Finke EH, et al. Automated-method for isolation of human pancreatic-islets. Diabetes 1988;37:413–20.
4. Ichii H, Ricordi C. Current status of islet cell transplantation. J Hepatobiliary Pancreat Surg 2009;16:101–12.
5. Shapiro AM, Ricordi C, Hering BJ, et al. International trial of the Edmonton protocol for islet transplantation. N Engl J Med 2006;355:1318–30.
6. National Center for Research Resources NIDDK and JDF: Human Pancreatic Islet Resources (ICRs): Request for application, http://grants.nih.gov/grants/guide/rfa-files/RFA-RR-01-002.html, accessed February 2010.

7. Ryan EA, Paty BW, Senior PA, et al. Five-year follow-up after clinical islet transplantation. Diabetes 2005;54:2060–9.

8. Hering BJ, Kandaswamy R, Ansite JD, et al. Single-donor, marginal-dose islet transplantation in patients with type 1 diabetes. JAMA 2005;293:830–5.

9. Gangemi A, Salehi P, Hatipoglu B, et al. Islet transplantation for brittle type 1 diabetes: the UIC protocol. Am J Transplant 2008;8:1250–61.

10. Merani S, Toso C, Emamaullee J, et al. Optimal implantation site for pancreatic islet transplantation. Brit J Sur 2008;95:1449–61.

11. Merchant FA, Diller KR, Aggarwal SJ, et al. Angiogenesis in cultured and cryopreserved pancreatic islet grafts. Transplantation 1997;63:1652–60.

12. Toso C, Oberholzer J, Ris F, et al. Factors affecting human islet of Langerhans isolation yields. Transplant Proc 2002;34:826–7.

13. Lakey JRT, Rajotte RV, Warnock GL,, et al. Human pancreas preservation before islet isolation – cold ischemic tolerance. Transplantation 1995;59:689–94.

14. Yamamoto T, Ricordi C, Messinger S, et al. Deterioration and variability of highly purified collagenase blends used in clinical islet isolation. Transplantation 2007; 84:997–1002.

15. Ault A. Edmonton's islet success tough to duplicate elsewhere. Lancet 2003;361: 2054.

16. Ichii H, Inverardi L, Pileggi A, et al. A novel method for the assessment of cellular composition and beta-cell viability in human islet preparations. Am J Transplant 2005;5:1635–45.

17. Hering BJ, Kandaswamy R, Harmon JV, et al. Transplantation of cultured islets from two-layer preserved pancreases in type 1 diabetes with anti-CD3 antibody. Am J Transplant 2004;4:390–401.

18. Lim F, Sun AM. (1980) Microencapsulated islets as bioartificial endocrine pancreas. Science 210, 908–10.

19. Calafiore R, Basta G, Luca G, et al. Microencapsulated pancreatic islet allografts into nonimmunosuppressed patients with type 1 diabetes: first two cases. Diabetes Care 2006;29:137–8.

20. Wang T, Adcock J, Kuhtreiber W, et al. Successful allotransplantation of encapsulated islets in pancreatectomized canines for diabetic management without the use of immunosuppression. Transplantation 2008;85:331–7.

21. Hering BJ, Walawalkar N. Pig-to-nonhuman primate islet xenotransplantation. Transplant Immunol 2009;21:81–6.

22. Hering BJ, Cooper DKC, Cozzi E, et al. The International Xenotransplantation Association consensus statement on conditions for undertaking clinical trials of porcine islet products in type 1 diabetes – executive summary. Xenotransplantation 2009; 16:196–202.

23. Ramsoondar J, Vaught T, Ball S, et al. Production of transgenic pigs that express porcine and endogenous retrovirus small interfering RNAs. Xenotransplantation 2009;16:164–80.

24. Borowiak M, Melton DA. How to make β cells? Curr Opin Cell Biol 2009; 21:727–32.

25. Dor Y, Brown J, Martinez OI, et al. Adult pancreatic beta-cells are formed by self-duplication rather than stem-cell differentiation. Nature 2004;429:41–6.

26. Nir T, Melton DA, Dor Y. Recovery from diabetes in mice by beta cell regeneration. J Clin Invest 2007;117:2553–61.

27. Meier JJ, Bhushan A, Butler AE, et al. Sustained beta cell apoptosis in patients with long-standing type 1 diabetes: indirect evidence for islet regeneration? Diabetologia 2005;48:2221–8.

28. Wang WD, Walker JR, Wang X, et al. Identification of small-molecule inducers of pancreatic beta-cell expansion. Proc Natl Acad Sci USA 2009;106:1427–32.

29. Kroon E, Martinson LA, Kadoya K,, et al. Pancreatic endoderm derived from human embryonic stem cells generates glucose-responsive insulin-secreting cells in vivo. Nat Biotechnol 2008;26:443–52.

30. Oliver-Krasinski JM, Stoffers DA. On the origin of the beta cell. Genes Dev 2008;22:1998–2021.

31. D'Amour KA, Agulnick AD, Eliazer S, et al. Efficient differentiation of human embryonic stem cells to definitive endoderm. Nat Biotechnol 2005;23:1534–41.

32. Xu D, D'Hoker J, Stange G, et al. Beta cells can be generated from endogenous progenitors in injured adult mouse pancreas. Cell 2008;132:197–207.

33. Rovira M, Scott SG, Liss AS, et al. Isolation and characterization of centroacinar/terminal ductal progenitor cells in adult mouse pancreas. Proc Nat Acad Sci USA 2010;107:75–80.

34. Okita K, Ischisaka T, Yamanaka S. Generation of germline-competent induced pluripotent stem cells. Nature 2007;448:313–7.

35. Zhou Q, Brown J, Kanarek A, et al. In vivo reprogramming of adult pancreatic exocrine cells to beta-cells. Nature 2008;455:627–32.

36. Yechoor V, Liu V, Espiritu C, et al. Neurogenin3 is sufficient for transdetermination of hepatic progenitor cells into neo-islets in vivo but not transdifferentiation of hepatocytes. Dev Cell 2009;16:358–73.

37. Berney T, Ferrari-Lacraz S, Buhler L et al. Long-term insulin-independence after allogenic islet transplantation for type 1 diabetes: over the 10-year mark. Am J Transplant 2009;9:419–23.

19 Stem Cells for Cardiac Repair

Ranil de Silva[1,2], Amish N. Raval[3], and John R. Pepper[1,2]

[1]Royal Brompton and Harefield NHS Foundation Trust, London, UK
[2]National Heart and Lung Institute, Imperial College London, London, UK
[3]University of Wisconsin School of Medicine and Public Health, Madison, WI, USA

Introduction

Cardiovascular disease is the leading cause of death in both the developed and developing world. Many patients have poor clinical outcomes and remain significantly limited by symptoms despite contemporary community and hospital-based treatments. New therapies are clearly required to address this important unmet clinical need. The heart shows inadequate ability to repair itself after myocardial infarction and other forms of heart disease, resulting in significant impairment of contractile function and adverse ventricular remodelling, which are the major determinants of adverse clinical outcome. Improvement of cardiac function through delivery of novel cellular therapies with the aim of replacing lost cells has therefore been a major strategic focus for the emerging field of regenerative medicine. Functional benefits of cell therapy for cardiovascular applications may arise from induction of angiogenesis, cardiomyogenesis, cardioprotection, or mechanical interstitial support. The first three modes of benefit may result from site-specific transdifferentiation of administered cells or by secretion of paracrine factors that may stimulate endogenous repair or protective mechanisms. On this basis, improvements in regional myocardial perfusion, systolic function, diastolic function, and adverse ventricular remodelling would be predicted. The additional mechanical interstitial support provided by cell administration may itself impact beneficially on the ventricular remodelling process. Clearly these potential benefits need to be weighed against the potential toxicity from cell therapy, such as exacerbation of atherosclerosis,

Tissue and Cell Clinical Use: An Essential Guide, First Edition. Edited by Ruth M. Warwick and Scott A. Brubaker.
© 2012 Blackwell Publishing Ltd. Published 2012 by Blackwell Publishing Ltd.

arrhythmogenesis (abnormal rhythm), inappropriate calcification, and local or ectopic tumor formation. In this chapter, we review the current status of cellular therapy for cardiovascular applications and highlight challenges that must be addressed before routine clinical use.

Skeletal myoblasts

Skeletal myoblasts are lineage-restricted progenitor cells that can be isolated from skeletal muscle biopsies and expanded ex vivo before delivery. These cells can adopt a striated muscle phenotype in the form of myotubes after engraftment, and have undergone extensive preclinical evaluation. These cells show evidence of contraction, but have limited capacity for electromechanical incorporation into the host myocardial syncytium. Recently, the first randomized placebo-controlled trial (MAGIC) [1], which involved the transepicardial injection of 4×10^8 or 8×10^8 myoblasts in 97 patients with ischemic cardiomyopathy and left ventricular ejection fraction (LVEF) less than 35% at the time of coronary artery bypass grafting (CABG), reported no improvement of contractile function, but did result in a trend for reduced left ventricular volumes in the high-dose group. An increased rate of ventricular tachyarrhythmia (rapid heart rhythm) was noted in patients randomized to myoblast administration, which is consistent with observations in previous non-randomized studies. These results have curbed enthusiasm for cellular cardiomyoplasty with skeletal myoblasts in patients with ischemic cardiomyopathy. However, the reduction in left ventricular volumes noted in the MAGIC trial is of interest and warrants further investigation of alternative strategies, including surgical transplantation of myoblasts embedded within a biological scaffold onto the epicardial surface of infarcted myocardium [2] and use of myoblasts transfected with gap junction protein connexin-43, which may facilitate electromechanical coupling, thereby reducing the risk of ventricular arrhythmia [3].

Bone marrow mononuclear cells

Unselected cell preparations
Preclinical studies have suggested the capacity for bone marrow-derived progenitor cells to undergo trans-differentiation into cells with myocardial and/or endothelial phenotypes, as well as to produce hemodynamic improvements in experimental models of acute non-re-perfused myocardial infarction [4]. Subsequent investigations challenged the notion that bone marrow

mononuclear cells (BMMNCs) can trans-differentiate into cardiac myocytes [5, 6], and have led to the concept that BMMNCs act predominantly through paracrine mechanisms which promote microcirculatory function and cyto-protection through prevention of apoptosis [7].

The early preclinical data provided the basis for rapid translation to phase I trials of unselected bone marrow mononuclear cells in patients with acute myocardial infarction and ischemic cardiomyopathy, delivered by intracoronary infusion and endomyocardial injection, respectively [8]. These studies confirmed procedural safety for the delivery methods and suggested no short-term toxicity arising from the delivered cells. All of these studies reported significant improvements in LVEF, despite significant variations in cell dose and timing of administration [8]. The magnitude of improvement in left ventricular function observed in these initial open-label, non-randomized, non-placebo controlled trials could not be replicated in the first generation randomized clinical trials in patients with acute electrocardiographic ST elevation myocardial infarction (STEMI). In the randomized trials so far, BMMNC were administered by intracoronary infusion 1–12 days after re-perfusion for acute STEMI. Recent meta-analyses have suggested that BMMNC administration in patients with acute STEMI is associated with an approximately 3% increase in LVEF, approximately 5 mL reduction in left ventricular end systolic volume and approximately 3.5% reduction in myocardial infarct size compared to placebo [9, 10]. These benefits are modest and have not translated into an overall reduction in major adverse clinical events [9]. However, local BMMNC administration offers a trend to more benefit in the subset of patients with greatest impairment in ventricular function [11, 12]. Several factors have been suggested to contribute to the variability of results reported in the clinical trials, which include trial design, cell preparation protocol, timing of cell delivery, cell dose, and method for measurement of functional change. Some of these will be addressed in the next generation of BMMNC therapy trials in acute STEMI (Table 19.1). These trials stem from initial studies that showed BMMNC therapy to be safe and associated with an improvement in LVEF of similar magnitude to other treatments such as re-perfusion, ACE inhibition, and beta blockade after acute STEMI [13].

BMMNCs have also been administered to patients with chronic myocardial infarction and ischemic cardiomyopathy, either by intracoronary infusion or direct myocardial injection. The latter can be performed trans-epicardially at the time of CABG or trans-endocardially using a percutaneous endomyocardial injection catheter. Open label studies in this patient group have demonstrated significant improvements in LVEF, myocardial perfusion, and cardiopulmonary exercise testing. In general, these studies have enrolled small numbers of patients. In the surgical studies with concomitant coronary bypass revascularization, it has been difficult to distinguish the effects of the injected cells from the potential confounding effects of revascularization on

Table 19.1 Recently reported or ongoing cardiovascular cell therapy trials. (Reproduced from Wollert KC, Drexler H. Nat Rev Cardiol.7(4):204–215.)

Study identifier	Trial name	Number of patients	Cells	Primary end point	Route of cell delivery
Non-ST-elevation acute coronary syndrome					
Clinical trial NCT00711542	REPAIR-ACS	100	Bone marrow-derived progenitor cells	Coronary flow reserve	Intracoronary
Acute myocardial infarction					
Controlled trial ISRCTN17457407	BOOST-2	200	Bone marrow cells Low vs high cell number Nonirradiated vs irradiated cells	LVEF	Intracoronary
Clinical trial NCT00355186	SWISS-AMI	150	Bone marrow-derived stem cells	LVEF	Intracoronary Day 5–7 vs day 21–28
Clinical trial NCT00684021	TIME	120	Bone marrow mononuclear cells	LVEF	Intracoronary Day 3 vs day 7 post AMI
Clinical trial NCT00684060	Late TIME	87	Bone marrow mononuclear cells	LVEF	Intracoronary 2–3 weeks post AMI
Clinical trial NCT00501917	MAGIC Cell-5	116	Peripheral blood stem cells mobilized with G-CSF vs G-CSF with darbepoetin	LVEF	Intracoronary
Clinical trial NCT00877903	—	220	Allogeneic mesenchymal stem cells	LVESV	Intravenous
Clinical trial NCT00677222	—	28	Allogeneic mesenchymal stem cells	Safety	Perivascular
Ischemic heart failure					
Clinical trial NCT00526253	MARVEL	390	Skeletal myoblasts	6m in walk test, QOL, LVEF	Transendocardial

Trial ID	Trial name	N	Cell type	Endpoint	Delivery
Clinical trial NCT00824005	FOCUS	87	Bone marrow mononuclear cells	MVO_2, LVESV, Ischemic area	Transendocardial
Clinical trial NCT00747708	REGENERATE-IHD	165	G-CSF-stimulated bone marrow-derived stem/progenitor cells	LVEF	Transendocardial vs Intracoronary
Clinical trial NCT00326989	Cellwave	100	Bone marrow mononuclear cells	LVEF	Extracorporal shock wave, then intracoronary cell therapy
Clinical trial NCT00285454	—	60	Bone marrow mononuclear cells	Safety, perfusion Systolic function	Retrograde coronary venous delivery
Clinical trial NCT00462774	Cardio133	60	CD133+ bone marrow cells	LVEF	Transepicardial during CABG
Clinical trial NCT00810238	C-Cure	240	Bone marrow-derived cardiopoietic cells	LVEF	Transendocardial
Clinical trial NCT00768066	TAC-HFT	60	Bone marrow cells vs mesenchymal stem cells	Safety	Transendocardial
Clinical trial NCT00644410	—	60	Mesenchymal stem cells	LVEF	Transendocardial
Clinical trial NCT00587990	PROMETHEUS	45	Mesenchymal stem cells	Safety	Transendocardial during CABG
Clinical trial NCT00721045	—	60	Allogeneic mesenchymal precursor cells	Safety	Transendocardial
Clinical trial NCT00474461	—	40	Cardiac stem cells harvested from right atrial appendage	Safety	Intracoronary

Unless stated, autologous cell sources are used. AMI, acute myocardial infarction; CABG, coronary artery bypass grafting; G-CSF, granulocyte colony-stimulating factor; LVEF, left ventricular ejection fraction; LVESV, left ventricular end systolic volume; MVO_2, myocardial oxygen consumption; QOL, quality of life.

changes in regional and global ventricular function. The largest randomized studies so far have shown that intracoronary infusion of BMMNCs into the epicardial artery supplying the most poorly functioning akinetic/dyskinetic myocardial segment produced an approximately 3% increase in LVEF at three-month follow-up [14]. Interestingly either intracoronary or myocardial injection into chronically infarcted regions at the time of CABG produced no increase in either regional or segmental ventricular function [15]. Several ongoing investigations will further evaluate the potential benefits of BMMNC for treating ischemic cardiomyopathy (Table 19.1).

Selected hematopoietic stem cell preparations

More recently, investigators have reported the use of selected cell populations from bone marrow, including CD133[+] and CD34[+] cells, for the treatment of patients with both acute STEMI and refractory angina. This is based upon preclinical literature which suggests that these cells can (1) differentiate into an endothelial cell and cardiac myocyte phenotype [16], (2) promote neovascularization through paracrine mechanisms, and (3) improve left ventricular function in animal models of myocardial infarction.

In an open label study [12], CD34[+] CXCR4[+] progenitor cells, which have been reported to be mobilized from bone marrow after an acute STEMI, were isolated from bone marrow aspirates using immunomagnetic bead selection and administered by intracoronary infusion to 80 patients with acute STEMI involving the left anterior descending coronary artery. Baseline and six-month follow-up assessment of LVEF and ventricular volumes by cardiovascular magnetic resonance (CMR) were available in only 51 patients. LVEF in patients receiving CD34[+] CXCR4[+] progenitor cells increased from 35 to 38%. This was not significantly different from patients receiving either unselected BMMNC or no cell therapy. Furthermore, cell therapy was not associated with attenuation of adverse left ventricular remodelling. There was a trend to benefit from cell therapy in patients with baseline LVEF less than 37% and patients with delayed re-perfusion, though interpretation of these data is difficult owing to limited study power and significant loss to follow-up. In addition, CD34[+] cells have been selected from apheresis product after granulocyte colony-stimulating factor (G-CSF) mobilization and administered by percutaneous endomyocardial injection in 24 patients with refractory angina [17]. This study reported improved angina frequency and exercise capacity in the group receiving CD34[+] cells and no significant safety concerns. The results of the completed randomized phase II study in 167 patients have recently been published [18], and show significant reductions in weekly frequency of angina (6.3 ± 1.2 versus 11.0 ± 1.2, $p = 0.035$) and improved exercise time (140 ± 171 versus 58 ± 146 seconds, $p = 0.017$) at 12 months. Interestingly, there were no significant differences in these parameters in the groups receiving either 1×10^5 or 5×10^5 cells per kilogram. Of note, the authors did report an increased rate of cardiac enzyme elevation associated with progenitor cell mobilization and collection. A phase 3 trial of this approach is currently planned.

CD133$^+$ progenitor cells ($12.6 \pm 2.2 \times 10^6$) selected from bone marrow aspirates, have been infused into infarct-related epicardial coronary arteries in 19 out of 35 patients, approximately 12 days after acute STEMI [19]. At four months, patients receiving CD133$^+$ cells had improved segmental wall motion and regional myocardial perfusion, but had an increased risk of developing stent occlusion, in-stent restenosis, or development of de novo coronary lesions. Other feasibility studies have been reported in patients receiving intramyocardial injection of CD133$^+$ cells at the time of CABG [20], with further larger trials currently underway (Table 19.1).

Mesenchymal stem cells

Mesenchymal stem cells (MSCs) are a self-renewing population of cells found in bone marrow which may have the capacity to transdifferentiate into several cell types, including cardiac myocytes [21] and can be stimulated to be directed to infarcted myocardium through the CXCL12/CXCR4 chemokine axis [22]. In addition, MSCs are potent sources of angiogenic and immunomodulatory cytokines. Furthermore, MSCs may be used for allogeneic administration without the need for concomitant immunosuppressive therapy, owing to the absence of major histocompatibility and co-stimulatory antigens on the cell surface. On the basis of these preclinical observations, a phase I double-blind placebo-controlled dose-escalation safety study of 0.5×10^6 to 5×10^6 allogeneic MSCs administered intravenously to patients with acute STEMI has recently reported [23], which showed no deterioration in pulmonary function tests or increased ventricular ectopy. In a subset of patients undergoing CMR (20 MSC treated compared with 14 placebo treated), these investigators reported a significant and sustained increase in LVEF in the MSC treated group ($5.2 \pm 8.5\%$ compared with $1.8 \pm 6.7\%$) as well as attenuation in adverse left ventricular remodelling. However, these data should not be over-interpreted, as the placebo-treated subjects in the CMR subgroup appeared to have larger infarctions and, in the analysis of the entire study group, echocardiographic measurement of LVEF and exercise time were no different in the MSC and placebo treated groups. Overall these data are promising and further investigation of allogeneic administration of MSCs is warranted.

Multipotent adult progenitor cells (MAPCs) are another population present at low frequency in bone marrow stroma, which are capable of self renewal and differentiation into cells of all three germinal layers after long-term expansion under stringent culture conditions [24]. Initial experiments in a swine model showed that intramyocardial injection of 50×10^6 allogeneic MAPC into the infarct border one hour after the application of coronary ligation resulted in improved regional and global contractile function by CMR. Interestingly, only about 3% and 2% of the cells developed an endothelial or cardiomyocyte phenotype, suggesting that most functional benefit may be achieved through a paracrine mechanism [25]. Similar observations have been reported in a rat hindlimb ischemia model, in which none of the engrafted cells adopted an endothelial or vascular smooth muscle phenotype [26]. MAPCs may also be considered for clinical evaluation pending future successful efficacy and safety studies.

Future cell preparations

BMMNCs transdifferentiate into a cardiac myocyte phenotype with very low efficiency and seem to confer functional benefit principally through angiogenesis. This has translated to modest improvements in left ventricular systolic function in clinical trials. Much attention has therefore focused on identification of cell preparations that can be differentiated efficiently into functioning cardiac myocytes, which may translate to greater improvement in cardiac contractile function.

Resident cardiac stem cells

Although it was previously held that the heart had no ability to self renew, it has now become apparent that there is a population of resident cardiac stem cells responsible for basal turnover of cardiac myocytes in the adult and fetal heart. These cells can be identified by several surface markers, including *Kit*, *SCA-1*, *MDR-1*, *ISL-1*, or *ABCG-2* [27]. In addition, investigators have identified stem cells that can be isolated from suspension cultures of myocardial biopsy tissue, which are known as cardiosphere-derived cells. Bench studies have shown that these cells can be differentiated in to cardiac myocytes and endothelial cells and can be successfully engrafted into animal models of myocardial infarction [28]. Recently, a phase I dose-escalation clinical trial (CADUCEUS) has reported in which 25 patients were randomized 2:1 to receive 12.5×10^6 to 25×10^6 autologous cardiosphere-derived cells from endomyocardial biopsy tissue administered by intracoronary infusion into patients with recent acute myocardial infarction and impaired left ventricular function [29] (Table 19.1). These preliminary data suggest that cardiosphere derived cells can mediate significant improvements in regional contractile function and reductions in ventricular scar assessed by cardiac MRI. No limiting toxicity was observed. Similarly, the open label SCIPIO trial [30], which is a phase I trial of intracoronary infusion of 1×10^6 c-kit positive cardiac stem cells administered 113 days after coronary bypass surgery, has also reported improved left ventricular systolic function and reduced infarct size without a significant increase in adverse events. Phase II trials of both these and other approaches are either in development or in progress. Other cardiac stem cell populations are currently undergoing preclinical testing.

Embryonic stem cells

Embryonic stem (ES) cells are self-renewing totipotent cells that have been successfully differentiated to beating cardiac myocytes in vitro. Successful engraftment of ES cells and ES-cell-derived cardiac myocytes has been achieved in animal models of myocardial infarction [31]. However, aside from the ethical issues surrounding gaining access to ES cells, several practical obstacles to clinical use remain, including immunogenicity, teratoma formation, and availability of safe clinical-grade culture reagents required for ex vivo expansion [27]. Currently, ES cell research remains confined to the laboratory setting and clinical applications in cardiology are unlikely in the near term.

Induced pluripotent stem cells

Recently, researchers have reported that human skin fibroblasts can be reprogrammed into pluripotent stem cells, through overexpression of the transcription factors *OCT4, SOX2, Nanog*, and *Lin28,* which can differentiate into cell types of all three germinal layers [32]. These are known as induced pluripotent stem cells (iPS) and share many of the characteristics and risk profile of ES cells. This protocol has recently undergone significant refinement. iPS cells circumvent many of the ethical concerns surrounding the use of ES cells and may offer a unique autologous cell source for chronic heart conditions. Tumorigenicity and a recent report that iPS cells may be inferior to ES cells in terms of differentiation capacity [33] may be problematic moving forward. Recent studies have evaluated iPS cells in murine models of myocardial infarction [34], but considerable further efficacy and safety studies are required before iPS can be considered for autologous grafting in humans.

Progenitor cell mobilization

Rodent studies have previously demonstrated that cytokine mobilization of progenitor cells from bone marrow may confer hemodynamic benefits in a murine model of acute coronary artery ligation [35]. Recent clinical data of G-CSF mobilization in patients with severe symptomatic coronary disease and previous myocardial infarction have not demonstrated improvements in regional or global left ventricular dimensions, contractile function, or perfusion [36]. Several clinical studies have also examined administration of G-CSF in patients with re-perfused acute STEMI. These have been the subject of a recent meta-analysis, which concluded that G-CSF administration confers no functional benefit to patients with acute STEMI [37]. Recent studies showing that combination cytokine therapy with the competitive CXCR4 receptor antagonist, AMD3100, and vascular endothelial growth factor (VEGF) may selectively mobilize endothelial and stromal progenitor cells while suppressing the release of hematopoietic stem cells and neutrophils from bone marrow, warrant further evaluation of the therapeutic potential of this approach [38].

Outstanding issues for clinical translation

It is noteworthy, that the magnitude of benefit observed in randomized clinical trials has been considerably less than would have been predicted on the basis of the results of preclinical experiments and phase I clinical trials. In our view, this discrepancy provides several important lessons.

Preclinical evaluation of new cell preparations

The optimal cell preparation for each cardiovascular application remains to be determined. It cannot be assumed that a single-cell preparation will be equally efficacious for all clinical applications, and different cell preparations may have varying toxicity profiles. Indeed, it is unclear if administration of a highly selected cell population is preferable to a heterogeneous unselected or combination cell product. Other unresolved issues include determination of the optimal number of cells to be delivered, timing and route of cell administration, importance of growth factor preconditioning of cellular products before administration, effects of ex vivo cell expansion and prolonged cell culture before administration, and the use of allogeneic rather than autologous cell preparations.

In our view, preclinical proof of concept studies designed to demonstrate the efficacy of a new cell product should include randomization, blinding, and measurement of clinically relevant endpoints. A cellular control should be adopted where possible. In addition, proof of concept studies should be performed in both rodent and large animal models. The latter provides the opportunity to test the combination of the desired cell product and planned method of clinical cell delivery in clinically relevant disease models, for example re-perfused myocardial infarction. Clinically relevant outcome measurements can be made using the same accurate, reproducible, and validated techniques as used in clinical trials, such as CMR and positron emission tomography, which can also be performed in rodent models (Figure 19.1). When this approach is used, some of the negative results observed in randomized clinical trials may have been predicted [39–41]. These experiments are lengthy and costly to perform, which will hopefully be recognized by grant-awarding bodies when considering future applications to evaluate novel cell preparations.

Once the efficacy of a cell preparation has been established in preclinical testing, further in vivo toxicity testing, bespoke to the planned clinical trial, should be undertaken. Discussions with regulatory authorities can be invaluable in planning the design and conduct of these studies. Ideally, cells

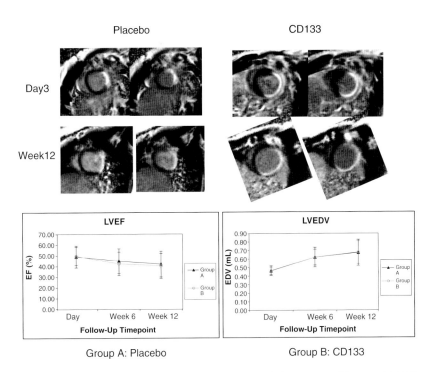

Figure 19.1 CMR to assess the effects of intramyocardial injection of human CD133⁺ cells in an athymic nude rat myocardial infarction model. The upper panels show late gadolinium enhancement images, which demonstrate that CD133 cell injection at the time of coronary ligation fails to prevent infarct thinning and expansion. The lower panels show quantitative measurements of left ventricular ejection fraction (LVEF, %) and left ventricular end diastolic volume (LVEDV, in milliliters). These data indicate that intramyocardial CD133 injection neither prevents reduction in LVEF nor attenuates adverse LV remodelling.

should be prepared using methods and reagents identical to the planned clinical trial. The biological activity of these cells should be assessed, such as by persistence of cell-surface markers, colony formation, or migration assays. Cell products that require prolonged ex vivo expansion should undergo detailed cytogenetic analysis, including fluorescence in situ hybridization to exclude balanced translocations. These studies are important as it has been shown that variation in the biological activity of cells arising from variations in the cell processing protocol may account for the differences in the outcomes observed in clinical trials [42]. The experimental design should include randomization, blinding, dose escalation, and, where possible, implement the same delivery method or route as in the planned clinical trial. These experiments would normally be undertaken in a large animal model, using either the animal homologue of the planned cell product, or may use the human cell product in an immunosuppressed animal model. Alternatively, for human cell preparations for which there is no animal homolog (e.g., CD133$^+$ cells), xenogeneic transplantation of the human cell product into an immunodeficient rodent model, such as the athymic nude rat, can be performed (Figure 19.2).

Cell delivery

For therapeutic purposes, cells should be delivered to the target tissue of interest in sufficient number to confer functional benefit with minimal toxicity to the patient. Although preclinical and clinical studies have suggested that systemic delivery of cell products can yield functional benefits, we are of the view that local cell delivery is theoretically more attractive in that larger numbers of cells may potentially be administered to specific regions of interest within the target organ. Clinically, local cell delivery can be achieved by direct myocardial injection at the time of CABG or percutaneously by catheter-guided intracoronary or retrograde venous infusion, or intrapericardial or intramyocardial injection. Whichever of these methods is chosen, biocompatibility of the cell product with the delivery system must be tested to ensure that the biological activity of the cell product is not altered as a result of passage through the delivery system. These experiments should test the effects of variations in injection speed, dwell time, and cell concentration on the biological activity concentration of the cells after passage through the delivery system.

The optimal delivery method remains to be established and will depend critically on the planned clinical application. There are few quantitative data addressing cell distribution and cell retention as a function of the mode of cell delivery. Biodistribution studies using technetium-99m-labelled bone-marrow-derived mesenchymal stromal cells in recently infarcted rats suggest that, after intravenous infusion, most infused cells are entrapped in the lungs with little distribution to the heart [43]. The number of cells in the heart was increased by infusion of cells directly into the left ventricular cavity, which simulates intra-arterial infusion. Other preclinical data suggest that at best only 30–40% of particulate material is retained within the myocardium after a successful endomyocardial injection [44], but this approach was found to be more efficient than either intracoronary or retrograde venous cell infusion [45].

Direct myocardial injection has the advantage of enabling delivery of therapies to myocardium supplied by occluded inflow epicardial coronary arteries and can be successfully performed either at the time of cardiac surgery or by a minimal access percutaneous approach using specialized catheters. Targeted delivery of cells to regions bordering infarcted myocardium is thought to provide the optimal chance of achieving clinically important treatment effects. The ease, safety, and success of this interventional

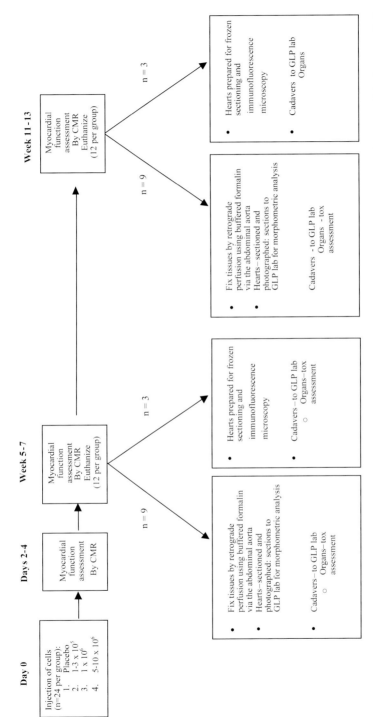

Figure 19.2 Experimental protocol to assess the efficacy and toxicity of human CD133+ cells in an athymic nude rat model of myocardial infarction by coronary ligation. The protocol includes randomization, blinding, use of an independent GLP laboratory for toxicity assessment, as well as functional and mechanistic assessments.

procedure is optimized by the use of guidance systems that allow identification of treatment targets according to their tissue properties as well as their anatomical location (Plate 19.1). Although surgical exposure is excellent for performing intramyocardial cell injection targeted to infarct borders under direct vision, it is unlikely to find widespread clinical application for the sole purpose of targeted cell delivery, and when performed as an adjunct to CABG, suffers from the uncertainty of whether any improvement in function is due to the administration of cells or from coronary revascularization. Surgical approaches designed to improve retention and engraftment by epicardial placement of cells embedded within biological scaffolds are currently under preclinical evaluation.

Future clinical trials

Clinical trials of newer cell therapies should be underpinned by robust preclinical efficacy and toxicity data. Ongoing clinical trials are summarized in Table 19.1. Randomization and blinding should be implemented at the earliest stages of clinical evaluation [23]. For autologous cell products, biological assays of an aliquot of the administered cells are highly desirable to understand the contribution of variation in biological potency of a cell product, which can clearly vary from individual to individual, to any observed variability in trial efficacy and safety endpoints. This may require the development of "potency"-based release assays for cellular products and clearly poses significant challenges to clinical good manufacturing practice protocols for processing of cellular products for cardiovascular applications. We would favor the routine use of CMR for measurement of regional and global left ventricular function, remodelling and myocardial infarct size, owing to the accuracy and reproducibility of this method. This will help minimize the sample size required for these studies.

Conclusions

Many obstacles remain along the path to successful routine clinical application of cardiovascular cell therapy. Much has been learned from the initial clinical experience, but in our view the emphasis should now be on further preclinical work to evaluate the efficacy and toxicity profiles of the next generation of cell preparations, rather than moving forward to additional clinical trials. This will be a lengthy and complex process, the success of which will require an integrated multidisciplinary collaboration between basic scientists, cardiologists, cardiac surgeons, hematologists, cell-processing experts, and industry.

Acknowledgments

Dr de Silva and Professor Pepper are supported by the NIHR Cardiovascular Disease Biomedical Research Unit at the Royal Brompton and Harefield NHS Foundation Trust and Imperial College London.

KEY LEARNING POINTS

- The heart shows inadequate ability to repair itself after myocardial infarction and other forms of heart disease, resulting in significant impairment of contractile function and adverse ventricular remodelling, which are the major determinants of adverse clinical outcome.

- Functional benefits of cell therapy for cardiovascular applications may arise from induction of angiogenesis, cardiomyogenesis, cardioprotection, or mechanical interstitial support.

- So far, most randomized clinical trials have evaluated autologous bone marrow mononuclear cell administration after acute myocardial infarction, and collectively have shown only marginal improvements in left ventricular function. No major safety concerns have been highlighted.

- New cell preparations are under evaluation. The optimal cell type, dose, route of administration, and timing of delivery for individual cardiovascular clinical applications remain undefined.

- Although much has been learned from initial clinical experiences, in our view the emphasis should now be on further preclinical work to evaluate the efficacy and toxicity profiles of next generation cell preparations, rather than moving directly to additional clinical trials.

References

1. Menasche P, Alfieri O, Janssens S, et al. The Myoblast Autologous Grafting in Ischemic Cardiomyopathy (MAGIC) trial: first randomized placebo-controlled study of myoblast transplantation. Circulation 2008;117:1189–200.
2. Siepe M, Giraud MN, Liljensten E, et al. Construction of skeletal myoblast-based polyurethane scaffolds for myocardial repair. Artif Organs 2007;31:425–33.
3. Roell W, Lewalter T, Sasse P, et al. Engraftment of connexin 43-expressing cells prevents post-infarct arrhythmia. Nature 2007;450:819–24.
4. Orlic D, Kajstura J, Chimenti S, et al. Bone marrow cells regenerate infarcted myocardium. Nature 2001;410:701–5.
5. Balsam LB, Wagers AJ, Christensen JL, et al. Haematopoietic stem cells adopt mature haematopoietic fates in ischaemic myocardium. Nature 2004;428:668–73.

6. Murry CE, Soonpaa MH, Reinecke H, et al. Haematopoietic stem cells do not transdifferentiate into cardiac myocytes in myocardial infarcts. Nature 2004; 428:664–8.

7. Korf-Klingebiel M, Kempf T, et al. Bone marrow cells are a rich source of growth factors and cytokines: implications for cell therapy trials after myocardial infarction. Eur Heart J 2008;29:2851–58.

8. Wollert KC, Drexler H. Clinical applications of stem cells for the heart. Circ Res 2005;96:151–63.

9. Kang S, Yang YJ, Li CJ, Gao RL. Effects of intracoronary autologous bone marrow cells on left ventricular function in acute myocardial infarction: a systematic review and meta-analysis for randomized controlled trials. Coron Artery Dis 2008; 19:327–35.

10. Martin-Rendon E, Brunskill SJ, Hyde CJ, et al. Autologous bone marrow stem cells to treat acute myocardial infarction: a systematic review. Eur Heart J 2008;29: 1807–18.

11. Schachinger V, Erbs S, Elsasser A, et al. Intracoronary bone marrow-derived progenitor cells in acute myocardial infarction. N Engl J Med 2006;355:1210–21.

12. Tendera M, Wojakowski W, Ruzyllo W, et al. Intracoronary infusion of bone marrow-derived selected CD34+CXCR4+ cells and non-selected mononuclear cells in patients with acute STEMI and reduced left ventricular ejection fraction: results of randomized, multicentre Myocardial Regeneration by Intracoronary Infusion of Selected Population of Stem Cells in Acute Myocardial Infarction (REGENT) Trial. Eur Heart J 2009;30:1313–21.

13. Reffelmann T, Konemann S, Kloner RA. Promise of blood- and bone marrow-derived stem cell transplantation for functional cardiac repair: putting it in perspective with existing therapy. J Am Coll Cardiol 2009;53:305–8.

14. Assmus B, Honold J, Schachinger V, et al. Transcoronary transplantation of progenitor cells after myocardial infarction. N Engl J Med 2006;355:1222–32.

15. Ang KL, Chin D, Leyva F, et al. Randomized, controlled trial of intramuscular or intracoronary injection of autologous bone marrow cells into scarred myocardium during CABG versus CABG alone. Nat Clin Pract Cardiovasc Med 2008;5:663–70.

16. Shmelkov SV, Meeus S, Moussazadeh N, et al. Cytokine preconditioning promotes codifferentiation of human fetal liver CD133+ stem cells into angiomyogenic tissue. Circulation 2005;111:1175–83.

17. Losordo DW, Schatz RA, White CJ, et al. Intramyocardial transplantation of autologous CD34+ stem cells for intractable angina: a phase I/IIa double-blind, randomized controlled trial. Circulation 2007;115:3165–72.

18. LosordoDW, Henry TD, Davidson C, et al., CT34-CMI Investigators intramyocardial, autologous CD34+ cell therapy for refractory angina. Circ Res 2011;109:428–36.

19. Bartunek J, Vanderheyden M, Vandekerckhove B, et al. Intracoronary injection of CD133-positive enriched bone marrow progenitor cells promotes cardiac recovery after recent myocardial infarction: feasibility and safety. Circulation 2005;112(9 Suppl):I178–83.

20. Stamm C, Kleine HD, Choi YH, et al. Intramyocardial delivery of CD133+ bone marrow cells and coronary artery bypass grafting for chronic ischemic heart disease: safety and efficacy studies. J Thorac Cardiovasc Surg 2007;133:717–25.

21. Pittenger MF, Mackay AM, Beck SC, et al. Multilineage potential of adult human mesenchymal stem cells. Science 1999;284:143–7.

22. Askari AT, Unzek S, Popovic ZB, et al. Effect of stromal-cell-derived factor 1 on stem-cell homing and tissue regeneration in ischaemic cardiomyopathy. Lancet 2003;362:697–703.

23. Hare JM, Traverse JH, Henry TD, et al. A randomized, double-blind, placebo-controlled, dose-escalation study of intravenous adult human mesenchymal stem cells (prochymal) after acute myocardial infarction. J Am Coll Cardiol 2009;54:2277–86.

24. Jiang Y, Jahagirdar BN, Reinhardt RL, et al. Pluripotency of mesenchymal stem cells derived from adult marrow. Nature 2002;418:41–9.

25. Zeng L, Hu Q, Wang X, Mansoor A, et al. Bioenergetic and functional consequences of bone marrow-derived multipotent progenitor cell transplantation in hearts with postinfarction left ventricular remodeling. Circulation 2007;115:1866–75.

26. Wragg A, Mellad JA, Beltran LE, et al. VEGFR1/CXCR4-positive progenitor cells modulate local inflammation and augment tissue perfusion by a SDF-1-dependent mechanism. J Mol Med 2008;86:1221–32.

27. Passier R, van Laake LW, Mummery CL. Stem-cell-based therapy and lessons from the heart. Nature 2008;453:322–9.

28. Johnston PV, Sasano T, Mills K, et al. Engraftment, differentiation, and functional benefits of autologous cardiosphere-derived cells in porcine ischemic cardiomyopathy. Circulation 2009;120:1075–83.

29. Makkar RR, Smith RR, Cheng K, et al. Intracoronary cardiosphere-derived cells for heart regeneration after myocardial infarction (CADUCEUS): a prospective, randomised phase 1 trial. Lancet 2012;379:895–904.

30. Bolli R, Chugh AR, D'Amario D, et al. Cardiac stem cells in patients with ischaemic cardiomyopathy (SCIPIO): initial results of a randomised phase 1 trial. Lancet 2011;378:1847–57.

31. Singla DK, Lyons GE, Kamp TJ. Transplanted embryonic stem cells following mouse myocardial infarction inhibit apoptosis and cardiac remodeling. Am J Physiol Heart Circ Physiol 2007;293:H1308–14.

32. Yu J, Vodyanik MA, Smuga-Otto K, et al. Induced pluripotent stem cell lines derived from human somatic cells. Science 2007;31:1917–20.

33. Hu BY, Weick JP, Yu J, et al. Neural differentiation of human induced pluripotent stem cells follows developmental principles but with variable potency. Proc Natl Acad Sci U S A 107:4335–40.

34. Nelson TJ, Martinez-Fernandez A, Yamada S, Perez-Terzic C, Ikeda Y, Terzic A. Repair of acute myocardial infarction by human stemness factors induced pluripotent stem cells. Circulation 2009;120:408–16.

35. Orlic D, Kajstura J, Chimenti S, et al. Mobilized bone marrow cells repair the infarcted heart, improving function and survival. Proc Natl Acad Sci U S A 2001;98:10344–9.

36. Hill JM, Syed MA, Arai AE, et al. Outcomes and risks of granulocyte colony-stimulating factor in patients with coronary artery disease. J Am Coll Cardiol 2005;46:1643–8.

37. Zohlnhofer D, Dibra A, Koppara T, et al. Stem cell mobilization by granulocyte colony-stimulating factor for myocardial recovery after acute myocardial infarction: a meta-analysis. J Am Coll Cardiol 2008;51:1429–37.

38. Pitchford SC, Furze RC, Jones CP, Wengner AM, Rankin SM. Differential mobilization of subsets of progenitor cells from the bone marrow. Cell Stem Cell 2009;4:62–72.

39. de Silva R, Raval AN, Hadi M, et al. Intracoronary infusion of autologous mononuclear cells from bone marrow or granulocyte colony-stimulating factor-mobilized apheresis product may not improve remodelling, contractile function, perfusion, or infarct size in a swine model of large myocardial infarction. Eur Heart J 2008; 29:1772–82.

40. Traverse JH, Henry TD, Ellis SG, et al., Cardiovascular Cell Therapy Research Network. Effect of intracoronary delivery of autologous bone marrow mononuclear cells 2 to 3 weeks following acute myocardial infarction on left ventricular function: the LateTIME randomized trial. JAMA 2011;306:2110–9.

41. Perin EC, Willerson JT, Pepine CJ, Henry TD, et al., Cardiovascular Cell Therapy Research Network. Effect of transendocardial delivery of autologous bone marrow mononuclear cells on functional capacity, left ventricular function, and perfusion in chronic heart failure: the FOCUS-CCTRN trial. JAMA 2012; March 24, [Epub ahead of print].

42. Seeger FH, Tonn T, Krzossok N, Zeiher AM, Dimmeler S. Cell isolation procedures matter: a comparison of different isolation protocols of bone marrow mononuclear cells used for cell therapy in patients with acute myocardial infarction. Eur Heart J 2007;28:766–72.

43. Barbash IM, Chouraqui P, Baron J, et al. Systemic delivery of bone marrow-derived mesenchymal stem cells to the infarcted myocardium: feasibility, cell migration, and body distribution. Circulation 2003;108:863–8.

44. Grossman PM, Han Z, Palasis M, Barry JJ, Lederman RJ. Incomplete retention after direct myocardial injection. Catheter Cardiovasc Interv 2002;55:392–7.

45. Hou D, Youssef EA, Brinton TJ, et al. Radiolabeled cell distribution after intramyocardial, intracoronary, and interstitial retrograde coronary venous delivery: implications for current clinical trials. Circulation 2005;112(9 Suppl):I150–6.

20 Use of Donated Gametes in Assisted Reproduction

Tarek El-Toukhy[1,2] and Mauro Costa[3]

[1]Guy's and St. Thomas' Hospital NHS Foundation Trust, London, UK
[2]Cairo University, Cairo, Egypt
[3]Galliera Hospital, Genoa, Italy

The past

History of development of assisted reproduction: what is assisted reproductive technology?

Infertility is a common condition affecting one in six couples. It has important medical and psychological implications. It is defined as the inability to conceive after one year of regular intercourse without contraception. It is not a disease but the symptom of many pathological conditions that can affect one or both partners. Some of these conditions are treatable with surgical or medical therapies but many have remained untreatable until the advent of in vitro fertilization (IVF) and related techniques, collectively known as assisted reproductive technology (ART).

The term "ART" includes all treatments or procedures that include the in vitro handling of both human oocytes and sperm, or embryos, for establishing a pregnancy. This includes, but is not limited to, IVF and embryo transfer, gamete intrafallopian transfer, zygote intrafallopian transfer, tubal embryo transfer, gamete and embryo cryopreservation, oocyte and embryo donation, and gestational surrogacy. The internationally accepted definition of ART does not include assisted insemination (artificial insemination) using sperm from either a woman's partner or a sperm donor [1].

Artificial insemination is the simplest and oldest form of assisted reproduction. Hunter reported the fist human pregnancy obtained in a couple with a male affected by hypospadias, after the vaginal insemination of the male semen. Pancoast reported the first case of human donor insemination

Tissue and Cell Clinical Use: An Essential Guide, First Edition. Edited by Ruth M. Warwick and Scott A. Brubaker.
© 2012 Blackwell Publishing Ltd. Published 2012 by Blackwell Publishing Ltd.

in 1884 and Bunge and Sherman published the first insemination with cryopreserved semen in 1953. The use of artificial insemination has progressively increased until the advent of IVF in 1978 and donor insemination has remained the main therapy for severe male factor infertility until the application of intracytoplasmic sperm injection (ICSI) technique in 1992.

Since the first report of a successful human pregnancy, IVF had received a prominent role in the clinical management of infertility. These techniques involve the laboratory preparation of gametes (oocytes and sperm) and artificially approximating them, thus increasing the chances of conception. With the major technological advances over the past three decades, the demand for ART services has grown substantially. Worldwide, an estimated 3.5 million children have been born using ART. In the UK, 36,861 women had 46,829 cycles of IVF treatment in 2007, an increase of nearly 6% on the previous year, resulting in the birth of 13,672 babies [2]. In the USA, a total of 138,198 ART procedures were reported in 2006. These procedures resulted in 41,343 live-birth deliveries, and 54656 infants, representing approximately 1% of US infants born in 2006 [3]. In 20 European countries, where all clinics reported to the IVF register, a total of 359,110 ART cycles were performed in 2006 in a population of 422.5 million, corresponding to 850 cycles per million inhabitants. European data on intrauterine insemination (IUI) using husband/partner's (IUI-H) and donor (IUI-D) semen were reported from 22 countries. A total of 134,261 IUI-H and 24,339 IUI-D cycles were included [4]. Trounson and colleagues reported the first pregnancy of a donated oocyte fertilized in vitro in 1983.

Current ART practices (Figure 20.1)

General indications for ART
1. Tubal damage
Tubal disease accounts for about a quarter of all cases of infertility and represents more than half of infertility causes in the female. IVF is considered the treatment of choice for women with severe tubal damage and in those where previous tubal surgery has failed.

2. Endometriosis
The pathophysiology of endometriosis may have an associated infertility, which entails a combination of factors, including distortion of pelvic anatomy by adhesions, locally increased prostanoid production, an increase in peritoneal macrophages, and impaired folliculogenesis. Where endometriosis is associated with infertility unresponsive to medical suppression or surgical ablation of endometriotic implants, ART can provide a realistic chance of achieving a pregnancy.

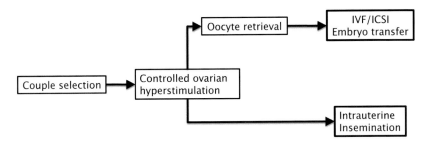

Figure 20.1 An overview of ART techniques.

3. Male factor infertility

A male factor is causative of infertility in approximately 50% of infertile couples. Categories of abnormal semen include oligozoospermia (low sperm count), asthenozoospermia (reduced motility), teratozoospermia (increased abnormal forms), a combination of these (oligo-astheno-teratozoospermia), or azoospermia (no spermatozoa in the ejaculate). In most cases impaired semen quality is not correctable medically or surgically. For mild abnormalities in sperm parameters (e.g., a sperm count between 15–20 million per milliliter), IUI may be useful. However, when a severe male factor exists, IVF and ICSI should be considered [5].

4. Unexplained infertility

Unexplained infertility affects 10–25% of infertile couples and is defined as lack of conception after one year in couples for whom the results of a standard infertility evaluation, including a semen analysis, examination of tubal patency, and documentation of ovulation, are normal. Superovulation (induced with clomiphene citrate or gonadotrophins) combined with timed intercourse or IUI can yield good results with most pregnancies occurring within four months of therapy. However, if pregnancy is not achieved after four to six months of stimulated IUI, IVF should be considered [6, 7].

Insemination technique

Insemination can be performed with the partner semen or with donor semen (donor insemination).

Insemination of semen can be performed without semen preparation (intracervical insemination) directly inserting a small amount of semen in the uterine cervix. This technique is today limited to cases of donor insemination, but it is preferable to treat semen to remove all the undesired components (bacteria, leukocytes, debris, prostaglandins).

IUI involves a laboratory procedure to separate and concentrate fast moving spermatozoa with normal morphology. A drop of culture medium with selected spermatozoa is introduced in the uterine cavity with a soft catheter at the moment of spontaneous or induced ovulation.

IVF Technique
Ovarian stimulation in IVF:
1. Controlled ovarian hyperstimulation
Superovulation or controlled ovarian hyperstimulation regimes are designed to induce the woman to produce a larger number of oocytes than the one or two required for normal ovulation induction programs. Some of the oocytes can be saved for use in oocyte donation programs. Multifollicular development allows the production in vitro of sufficient embryos to allow two quality embryos to be transferred to the uterus and may leave surplus embryos for cryopreservation for future use by the patient for her own use or for donation. This improves the likelihood of pregnancy for each cycle of stimulation while reducing the need for further superovulation cycles. The role of exogenous follicular stimulating hormone (FSH) injections in this process is essential whereas luteinizing hormone plays a less important role.

2. The use of gonadotrophin releasing hormone agonists in controlled ovarian hyperstimulation
One of the most significant advances in IVF techniques has been the adoption of superovulation regimens which control endogenous secretion of luteinizing hormone by the use of gonadotrophin releasing hormone (GnRH) agonists to induce a state of pituitary desensitization and prevent premature surge of luteinizing hormone. GnRH agonists have increased stability and potency and a higher binding affinity to GnRH receptors than does the native molecule. This high binding affinity causes a suppression of pituitary gonadotrophin production with continued administration and a decrease in the number of GnRH receptors (desensitization or downregulation). This pituitary blockade persists during the agonist treatment but is completely reversible after cessation of therapy.

Use of GnRH agonists to suppress endogenous gonadotrophin production allows ovarian stimulation using exogenous FSH injections to continue until a sufficient number of follicles reach an adequate size without the fear of an endogenous surge of luteinizing hormone and premature ovulation. Different treatment protocols using GnRH agonists and gonadotrophins are now used, including the "long" and "short" protocols.

3. The use of GnRH antagonists in controlled ovarian hyperstimulation
The long agonist protocol is generally the most commonly used because it allows total cycle control, but has a relatively long lead-up time until pituitary desensitization is achieved. The role of GnRH antagonists in ovarian stimulation for IVF is well established. GnRH antagonists competitively bind and directly block pituitary GnRH receptors. In doing so, they immediately

prevent the action of native GnRH without the initial flare response characteristic of the agonist. Administration of GnRH antagonist during the late-follicular phase (i.e., starting on day six of stimulation) effectively prevents a premature rise in luteinizing hormone during controlled ovarian hyper-stimulation and is associated with similar live birth rates and significantly reduced treatment burden in terms of duration of ovarian stimulation, incidence of ovarian stimulation syndrome and treatment drop-out rates, compared with the agonist long protocols [8].

Oocyte retrieval

Transvaginal ultrasound guided oocyte retrieval is the norm and is usually performed under light sedation and analgesia. The procedure is relatively short (about 20 minutes) with the oocyte donor able to go home within two hours. The vaginal ultrasound probe mounted with a needle-guide is so positioned to be as close as possible to the ovary. A single lumen needle attached to a gentle electric pump is passed through the vaginal fornix into the ovary to aspirate the follicular fluid, which is then examined under the microscope to confirm oocyte retrieval.

Insemination and ICSI

Insemination of the oocytes with sperm prepared from a masturbated semen sample takes place two to six hours after retrieval. Motile spermatozoa are placed with the oocytes (placed either individually or in groups) at a concentration of 50,000–100,000 per milliliter and generally left overnight for fertilization to occur, although a short two-hour protocol is used in some centers. The oocytes are examined at 14–16 hours after insemination to identify the presence of two pronuclei, indicating that normal fertilization has taken place.

IVF as a treatment for severe male factor infertility is associated with lower fertilization and pregnancy rates than for other indications. Intracytoplasmic injection of a single sperm into the oocyte (ICSI) was a major milestone in obviating male infertility as it can be used for men with profound oligo-zoospermia, athenoteratozoospermia, or even azoospermia, provided that some sperm can be aspirated or microsurgically retrieved from either the epididymis (PESA) or testis (TESE). ICSI now provides the possibility of a pregnancy for couples who previously might have opted for the use of donor sperm. Fertilization, implantation, as well as pregnancy rates after ICSI are similar to IVF and are independent of whether the sperm was ejaculated or surgically retrieved [9]. In addition, patients who have experienced repeated fertilization failures after conventional IVF may also benefit from ICSI with fertilization, and pregnancy rates comparable to patients with abnormal sperm parameters. If surgical sperm retrieval and/or ICSI are not successful then donated sperm may be indicated.

Embryo transfer

The fertilized embryos are left in culture for two or three days until they have cleaved to the four- (day two) or eight- (day three) cell stage. Embryo transfer is generally performed by depositing the tiny (30 μl) droplet of culture fluid containing the embryos at a defined length from the internal os of the cervix. The presence of a full bladder may help straighten the natural curve at the level of the internal os. Transabdominal ultrasound guidance may be helpful in placing the catheter and depositing the fluid in the endometrial cavity.

Blastocyst culture and transfer

One of the main drawbacks of transferring cleavage-stage embryos is the difficulty in establishing the developmental potential of such embryos, because only a small percentage of embryonic genes have been activated at that stage. One way of identifying the implantation potential of cleavage-stage embryos is through extended culture. Embryos with limited or no developmental potential will cease to divide, whereas those embryos more likely to be developmentally "competent" will continue to grow to reach the next developmental milestone – the blastocyst. Approximately, half of the embryos judged to be suitable for transfer on day three of culture will progress to the blastocyst stage whereas the remaining embryos will arrest.

Additionally, human embryos normally reside in the fallopian tube in their early stages of development and do not reach the uterus and implant until just before blastocyst formation. Hence, premature placement of cleavage-stage embryos into the uterus potentially could result in embryonic–maternal asynchrony and metabolic stress.

Therefore, transfer of embryos after in vitro culture to the blastocyst stage seems to offer a means of transferring more developmentally competent embryos when they are more metabolically compatible with the uterine environment. This synchronization between the transferred embryos and the maternal reproductive tract should translate into higher implantation rates, which may in turn lead to the transfer of fewer embryos, if not only one, to reduce the risk of multiple pregnancy, which is the most common and preventable complication of assisted conception treatment [10]. Multiple pregnancies carry higher risks of hypertensive disorders, anemia, and hemorrhage during pregnancy. The risk of neonatal death in twins is seven times that of singletons. Infants are more likely to be born prematurely and with a lower birthweight than babies from singleton pregnancies, with an increased risk of long-term medical and developmental problems, in particular neurological impairment.

Luteal support

As the hormonal milieu in stimulated cycles is unbalanced toward a prevalence of estrogens, and progesterone production may be impaired with some stimulation protocols, a luteal progesterone supplementation is necessary. Luteal support is continued for two to three weeks after embryo transfer to enhance the chance of embryo implantation and then stopped even if the pregnancy test is positive as further progesterone supplementation is not necessary. Luteal support is commonly achieved with vaginal natural progesterone pessaries (400 mg daily) or progesterone in oil (25–50 mg/day intramuscularly), but can also be provided by hCG injection (2500 IU per three to five days). Both therapeutic regimens appear to be equally effective. HCG should not be given if there is any increased risk of ovarian hyperstimulation syndrome. Ovarian hyperstimulation syndrome (OHSS) is a serious and potentially fatal iatrogenic event due to an ART cycle. The cardinal event of this syndrome is a third space fluid shift related to the ovarian production of substances that increase vascular permeability. OHSS may be mild, moderate, or severe, and the clinical impact of the syndrome depends on the variety of symptoms caused by development of ascites, pleural effusions, hemoconcentration, reduced renal perfusion, and thrombotic complications. The frequency of severe OHSS is around 1% after multiple ovulation induction and occasionally leads to death due to thromboembolism, renal failure, or adult respiratory distress syndrome. The mortality rate has been estimated between 1 in 45,000 and 1 in 500,000. The European IVF monitoring consortium reports that in a total number of 459,170 ART cycles, 2753 cases of OHSS were recorded, corresponding to a risk of OHSS of 0.8% of all stimulated cycles in year 2006.

Preservation of human gametes and embryos for later use (autologous or homologous donation)

The ability to cryopreserve and store the structure and function of biological cells and tissue plays a pivotal role in many areas of clinical medicine. The role of cryopreservation in human-assisted reproduction was recognized at an early stage in the development of the technology and has increased in importance as a result of a range of clinical and ethical considerations. Embryo or gamete (sperm and oocytes) cryopreservation has been a proven method to enhance the effectiveness of ART by increasing the number of embryo transfers that could follow one ovarian stimulation cycle. Cryopreserved gamete and embryos are also used in donation programs.

In addition the cryopreservation of embryos or gametes before initiation of gonadotoxic treatment in patients affected with neoplastic disease allows the partial preservation of reproductive potential. Ovarian tissue cryopreservation is also a promising experimental clinical technique because it avoids ovarian stimulation and provides the opportunity for preserving gonadal function in postpubertal patients and it is hoped it will allow the same for prepubertal patients.

Embryo freezing

The demonstration that cryopreserved human embryos could give rise to live offspring after thawing and intrauterine transfer opened the door to the possible application of this technology in clinical ART. Soon after the introduction of IVF, this methodology, based on the use of slow cooling and rapid thawing in the presence of the cryoprotectant dimethyl sulfoxide (DMSO) or more recently 1,2 propanediol (PROH) and sucrose, was applied to human early cleavage stage embryos and resulted in the first reports of pregnancy and live birth from human cryopreserved embryos. Although embryo loss can occur in a proportion of cryopreserved embryos, the application of embryo cryopreservation within an assisted reproduction program can have a profound impact on treatment strategy and success rates [11].

Oocyte freezing

Oocyte freezing is an attractive strategy to preserve female fertility using standard IVF stimulation protocols. Until recently, pregnancy rates achieved after transfer of embryos derived from frozen oocytes had been low (around 2–3%). This was due to low oocyte survival rates (25–40%), and low fertilization rates after traditional IVF due to freezing-induced zona hardening and poor implantational ability of the resulting embryo. However, more recent studies have reported better post-thaw oocyte survival and pregnancy rates after vitrification (rapid cooling) and fertilization using ICSI. In addition, the incidence of chromosomal abnormalities in human embryos obtained from cryopreserved oocytes has been shown to be similar to that of embryos created using fresh oocytes.

Sperm or testicular tissue freezing

Successful achievement of live births using human cryopreserved semen was first reported in the 1950s and has been widely applied in several clinical situations, mainly in treatment of azoospermic men (donor insemination) or for preservation of fertility in men affected with cancer and at risk of losing their fertility as a result of exposure to cytotoxic treatment. Therefore, this approach is now in widespread use for storage and quarantine of donated sperm and storage of reproductive potential when loss of fertility is imminent. It is also useful in the context of confirmation of seronegativity for sexually transmitted diseases in semen storage before sperm donation. Consequently, fresh sperm use for donor insemination has been abandoned because of the window period of seroconversion of many viral transmissible diseases.

Pre-implantation genetic diagnosis and gender selection

The utilization of donated gametes and embryos to prevent genetic disease transmission has recently been restricted by the possibility to apply diagnostic techniques directly to the embryo. The successful application of pre-implantation genetic diagnosis (PGD) can contribute to reduced need for the use of donated gametes in couples at risk of transmitting a serious genetic condition to their child [12]. However, if PGD is not successful or not applicable to a certain disease, or the patients do not accept its low rate of error, then the use of donated gametes could be an alternative.

PGD describes the detection of genetic information in an embryo fertilized in vitro by examining a representative sample taken at the pre-implantation stage of development, to identify embryos that are free of a serious genetic disorder. Significant genetic diseases may be inherited as autosomal recessive or autosomal dominant conditions, may be sex-linked, or in some cases involves a rearrangement of the chromosomes (e.g., a reciprocal or Robertsonian translocation).

PGD has become a viable alternative to prenatal diagnosis (PND) and termination of affected pregnancy for couples at risk of conceiving a pregnancy affected by a known genetic disorder. Patients may choose PGD if they have or have lost an affected child, had several terminations of affected pregnancies and hope for favorable odds in future pregnancies, or have cultural or religious objections to termination of pregnancy. In a cleavage-stage (day three after fertilization) embryo, each blastomere is expected to be genetically representative of the whole embryo. Obtaining this cell by embryo biopsy and subjecting its nucleus to genetic diagnostic techniques constitutes the main step in PGD.

PGD is an expensive and labor-intensive procedure comprising many stages and involving a multidisciplinary team of health professionals. Therefore, it is offered only in a limited number of specialized centers worldwide. Centers offering PGD treatment should deliver a comprehensive service to patients including non-directive counseling and patient support before, during, and after a treatment cycle by an appropriately qualified professional.

The practice of PGD has developed dynamically over the past two decades. After being first introduced for sexing embryos in the case of X-linked genetic disorders in 1990, the first case of a live birth after successful PGD for the single gene disorder, cystic fibrosis, was reported in 1992. This was followed by a report of the birth of a non-carrier female after PGD for Duchenne muscular dystrophy to detect the dystrophin gene deletion in 1995. Since then the worldwide development of PGD has expanded to offer testing for over 200 single gene and chromosomal disorders [13]. With the development of genetic probes that allowed identification of specific regions of chromosomes with tagged fluorescent dyes (fluoresence in situ hybridization, FISH), and the ability to amplify tiny amounts of DNA reliably using the polymerase chain reaction (PCR), a raft of applications to specific clinically relevant genetic conditions became available. The technique has also diversified to include embryo testing for human lymphocytic antigen (HLA) matching for sick siblings. Future developments will possibly include comparative genomic hybridization (CGH) microarray technology, which would enable testing for full chromosome aneuploidy and monogenic disorders from a single embryo biopsy [14].

PGD has a low risk of misdiagnosis. The European Society of Human Reproduction and Embryology PGD Consortium has collected data on PGD cycles and deliveries since 1997. From 15 158 cycles, 24 misdiagnoses and adverse outcomes have been reported; 12 out of 2538 cycles after PCR and 12 out of 12 620 cycles after FISH. The causes of misdiagnosis include confusion of embryo and cell number, transfer of the wrong embryo, maternal or paternal contamination, allele dropout, use of incorrect and inappropriate probes or primers, probe or primer failure, and chromosomal mosaicism. Unprotected sex has been mentioned as a cause of adverse outcome not related to technical and human errors [15].

Gender selection

Currently, identification of the gender of pre-implantation embryos to avoid X-linked diseases is the third most common indication for PGD after chromosomal abnormalities and monogenic diseases.

Those who present for sex selection using PGD are usually carriers of an X-linked recessive condition, where male offspring have a 50% risk of being affected, or an X-linked dominant condition where females also have a 50% of being affected. Sex selection alone is inefficient because it excludes the 50% of male embryos that will be unaffected and cannot detect carrier females in X-linked recessive conditions, which owing to non-random X-chromosome inactivation may develop some clinical features. The use of PCR-based assays to detect specific mutations on the X chromosome alongside linked multiplex markers has been reported. Pre-implantation genetic haplotyping (PGH) has now improved the diagnosis for such families as the linked markers can distinguish affected from unaffected alleles within the X chromosomes, which means unaffected male embryos can also be diagnosed and considered for transfer. This means that on average in X-linked recessive conditions, 75% of the embryos can be considered for embryo transfer.

In the absence of a direct test, or where the specific mutation is not known, FISH provides a robust technique using commercially available centromeric probes for X and Y chromosomes, with an additional control probe on an autosome to determine ploidy.

PGD and HLA tissue typing (savior sibling): a special case of donation

PGD to determine the HLA tissue type (PGD-H) can be performed simultaneously with PGD for inherited hematologic disease such as β-thalassemia, sickle cell disease, hemophilia, Fanconi's anemia, and Diamond–Blackfan anemia. The combined purpose is to establish an unaffected pregnancy where the healthy child (savior sibling) may act as an HLA-matched donor

CASE STUDY 20.1

PGD for sickle cell disease and HLA matching resulting in a normal sibling and cord blood transplant for affected sibling

A couple approached their local fertility and PGD center for advice about their three-year history of infertility after the birth of their only son, who was found to suffer from sickle cell disease and was transfusion dependent. The couple were offered PGD and HLA matching. The treatment was successful and cord blood was taken from the newborn's umbilical cord. The sick son had the cord blood transfused into his body, resulting in a newborn free of sickle cell disease and a much healthier older sibling. The newborn was regarded as the savior of his brother. The parents were acutely aware that no other tissue (other than cord blood) would be obtained from the younger brother to use in his older brother's treatment.

for an existing sibling needing hematopoietic stem cell transplant (HSCT). PGD-H can also be performed with the sole intention of finding a source of HLA-matched stem cells for an existing sibling with a blood disorder that is not caused by an inheritable genetic disorder, when no other suitable source of stem cells can be found.

Follow-up of pregnancies and children born after ART and PGD

ART is associated with increased risks for medical complications during pregnancy (hypertension, diabetes) and obstetric complications (preterm delivery, operative delivery, antepartum hospitalization, premature rupture of membranes). Congenital malformations occur more frequently after ART. These adverse events have been initially attributed to a higher rate of multiple gestations, but when singleton pregnancies have been studied a less pronounced but still increased risk was found. Today it has been demonstrated that when infertile couples conceive without ART their risk for antepartum and perinatal complications is increased. This enforces the suggestion that the excess risk is associated with infertility itself rather than the ART [16].

Risks related to ICSI

Undoubtedly, ICSI has revolutionized the treatment of severe male factor infertility. However, there have been concerns about its safety, owing to the loss of natural sperm selection. The potential for ICSI to transmit genetic defects that may cause male infertility has been studied. About 10–15% of azoospermic and 5–10% of severely oligozoospermic men have microdeletions of the long arm of the Y chromosome. Male infants born to these men could have the same microdeletions as their fathers [17]. Some studies have reported an increased risk of sex chromosomal abnormalities (0.8%) in children born after ICSI. There is a significantly higher aneuploidy and diploidy rate found in spermatozoa from patients with severely oligoteratozoospermic men compared with controls.

Controversy surrounding the issue of an increased incidence of malformations has not been resolved yet, but several studies have reported reassuring outcome of children born after ICSI [18, 19].

A meta-analysis of four prospective cohort studies found no significant additional risks of ICSI procedure in addition to the risk involved in standard IVF for any of the following categories of major birth defects: cardiovascular defects, musculoskeletal defects, hypospadias, neural tube defects, or oral clefts [20].

The last published large, population-based study failed to find any difference in outcomes when comparing IVF with ICSI [21].

Risks related to PGD

Preliminary evidence suggests that human embryo development in vitro is not affected by biopsy at the eight-cell stage. However, monitoring of pregnancies by ultrasound scanning for evidence of fetal abnormality and of children after birth remains crucial to establish reliably the safety of ART and PGD.

Regulation of ART and PGD

The regulation of ART and PGD varies widely worldwide as well as within European Union Member States. Patients travel outside their own Member States for treatment because of local legal restrictions, cheaper treatment elsewhere, or the ART or PGD technology not being available in the home State. This practice has implications for ongoing care of patients and the children born through treatment, as well as the potential difficulties of undertaking a complex process at a distance from the treatment center and the possibility of language barriers.

In many countries where ART is regulated, the same bodies responsible for ART will regulate PGD. In the UK, ART and PGD are licensed by the Human Fertilisation and Embryology Authority, a statutory nongovernmental regulatory body which was established in 1991. Contrary to the situation in the UK, regulation of ART and PGD in the rest of Europe is limited and patchy with varied legislation. For instance, PGD is allowed in Spain, Sweden, Denmark, and Finland, whereas it is prohibited in Ireland and Austria. In Portugal, there is no specific law that opposes PGD. In France it is allowed in a limited number of centers. In July 2011 the German parliament passed a law allowing PGD for some conditions, such as when the parents have the likelihood of passing on a genetic defect and if the risk of miscarriage or stillbirth is high for genetic reasons. The patient must undergo preliminary counseling and their case is required to be examined by an ethics committee before PGD is allowed. In Norway, it is allowed but only in special cases of sex-linked hereditary conditions. In the USA, professional self regulation prevails.

The advantages of public regulation in the area of PGD and ART in general include quality control, accountability, transparency of the process, and collecting data about use, safety, and implications of ART and PGD. It also promotes public debate of the ethical issues embraced by ART and PGD technology.

The role of using donated gametes in ART

Gamete donation is now an integral part of ART, allowing individuals previously considered sterile to conceive. In the UK in 2008, the number of new sperm and oocyte donors registered with the Human Fertilisation and Embryology Authority was 396 and 1150, respectively. In the same year, the number of births involving sperm, oocyte, or embryo donation in the UK was 1333 compared with 11,064 IVF births not involving donation, thus representing 11% of all births occurring as a result of assisted conception treatment. Similar statistics are reported from the USA. In Europe 13,029 cycles of egg donation and 24,339 cycles of donor insemination were performed in 2006.

Indications for gamete donation are different for male (Box 20.1) and female infertility (Box 20.2), with the exception of genetic indications in otherwise fertile couples.

Gonadal failure, in either the female or male, represents irrecoverable loss of fertility. It affects approximately 1% of females under the age of 40 and

---

Box 20.1 Indications for use of donor semen

1. Azoospermia, or significant male factor infertility (i.e., significant oligoasthenospermia or previous failure to fertilize after insemination in vitro, and ICSI is not elected or feasible also for economical reasons).
2. Other significant untreatable sperm or seminal fluid abnormalities.
3. Failure to recover any viable sperm after surgical sperm retrieval in azoospermic patients.
4. Untreatable ejaculatory dysfunction.
5. The male partner has a significant genetic defect or the couple previously has produced an offspring affected by a condition for which carrier status cannot be determined.
6. Sexually transmissible infection in the male, which cannot be eradicated.
7. Rh-negative female partner who is severely Rh-isoimmunized, and the male partner is Rh-positive.
8. Females without male partners.

> **Box 20.2 Indications for use of donor oocytes**
> 1. Gonadal failure with hypergonadotropic hypogonadism.
> 2. Women of advanced reproductive age.
> 3. Women with diminished ovarian reserve.
> 4. Women who are known to be affected by, or known to be the carrier of, a significant genetic defect or who have a family history of a condition for which carrier status cannot be determined.
> 5. Women with poor oocyte and/or embryo quality or multiple previous failed attempts to conceive by ART.

CASE STUDY 20.2

Frozen thawed sperm saved to treat infertility subsequent to teenage cancer treatment

A 17-year-old man was diagnosed with non-Hodgkin's lymphoma requiring systemic therapy. The man stored three samples of mature ejaculated sperm in the local fertility center before chemotherapy and used the frozen-thawed sperm later on in his wife's treatment. Fifteen years after complete recovery from the disease, the patient and his partner visited their general practitioner because of a one-year history of infertility. A sperm test revealed the presence of azoospermia. The couples were referred to their local fertility center. ICSI using the cryo-thawed sperm sample resulted in the couple's first child. Two surplus embryos were cryopreserved for future use. The couple returned to the fertility center two years later and used the frozen embryos. The treatment resulted in the couple's second child. The couple are now considering donating their surplus embryos to a couple who have been previously unsuccessful with IVF.

10% of infertile men. Whereas males with severe oligospermia can still procreate using gamete micromanipulation with ICSI and testicular spermatozoa are recovered in a good proportion of azoospermic patients, females with severe reduction of ovarian reserve are often advised to consider receiving an oocyte donation because of the very low chance of conception from ART using their own oocytes.

Survivors of childhood and adolescent malignancy are often suitable candidates for gamete donation if fertility preservation techniques were not applied before cancer therapy.

Gamete or embryo donation could be an option for couples who carry a genetic disease and are therefore at risk of conceiving a child affected with a serious genetic disease such as cystic fibrosis, Huntington's disease, spinal muscular atrophy and maternally inherited mitochondrial disease.

Couples who have repeatedly experienced IVF failure, owing to poor oocyte quality or declining fertility with age, could be advised to consider accepting gamete donation in an attempt to improve IVF success rate.

Egg donors may share their eggs with an egg recipient if the donor herself requires assisted conception, in return for subsidized treatment. This type of donation is known as "egg sharing" and represents about a third of egg donation cycles in the UK [2]. Egg donation may also be altruistic or commercial, because in some countries like USA the donor can be paid.

Embryo donation is a further possibility for all the previous male and female indications in the countries where it is permitted.

Donor selection

Selection criteria differ from country to country, and there are differences in economical aspects of donation (altruistic donation or financial remuneration); but there are common scientific concepts underlying the different international guidelines or legislations.

The donor should be of legal age and in a good health status, less than 40 years of age for sperm donation and 35 for egg donation, owing to the increase in cytogenetic risk and the decrease in pregnancy rate. He or she must undergo a thorough evaluation comprising screening and testing.

A genetic screening for heritable disease must be conducted for the exclusion of Mendelian disorders (autosomal and X-linked), major malformations, familial diseases with genetic component, and karyotype abnormality. Genetic testing must be conducted for some diseases (cystic fibrosis) or on the basis of regional prevalence of the disease (beta-thalassemia in Mediterranean populations, sickle cell disease in African and Afro-Caribbean populations, and Tay–Sachs disease in Jews of Eastern European descent). Blood and Rh types must be obtained, especially when there is the risk of potential rhesus incompatibility.

A full medical history must minimize the risk that the donor is infected with transmissible agents; the following items must be checked: sexually transmissible diseases, sexual habits, piercing, tattooing, or any behavior that could increase the risk of contracting HIV-I and -II, human T-lymphotropic virus (HTLV), and sexually transmitted diseases, transplants, transfusion of whole blood or clotting factors, previous contacts or risk of contact with hepatitis B or C virus, vaccinia virus, West Nile virus, and risks of transmissible spongiform encephalopathies such as Creutzfeldt–Jakob disease. The risks of these and other diseases are further reduced by a detailed donor physical examination.

Serological testing must include HIV-1 antibody as well as NAT, HIV-2 antibody, hepatitis C antibody and NAT, hepatitis B surface antigen, hepatitis B core antibody (IgG and IgM), serologic test for syphilis, HTLV-1 and HTLV-2, and cytomegalovirus (IgG and IgM). Semen, urine, or a urethral swab should be tested for *Neisseria gonorrhoeae*. Either urine or a urethral swab should be tested for *Chlamydia trachomatis*.

Specific evaluation for sperm donors

Donor fertility should be demonstrated or presumed by the examination of several semen samples, conducted in agreement with the World Health Organization guidelines.

Specific evaluation for oocyte donors

Assessment of ovarian reserve

The success of any IVF cycle depends substantially on adequate recruitment of ovarian follicles after gonadotrophin stimulation. In turn, this will depend on the number of primordial follicles available for recruitment in the ovary, known as ovarian reserve or the "biological" ovarian age. At birth, each ovary contains about one million primordial follicles. This number is reduced to about 250,000 at menarche and very few (about 1000) towards the end of the reproductive life (menopause). The steady loss of follicles accelerates around the age of 37, although the rate of follicle depletion varies widely. To avoid cycle cancellation because of failure to respond to stimulation, it is clinically and economically helpful to try to predict poor responders before starting an oocyte donation treatment cycle.

The age of the oocyte donor is an important factor in identifying ovarian reserve. Ideally, the age of oocyte donors should be under 35 at the time of the donation. In addition to age, ovarian reserve can be evaluated by measuring the anti-Müllerian hormone and basal (i.e., early follicular phase) FSH and estradiol (E2) levels. As the ovary ages and becomes depleted of responsive follicles, secretion of anti-Müllerian hormone declines and pituitary production of FSH increases. Both anti-Müllerian hormone and basal FSH measurements are currently the most commonly used markers for assessing ovarian reserve and have been found to be closely correlated with pregnancy rates following oocyte donation treatment [22]. Other parameters used to assess ovarian reserve include the antral follicle count as viewed by ultrasound before the start of IVF treatment [23]. Thorough evaluation of oocyte donors before starting an oocyte donation treatment is essential to determine the appropriateness of treatment and to tailor the IVF treatment protocol to each donor's needs, whether the donor is undergoing an IVF treatment herself or whether she is undergoing stimulation only to donate oocyte.

Patient selection and evaluation before starting an IVF donation cycle

The principles of use of donated oocytes are the same as when IVF is applied to a couple undergoing IVF using their own gametes. The IVF process should be thoroughly reviewed at the initial visit including a detailed explanation of what is involved in a typical IVF cycle, the envisaged success rate for the oocyte recipient (and the donor in shared programs) and the potential risks and stresses associated with treatment for the donor. Finally, a pelvic examination and ultrasound pelvic scanning is performed for all donors. For both, the donor and recipient, optimization of the woman's body mass index to be in the range of 18.5–29 is critical. Being overweight or underweight can affect the response to ovarian stimulation and reduce the overall success rate of oocyte donation treatment [24].

Recipient evaluation and treatment

Whether the treatment is a donor sperm insemination or an oocyte donation, the recipient should have normal genital apparatus to allow a pregnancy. A regular uterine cavity should be a prerequisite before starting treatment, as polyps, submucous fibroids, or uterine anomalies (such as a uterine septum, bicornuate uterus, or T-shaped cavity) may impair implantation. Further evaluation of the uterine cavity with hysterosonography and/or hysteroscopy with possible surgical correction (e.g., transcervical resection) may be necessary.

In cases of donor oocyte IVF, basic to the initial evaluation is a look at the partner's semen quality in the IVF unit's laboratory to determine the appropriate method for sperm preparation and to advise the most appropriate assisted conception technique (i.e., IVF or ICSI) likely to be needed.

Donor insemination treatment

The patient undergoes either serial ultrasound monitoring in order to identify the day of ovulation or controlled ovarian stimulation. When the leading follicle has a diameter of 17–18 mm, ovulation is pharmacologically induced. The insemination of the selected spermatozoa is easily performed with a soft catheter in the hours that the follicle is presumed to ovulate. In case of ovarian stimulation, it is useful to prescribe a luteal support therapy, as previously explained.

Oocyte or embryo donation treatment

The treatment protocol differs, depending on whether fresh or cryopreserved material is used. If the recipient uses the donated oocyte at the same time that the donor undergoes the treatment, the two cycles have to be pharmacologically coordinated so as to ensure that the recipient's endometrium is synchronous with the donor's. If cryopreserved material (oocytes or embryos) is used, the endometrial preparation of the recipient can be induced at any time and the oocytes or embryos will be thawed when the endometrium has the ideal conformation. The IVF procedure is conducted in the usual way after the oocyte's fertilization.

Recipient's endometrial preparation

The technique commonly used for endometrial preparation to facilitate implantation is simple. It involves the use of estradiol valerate 6 mg daily commenced orally on day one or two of menstruation after previous pituitary suppression and continued for approximately 14 days, after which endometrial thickness is evaluated. If endometrial thickness is less than 7mm, the daily dose of the estradiol valerate is increased to 8 mg for a further seven days. Progesterone supplementation, usually in the form of micronized progesterone pessaries, is commenced when endometrial thickness of 7 mm or more is achieved and embryo transfer is scheduled two to five days later. Hormonal supplementation is continued until 12 weeks' gestation.

Specific risks and adverse reactions associated with gamete donation in ART

These risks can be broadly divided into those associated with the ART treatment itself and those related to gamete donation *per se*.

ART risks

Risks to the donor

Oocyte donors receive exogenous FSH injections for multifollicular ovarian stimulation. This process carries a risk of OHSS (see earlier in this chapter). The fact that the oocyte donor does not receive an embryo transfer does not eliminate completely the risk of OHSS. In addition, the procedure of oocyte retrieval could cause injury to pelvic structures, ovarian torsion, or bleeding and could introduce infection leading to ovarian infection and pelvic abscess formation. Although the literature is replete with case reports of such complications, the overall risk of serious morbidity is below 1%. Oocyte retrieval is often performed under deep sedation or general anesthesia, which also carry a certain risk of morbidity [25]. In the European IVF Monitoring Consortium by ESHRE, the frequencies of complications in 2006 were as follows: all complication 0.2%, bleeding 0.1%, infection 0.009% [4].

There is also a theoretical risk of loss of ovarian function after repeated cycles of oocyte donation because of oocyte depletion. However, recent studies reported no deterioration in ovarian reserve after up to three cycles of oocyte donation. Beyond three cycles, it is difficult to ascertain the effect of oocyte donation on the ovarian reserve of the donor because of confounding by the increasing age of the donor.

Risks to the recipient

Oocyte recipients are generally women with ovarian failure or older women with declining ovarian reserve. On the basis of the recipient's age alone, oocyte donation pregnancies are at higher risk of developing hypertension, gestational diabetes, antenatal bleeding, premature delivery, hospitalization, and operative obstetric interventions. Pregnancy induced by the use of donated oocytes could pose additional risks beyond those expected based on the recipient's age alone. For example, these pregnancies are at a higher risk of placental dysfunction, further increasing the risk of pregnancy-induced hypertension, fetal growth restriction, low birthweight, and premature delivery. All these complications can, of course, be made worse if the pregnancy established after oocyte donation results in a multiple pregnancy as a result of multiple embryo transfer.

In addition, women affected with Turner's syndrome and who conceive after oocyte donation are at particular risk of progressive aortic root dilatation and aortic dissection, which is a potentially fatal complication of pregnancy induced hypertension in those patients, and requiring close and careful monitoring throughout pregnancy [26].

Specific risks related to the gamete donation procedure
Transmission of genetic conditions
Despite screening donors for common genetic conditions before starting gamete donation cycles, it is theoretically possible for a genetic trait unrecognized by the donor and not tested for routinely to be transmitted to the offspring by the treatment. Although gamete banks can effectively test for the commoner genetic conditions such as cystic fibrosis, rarer conditions with an asymptomatic donor can only be prevented after an index case by meticulous vigilance and surveillance with reporting back to the gamete facility by clinicians caring for ART-conceived offspring. This can be difficult in some circumstances because not all recipients of donated gametes declare the origin of the conception. Clinicians who may be aware of the mode of conception using donated gametes for use in others can prevent further cases from occurring if they recognize a genetic disease in the offspring and report it back to the facility that provided the gametes.

Up to now there have been cases of genetic disease transmission including hypertrophic cardiomyopathy (see Case Study 20.3) [27] and severe congenital neutropenia, a genetic illness that is so rare that it is not considered to be cost effective to screen all donors routinely for this condition. A cluster of five affected children from four families in Michigan has been reported [28]. Other genetic diseases have been described in infants after gamete donation: fragile X syndrome, autosomal dominant cerebellar ataxia, and Opitz syndrome.

There have also been cases of alloimmune hemolytic disease of the fetus and newborn and of neonatal alloimmune thrombocytopenia, with the suggestions that screening of surrogate carriers and gamete donors for blood group antigens may be applicable [29–31].

Other cases of hemolytic disease of the fetus and newborn have been described, raising the issue of whether blood group compatibility should be considered in cases of donated gametes for ART [32–35].

CASE STUDY 20.3

Genetic disease transmissions by sperm donation and the need for surveillance and vigilance by clinicians caring for ART conceived offspring

An apparently well 23-year-old male was shown to be negative for markers of infectious diseases and donated sperm for 2 years. He was subsequently shown to have a novel β-myosin heavy-chain mutation which causes hypertrophic cardiomyopathy. One of his offspring was clinically diagnosed with this condition. The donor was known to have fathered 24 children, including 22 who were conceived through ART using his sperm donation, and he fathered two children conceived with his own wife. Of all these offspring, nine have been shown to be genetically affected with hypertrophic cardiomyopathy. Three of the nine gene-positive children were reported to have the expressed phenotypic evidence of it. One died at age 2 years owing to heart failure associated with the condition, and there are two others with extreme left ventricular hypertrophy at age 15 years. These two cases and the donor are considered likely to be at increased risk for sudden death.

CASE STUDY 20.4

Alloimmune hemolytic disease of the fetus and newborn after undisclosed oocyte donation

In one case, a mother with blood group O did not disclose the donated oocyte when she delivered dizygotic twins, which were both blood group AB and had hemolytic disease of the fetus and newborn requiring phototherapy. The first flag of suspicion was raised by the AB blood group status of both neonates. In this case the genotype of the affected mother and infants did not match the presumed parents, which prompted a more detailed investigation of the obstetric history of the mother. This history revealed that ART had been performed with donated oocytes, a fact that the mother was reluctant to admit.

The future

Oocyte and sperm donation for fully sterile patients, where fertility is compromised owing to age or absent gametes, will remain necessary until the development of gametes from stem cells or cloning is available. Patients with transmissible disease will benefit more from PGD techniques. PGD is rapidly advancing, with future improvements expected in both availability and accuracy. The list of genetic disorders for which PGD is applicable will expand beyond the current 200.

KEY LEARNING POINTS

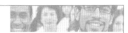

- Gamete donation is now an integral part of assisted reproductive technology (ART), allowing individuals previously considered sterile to conceive. ART accounts for 11% of all births in the UK.

- Gonadal failure, in the female or male, represents irrecoverable loss of fertility and affects approximately 1% of females under the age of 40 and 10% of infertile men so that gamete donation would be required for ART.

- Survivors of childhood and adolescent malignancy are often suitable candidates for gamete donation if fertility preservation techniques were not applied before cancer therapy.

- Gamete or embryo donation is an option for couples who carry a genetic disease and or who have repeatedly experienced in vitro fertilization failure.

- Oocyte donors may share their eggs with an egg recipient if the donor herself requires assisted conception, in return for subsidized treatment.

- Rarely, disease transmission by gamete donors may occur and vigilance and surveillance of ART conceived offspring can alert donor clinics to investigate implicated donors and to quarantine any additional donations in their facility from the same donor.

References

1. Zegers-Hochschild F, Adamson GD, de Mouzon J, et al. International Committee for Monitoring Assisted Reproductive Technology (ICMART) and the World Health Organization (WHO) revised glossary of ART terminology, 2009. Hum Reprod 2009;24:2683–87.
2. www.hfea.gov.uk/docs/2010-1124_Facts_and_Figures_2007_Publication_updated_November_2010_FINAL_pdf. 2010; available from: www.hfea.gov.uk/docs/2010-11.
3. Sunderam S, Chang J, Flowers L, et al. Assisted reproductive technology surveillance – United States, 2006. MMWR Surveill Summ 2009;58:1–25.
4. Nyboe Andersen A, V. Goossens L, Gianaroli R, et al. Assisted reproductive technology in Europe, 2003. Results generated from European registers by ESHRE. Hum Reprod 2007;22:1513–25.
5. Bonduelle M, Camus M, De Vos A, et al. Seven years of intracytoplasmic sperm injection and follow-up of 1987 subsequent children. Hum Reprod 1999;14 (Suppl 1):243–64.
6. Aboulghar M, Mansour R, Serour G, et al. Controlled ovarian hyperstimulation and intrauterine insemination for treatment of unexplained infertility should be limited to a maximum of three trials. Fertil Steril 2001;75:88–91.
7. Reindollar RH, Regan MM, Neumann PJ, et al. A randomized clinical trial to evaluate optimal treatment for unexplained infertility: the fast track and standard treatment (FASTT) trial. Fertil Steril 2010;94:888–99.

8. Verberg MF, Eijkemans MJ, Heijnen EM, et al. Why do couples drop-out from IVF treatment? A prospective cohort study. Hum Reprod 2008;23:2050–5.

9. Tarlatzis BC, Bili H. Intracytoplasmic sperm injection. Survey of world results. Ann N Y Acad Sci 2000;900:336–344.

10. El-Toukhy T, Khalaf Y, Braude P. IVF results: optimize not maximize. Am J Obstet Gynecol 2006;194:322–31.

11. Edgar DH, Archer J, Bourne H. The application and impact of cryopreservation of early cleavage stage embryos in assisted reproduction. Hum Fertil (Camb) 2005;8:225–30.

12. Bickerstaff H, Flinter F, Yeong CT, et al. Clinical application of preimplantation genetic diagnosis. Hum Fertil (Camb) 2001;4:24–30.

13. Goossens V, Harton G, Moutou C, et al. ESHRE PGD Consortium data collection VIII: cycles from January to December 2005 with pregnancy follow-up to October 2006. Hum Reprod 2008;23:2629–45.

14. Preimplantation Genetic Diagniosis International Society (PGDIS) Guidelines for good practice in PGD: programme requirements and laboratory quality assurance. Reprod Biomed Online 2008;16:134–47.

15. Wilton L, Thornhill A, Traeger-Synodinos J, et al. The causes of misdiagnosis and adverse outcomes in PGD. Hum Reprod 2009;24:1221–8.

16. Jaques AM, Amor DJ, Baker HW, et al. Adverse obstetric and perinatal outcomes in subfertile women conceiving without assisted reproductive technologies. Fertil Steril 2010;94:2674–9.

17. Kamischke A, Gromoll J, Simoni M, et al. Transmission of a Y chromosomal deletion involving the deleted in azoospermia (DAZ) and chromodomain (CDY1) genes from father to son through intracytoplasmic sperm injection: case report. Hum Reprod 1999;14:2320–2.

18. Sutcliffe AG, Taylor B, Li J, et al. Children born after intracytoplasmic sperm injection: population control study. BMJ 1999;318:704–5.

19. Bonduelle M, Joris H, Hofmans K, et al. Mental development of 201 ICSI children at 2 years of age. Lancet 1998;351:1553.

20. Lie RT, Lyngstadaas A, Ørstavik KH, et al. Birth defects in children conceived by ICSI compared with children conceived by other IVF-methods; a meta-analysis. Int J Epidemiol 2005;34:696–701.

21. Finnström O, Källén B, Lindam A, et al. Maternal and child outcome after in vitro fertilization – a review of 25 years of population-based data from Sweden. Acta Obstet Gynecol Scand 2011;90:494–500.

22. Wang JG, Douglas NC, Nakhuda GS, et al. The association between anti-Müllerian hormone and IVF pregnancy outcomes is influenced by age. Reprod Biomed Online 2010;21:757–61.

23. Broer SL, Dólleman M, Opmeer BC, et al. AMH and AFC as predictors of excessive response in controlled ovarian hyperstimulation: a meta-analysis. Hum Reprod Update 2011;17:46–54.

24. Sathya A, Balasubramanyam S, Gupta S, et al. Effect of body mass index on in vitro fertilization outcomes in women. J Hum Reprod Sci 2010;3:135–8.

25. Bodri D, Vernaeve V, Figueras F, et al. Oocyte donation in patients with Turner's syndrome: a successful technique but with an accompanying high risk of hypertensive disorders during pregnancy. Hum Reprod 2006;21:829–2.

26. Boissonnas CC, Davy C, Bornes M, et al. Careful cardiovascular screening and follow-up of women with Turner syndrome before and during pregnancy is necessary to prevent maternal mortality. Fertil Steril 2009;91:e925–7.

27. Maron BJ, Lesser JR, Schiller NB, et al. Implications of hypertrophic cardiomyopathy transmitted by sperm donation. JAMA 2009;302:1681–4.

28. Boxer LA, Stein S, Buckley D, et al. Strong evidence for autosomal dominant inheritance of severe congenital neutropenia associated with ELA2 mutations. J Pediatr 2006;148:633–6.

29. Zuppa AA, Cardiello V, Lai M, et al. ABO hemolytic disease of the fetus and newborn: an iatrogenic complication of heterologous assisted reproductive technology-induced pregnancy. Transfusion 2010;50:2102–4.

30. Storry JR. Don't ask, don't tell: the ART of silence can jeopardize assisted pregnancies. Transfusion 2010;50:2070–2.

31. Curtis BR, Bussel JB, Manco-Johnson MJ, et al. Fetal and neonatal alloimmune thrombocytopenia in pregnancies involving in vitro fertilization: a report of four cases. Am J Obstet Gynecol 2005;192:543–7.

32. Freund GG, Finke C, Kirkley SA. Anomalous ABO inheritance explained by ovum transplantation. Transfusion 1995;35:61–62.

33. Mitchell S, James A. Severe hemolytic disease from rhesus anti-C antibodies in a surrogate pregnancy after oocyte donation. A case report. J Reprod Med 1996; 44:388–90.

34. Mair DC, Scofield TL. HDN in a mother undergoing in vitro fertilization with donor ova. Transfusion 2003;43:288–9.

35. Medicine PCoASfR, Technology PCoSfAR. 2008 Guidelines for gamete and embryo donation: a Practice Committee report. Fertil Steril 2008;90 (5 Suppl), S30–44.

Index

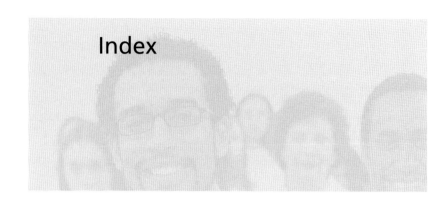

Tissue and Cell Clinical Use: An Essential Guide, First Edition. Edited by Ruth M. Warwick and Scott A. Brubaker.
© 2012 Blackwell Publishing Ltd. Published 2012 by Blackwell Publishing Ltd.